Brought to Bed

Brought to Bed

Childbearing in America 1750 to 1950

JUDITH WALZER LEAVITT

Oxford University Press
New York   Oxford

Oxford University Press

Oxford New York Toronto
Delhi Bombay Calcutta Madras Karachi
Petaling Jaya Singapore Hong Kong Tokyo
Nairobi Dar es Salaam Cape Town
Melbourne Auckland

and associated companies in
Beirut Berlin Ibadan Nicosia

Published by Oxford University Press, Inc.,
200 Madison Avenue, New York, New York 10016

Library of Congress Cataloging-in-Publication Data

Leavitt, Judith Walzer.
Brought to bed.

Includes index.
1. Obstetrics—United States—History—18th century. 2. Obstetrics—United States—History—19th century. 3. Obstetrics—United States—History—20th century. 4. Childbirth—United States—History—18th century. 5. Childbirth—United States—History—19th century. 6. Childbirth—United States—History—20th century. I. Title. [DNLM: 1. Delivery. 2. Labor. 3. Obstetrics—history. WQ 11 AA1 L46b]
RG518.U5L4 1986 618.2'00973 85-30967
ISBN 0-19-503843-6
ISBN 0-19-505690-6 (PBK)

4 6 8 9 7 5 3 1

Printed in the United States of America

To my children
SARAH and DAVID
with love

Acknowledgments

I have many people to thank for their help and encouragement over the years that I worked on this book. My mother, whose accounts of her harrowing taxi-cab ride while she was in labor with me and my over-eager arrival two months early, first sparked my interest in this subject, long before labor and delivery became events in my own life. Not only was her confinement experience spectacular, but Sally Walzer's entire life has been an important model in helping me to understand women's strength and abilities. My friend and colleague Susan Stanford Friedman gave most generously of her time to discuss with me the ideas raised in childbirth history and to read the manuscript when it was in its very rough form; her comments were of vital importance in helping me conceptualize the issues. My husband, Lewis A. Leavitt, provided, in addition to his thoughtful comments and medical insight, encouragement and support at each step in the development of this book. Our children, Sarah and David, born in 1970 and 1976, directly precipitated my writing on this subject; they provide me with an important connection to the women of the past and to the world of the future.

Elizabeth T. Black, Calvin Dexter, Evelyn Fine, Patricia Harris, Lisa MacPherson, Leslie Schwalm, and Whitney Walton provided excellent research assistance for this study: each of these scholars gave much energy and insight to my work. Whitney Walton wrote with me an article on death fears among birthing women, some of which is reproduced here as parts of Chapters 1 and 4. Edith Hoshino Altbach of Buffalo, Regina Morantz-Sanchez of the University of Kansas, and my colleagues at the University of Wisconsin—Ruth Bleier, Linda Gordon, and Ronald L. Numbers—contributed valuable criticisms of the manuscript and offered wonderful insights and encouragement. I am most grateful for the time they took out of their busy schedules to help. Jean Donnison of the Northeast London Polytechnic read a draft of Chapter 2 and offered thorough and careful advice for revision. Ann Gordon of the University of Massachusetts provided helpful commentary on one chapter.

I have been fortunate to have the research and teaching environment at the University of Wisconsin in both the History of Medicine Department and in the Women's Studies Program that allows scholars to share their ideas on a daily basis. In addition to my colleagues names above, I would like to thank particularly Rima Apple, Charlotte Borst, Douglas Campbell, Gerda Lerner, Florencia Mallon, Elaine Marks, Morris Vogel, and Mariamne Whatley for their intellectual challenges over the years. Judith Borodovko Walzer, of the New School for Social Research, offered critical insights at a particularly important time in the book's evolution. Comments from seminar participants at the Institute for the History of Medicine at Johns Hopkins University Medical School, the Institute for the Medical Humanities at the University of Texas Medical Branch, and at Indiana University were very helpful. Nancy Schrom Dye of the University of Kentucky read parts of two chapters in the course of our planning sessions on the history of childbirth at the American Historical Association and at the Berkshire Conference of Women Historians; her comments and camaraderie are much appreciated.

I would like to thank librarians and archivists at the University of Wisconsin Center for Health Sciences Library, particularly Dorothy Whitcomb and Blanche Singer; the State Historical Society of Wisconsin; the Sophia Smith Collection at Smith College; the Arthur and Elizabeth Schlesinger Library at Radcliffe College; and interlibrary loan officers and archivists at libraries around the country who facilitated my efforts to locate women's birth accounts.

A special thanks is due to the hundreds of women who took the time to respond to my Author's Query in the *New York Times Book Review* in July 1983. Their responses were informative and helpful for my understanding of twentieth-century childbirth experiences, but even more meaningful to me was the spirit in which they were given. I felt very much as if the letters marked a modern women's support network.

My support network in the History of Medicine Department is

headed by the cheerful assistance of Carolyn Hackler, who not only made this book possible but who contributes valued aid and encouragement daily. I hope my book will match—in spirit and in content—the generosity and the support of all the people who have helped make it possible.

My research efforts were facilitated by grants from the Brittingham Trust, the Graduate School of the University of Wisconsin, and the National Institutes of Health (grant # 1 RO1 LM 04217-01). Without this support, the project could not have been completed.

It has been a pleasure—and a learning experience—working with the editors at Oxford University Press. I would especially like to thank Sheldon Meyer for being a sympathetic and critical reader, beginning the day we sat on Bascom Hill on the University of Wisconsin campus and discussed the early ideas of the book through its revisions to its completion. Leona Capeless guided the manuscript through production and Lester Meigs and Stephanie Sakson-Ford offered helpful editorial suggestions.

I am grateful to the editors of *Feminist Studies, Journal of American History,* and *Signs* for permission to reprint previously published work. Parts of Chapter 5 appeared in *Signs,* Vol. 6, No. 1 (Autumn 1980) under the title "Birthing and Anesthesia: The Debate over Twilight Sleep." Parts of Chapter 2 appeared in the *Journal of American History,* Vol. 70, No. 2 (Sept. 1983) under the title " 'Science' Enters the Birthing Room: Obstetrics in America since the Eighteenth Century." Parts of Chapters 1 and 4 appeared in *Feminist Studies,* Vol. 12 (Spring 1986) under the title, "Under the Shadow of Maternity: American Women's Responses to Death and Debility Fears in Nineteenth-Century Childbirth."

Table of Contents

Brought to Bed

[The grandmother had ten children; each time] . . . preparing the layette for the newcomer by reusing the layette of those who, dead or alive, had come before, and, more discreetly, collecting each time in one of her dresser drawers bits and pieces of her own deathbed attire on which were pinned timid last wishes in case God would, on this occasion, call her to him . . .

Marguerite Yourcenar, *Souvenirs pieux.*
Translated by Elaine Marks.

Introduction

Childbirth is more than a biological event in women's lives. It is a vital component in the social definition of womanhood. Historically, women's physiological ability to bear children and men's inability to do so have contributed to defining the places each held in the social order. The sexual differentiation between men and women fostered a cultural division of labor based on these biological distinctions, a division that allocated the domestic sphere to women and the public sphere to men. Childbirth symbolizes this historical and cultural definition of women's essence: the bearing of children has represented women's most valued work.

This book focuses on the phenomenon of birth precisely because of its centrality to women's lives. By understanding childbirth we can understand significant parts of the female experience. Of course childbirth, like other human activities, has not remained static over the course of history, nor has women's relationship to childbirth remained constant. Both have undergone significant and revealing changes in America in the period from the middle of the eighteenth century—when male physicians began attending normal labor and delivery, introducing medical interventions into the birth process and for the first time challenging women's traditional domination over childbirth practices—to the middle of the twentieth century, when the majority of American women delivered their babies in hospitals under conditions set by health care professionals. Analysis of these changes in the American childbirth experience forms the bulk of my study. By examining closely the ways childbirth has changed, I hope to illuminate some basic aspects of women's lives in the past while at the same time analyzing the evolution of medical and social practices that influenced those lives.

My findings are stated quite simply: until childbirth moved to the hospital during the first third of the twentieth century, birthing women themselves were the most active agents of change in American childbirth history. Because they found their often repeated childbirths dangerous and burdensome, women created a way of fighting back, a means of reacting to the sometimes overwhelming difficulties of bearing children. By banding together in their common cause, women relied on the strengths and help of other women to face their problems. In their unity women developed coping mechanisms and consciously acted to keep childbirth within women's power when that power was being threatened by a medical profession growing in ability in the nineteenth and early twentieth century. By banding together to retain female traditions and values and to shape the events in their own birthing rooms, women acted in a way that acknowledged a specific women's agenda. Their activities were illustrative of what I think can be called a feminist impulse embedded within women's traditional experiences. Feminist inclinations and the collective behavior they fostered developed out of the basic and shared experiences of women's bodies at times, such as birthing, when the experience of those bodies seemed most confining and difficult.[1] The writings of women—in diaries, letters, and autobiographies—provide evidence of a powerful network that was in place and sustained by the process of childbirth. Childbirth, the symbol of traditional womanhood, served as the center of the network women built to overcome the constraints of tradition and ultimately to widen the female sphere.

The women's network that developed during these often repeated confinement experiences empowered birthing women to determine and to change events during their own and their friends' birthings. The process of changing childbirth experiences throughout American history incorporated the wishes and demands of the birthing women themselves; change occurred in large part when and how birthing women wanted it to happen. Traditionally, women held all the power to determine birth procedures, because men were excluded from birthing rooms. In America, male physicians first began attending normal childbirth in the middle of the eighteenth century, when women invited them as technical experts. Physicians then began the process of actively intervening in birth procedures, with instruments and with drugs, and they contributed to the creation of a changing attitude among large groups of Americans that birth could be manipulated and altered according to specific activities planned and executed by experts.

But male physicians, entering a traditional female environment in home birthing rooms, at first had relatively little power to dominate the management of labor and delivery. Childbirth was women's domain, and physicians' didactic training left them at a disadvantage in front of the birthing women's companions, most of whom had had considerable birthing room experience. Nineteenth-century confinements incorporated changing medical ideas and procedures, but at the same time they continued to reflect women's traditional practices. When childbirth entered the hospital, however, as it did in the twentieth century, physicians, armed with a stronger profession behind them and increasing practical as well as theoretical obstetric training, gained the power they had missed in their patients' homes and became key authorities over birth practices. With the move to the hospital, women lost their traditional hold over childbirth decision making and began their quest, continuing today, to recover some of that control. Over the two-hundred-year period examined in this book, birth changed from a woman-centered home event to a hospital-centered medical event. The process by which this occurred reflected the needs women felt to upgrade and to control their birthing experiences, as well as the increasing medical management of birth. Examination of the role women themselves played in bringing childbirth from a traditional happening that epitomized women's power to a hospital routine that represented the height of mid-twentieth-century medical power forms a major focus of this book.

My study of the history of childbirth grew both from my professional interests in the processes of change in nineteenth-century American health care and from my two personal experiences with pregnancy and childbirth. As a historian I was most fascinated with changes over time, and I wanted to understand the patterns of change in medical history and the factors that led to them. My book on the history of public health *(The Healthiest City: Milwaukee and the Politics of Health Reform)* had focused on questions of how public policy toward health care developed historically. I investigated in that study the political and economic context in which health policy emerged and the close relationship between medical and cultural events. My historical interests in the interactions between medicine and society developed into a specific interest in the history of childbirth as a direct result of my personal confinement experiences. During the hours of labor and delivery I understood and accepted a bond with biological womanhood and with all women in the past and present who had had this experience. I recognized that the powerful physicality of birth drew women together at least as much as the particular differences of their individual lives and confinements pushed them apart, and that this one part of womanhood held important historical keys to the past. This was an event that women shared with one another. It was also an event that elicited fears of pain and debility and the need for both familiar comforts and for the security of helpful experts. Going through the experience of labor and delivery connected me with issues in the history of medicine needing scholarly attention.

In investigating childbirth history, I wanted to continue to ask questions about change and choice that had influenced my earlier research. I wanted to explore the interactions between birthing women and their doctors, to understand the power balance between them, and to discover how childbirth had undergone such significant changes from the middle of the eighteenth century to my own era in the middle of the twentieth century. How much had birthing women contributed to changing childbirth patterns in this country? To what extent had women worked together to overcome some of the burdens of childbearing? How had birth attendants, specifically doctors, at whom social critics have been pointing the finger of blame for the overmedicalization of birth, contributed to changing practices? What kinds of interactions between birthing women and their physicians occurred that might explain some of the changes that are observable historically? What was the decision-making process in obstetrics practice in the traditional home environment? How did this change over time and prepare the way for the transition to the hospital in the twentieth century? How were birth events influenced by developments in medical science, including bacteriology, the use of anesthesia, and increasingly sophisticated instrumentation? Who had the power and the knowledge in America's birthing rooms, and how did that change over time? What did women want in their childbirth experiences, and to what extent did they bring those wishes to fruition? What did attending physicians want, and how did they increase their ability to make decisions in America's birthing rooms? These are some of the questions that I explore in this book.

Medical historians traditionally have focused on the profession of medicine; they have looked at what doctors wrote, how doctors were educated, how medical theory changed. Only recently have historians tried to examine the actual practice of medicine and the experience of the patients instead of the healers. The difficulty of finding evidence directly relevant to patients and to practice has delayed development in this area of medical history. My particular historical interests combined with my personal experience pushed me, despite the difficulties in locating sources, to write not a history of obstetrics, which could have been based largely on medical materials, but a history of childbirth, which required also uncovering the birthing women's sources and telling the story from both perspectives. I was helped along by events in women's history.

In the 1970s, while I was becoming a mother and simultaneously the ideas for this book were germinating, historians were uncovering a woman's cultural world of the nineteenth century that had at its core women's shared biological and social role experiences. Carroll Smith-Rosenberg's article in the first issue of *Signs* examining the "female world of love and ritual" and Linda Gordon's study of birth control within a broad cultural analysis of women's lives *(Woman's Body, Woman's Right)* were pivotal in helping me integrate my personal insights into my professional research. With the help of a whole community of scholars, my research led me to integrate my long-standing interest in the relationship between medicine and society with my newly understood experience of the importance of childbirth for understanding women's lives.[2]

The strengths women have exhibited—past and present—became the single most powerful agent propelling me forward in my work. Individually and collectively, women have endured enormous hardships in childbearing and have fought admirably against them. Childbirth has presented women with some of their most difficult moments, especially in terms of physical risks; but many women managed to turn the moments to their advantage, to overcome the worst, and to build from them a collective tradition of resistance. It is exhilarating to read in women's diaries and letters how they armed themselves against the fearful aspects of childbirth by seeking the support of other women who had passed through the experience successfully, and how they planned the events to meet their particular needs and expectations. Many women, of course, could not conquer their confinement problems, and they suffered and died under these extreme physical and psychological burdens. But my research has uncovered a large cache of what can best be described as a feminist vein of seeking improvements and working actively toward a vision of a better life deeply imbedded in women's traditional experiences. The realization of just how deep this female determination runs was the most exciting aspect of my research; the deeply rooted female strengths I uncovered reflect, I believe, a heritage that is both traditional and radical.

This study focuses on the birth experiences of middle- and upper-class women. This is not because I think these groups representative of all women. In fact, for most of American history the birth experiences of these women have been significantly different in many respects from those of all other women. The first reason for my emphasis on middle- and upper-class women is that the historical documentation exists in greater abundance for these groups than for poorer women. In trying to understand the dynamics of change in childbirth history, it was important for me to find evidence from women themselves, and the written record, in women's own voices, is significantly richer for the groups under focus here. But in the process of my research, an even more important reason for this emphasis emerged: the more affluent members of American society had, at each point in our history, more options available to them for their confinements and because of this, could be more active in changing practices to meet their needs as those needs developed. The middle- and upper-class women living in the urban centers along the East coast first invited physicians to attend them in their confinements; the same groups pioneered with various medical interventions, including anesthesia use, and they helped to navigate birth into the hospital in the twentieth century. Through an analysis of the experiences of the middle-class birthing women, particularly as they acted in conjunction with their medical attendants, we can best understand the forces that combined to change procedures in childbirth history. Those women who sought medical attendance and who encouraged obstetricians to employ increasing interventions were the vanguard of changing childbirth practices and procedures. The rest of the population inherited the changes that these groups initiated. Because this book analyzes the processes of change, the emphasis is rightfully on the most active agents of the changes, birthing middle- and upper-class women.

The physicians who delivered the babies of middle- and upper-class women provide the second major focus of this study. This is not to deny the importance of midwives throughout American history. In fact, midwives have probably over time set the stage for delivery more often than their medical counterparts. My decision to exclude midwives from the center of my analysis rested in part on the fact that other historians have studied this group specifically.[3] But also important to my decision was, again, my desire to focus on the processes of change. The changes that have led to our present obstetrical situation in this country have, I believe, involved physicians more than they have involved midwives, in large part because of the power imbalance between the two groups.

Midwives continued to be active in American birthing rooms until the twentieth century, but they were more often agents of tradition and conservatism in birth practices than agents of change. Beginning in the mid-eighteenth century, physicians represented the new, untried challenge of the future.

I do not at all mean to imply that the changes that occurred in childbirth history, many of which involved medical interventions, necessarily were good for women or that they moved on a singularly progressive march forward. In fact, as the evidence of this book reveals, many of the obstetric procedures introduced during the two hundred years of childbirth history examined here, particularly when they were new and practiced by inexperienced hands, worked to the detriment of women's health, not to their benefit. Change, progressive and retrogressive, is the focus of this book; middle- and upper-class women and their medical birth attendants as agents of that change thus appear prominently in my study. However, the legacies of the women who did not leave an accessible written record of their lives, most middle-class white women, the poor, the immigrant, and black women—the majority of the birthing women in America—and the midwife whose class, race, and ethnicity mirrored those of her patients, are extremely important for the historian. I have tried to incorporate the voices of these women whenever possible, but future research will have to examine more closely the extent to which my interpretation applies.

The evidence on which this study is based represents a cross matching of medical and women's sources. I have examined medical journals and texts and physicians' diaries and papers, and I have searched out thousands of women's birth accounts in letters, diaries, autobiographies, and family histories. I have put side by side the women's accounts with the physicians' accounts and have been struck more often by the congruence of the two rather than by their divergence. Both birthing women and their physicians voiced similar concerns about maternal safety; both evoked an increasing faith in medical science, and both provided evidence during the prehospital era of a true interactive negotiation process as the way to accomplish labor and delivery. This is not to suggest that women and physicians always agreed with each other. As this book documents, physicians frequently found their suggested interventions overruled by the women who had asked them to attend the deliveries and discovered that women sought medical expertise often only to bolster their own ideas about proper interventions. Even when they record violent disagreement over proposed interventions, the medical and women's sources written before childbirth moved to the hospital, if examined together, reveal a basic respect for the knowlege that both women and their doctors brought into the birthing room and a need to negotiate the final determination of events.

In addition to comparing medical and women's accounts, I have compared the prescriptive literature, which taught both doctors and women what they should do and set the standards for each era, with the empirical data, which described actual events around the birthing beds. Through this juxtaposition I have examined the ideology and the happening, and I have discovered the shortcomings of the prescriptive literature for understanding real events. Rarely were physicians able to accomplish what they were taught in theory they should accomplish; rarely could women achieve their ideal confinements. By focusing on actual birth accounts written by people in attendance or family members immediately concerned, I have tried to describe and analyze events as they occurred rather than events as they were predicted or prescribed. This focus has allowed me a perspective on the childbirth experience that is rooted in both the physicians' and the birthing women's points of view. It has led me to conclude that obstetric medicine in the prehospital era gained its ground through a communication involving all the parties and reflected, to a large degree, women's desires to change—again and again—obstetric procedures.[4]

Colonial women's diaries provided the title of the book. Women wrote often that their friends had been "brought to bed of a son," or that they themselves were "brought to bed of my darling daughter Elizabeth." The phrase suggests the simultaneously active and passive roles for women in the processes of childbirth at the same time as it records the differences in childbirth experiences over time. In traditional childbirth, women were brought to bed in their homes by a collection of their friends: birthing women were active in setting the environment and in picking the people to be with them at the same time as they were passive in receiving the ministrations of their helpers and in being at the mercy of those helpers' specific knowledge and abilities. While the particulars of the active and passive parts of women's participation in childbirth changed dramatically in the two hundred years from 1750 to 1950, this book argues that the conceptual division of the birth process into two parts, one of which a birthing woman could control and the other of which she could not, did not go away. Throughout American history, women focused on different parts of the experience to try to determine their own roles and to make birth safer, more comfortable, or more meaningful; but the dichotomy epitomized in the eighteenth-century phrase that conjures strength and weakness, control and lack of control, activity and passivity remained. Childbirth has portrayed the ambivalences of woman's larger social roles in the culture: both mistress of the hearth and thrall of the master.

This book is organized both chronologically and topically. Chapter 1 explores the prominence of repeated childbirth in women's lives and some of their responses to fears of death and debility associated with bearing children. It sets the stage for understanding why women tried so hard and so long to improve childbirth. Chapter 2 begins a review of male physicians' role in normal obstetrics. It focuses on the period when physicians first entered America's birthing rooms and examines particularly their use of the forceps, the first technology applied to aid complicated deliveries. Chapter 3 interrupts this chronological examination of changing birth procedures to describe the differences in women's childbirth experiences, particularly those determined by class and cultural distinctions. Its purpose is to help the reader interpret the variations evident in medical and women's descriptions of childbirth experiences. Chapter 4 analyzes the sex-specific influences on childbirth and the ways that women devised, within their own domestic traditions, to change the event to meet their needs for increased safety and comfort. The role that women physicians played in helping birthing women integrate traditional practices with some medical interventions is also examined. Chapter 5 picks up the chronological development again to analyze the greatest triumph of obstetrics: control of the pain of labor and delivery. The introduction of obstetrical anesthesia, from ether and chloroform to twilight sleep, illuminates how physicians and birthing women negotiated the specifics of childbirth practices. Chapter 6 examines other medical interventions in childbirth practices, particularly focusing on the use of drugs such as ergot, on procedures for suturing perineal tears, and on methods of coping with postpartum infections. The inability of doctors, even after they understood the role of bacteria, to stem the tide of postpartum infections reveals the particular difficulties physicians and birthing women confronted in the prehospital era. Chapter 7 moves the story into the twentieth century and analyzes the transition of childbirth to the hospital, a transition that caused the most significant changes in women's experiences. Chapter 8 analyzes all the changes described in the book and suggests a framework for understanding the factors that fostered

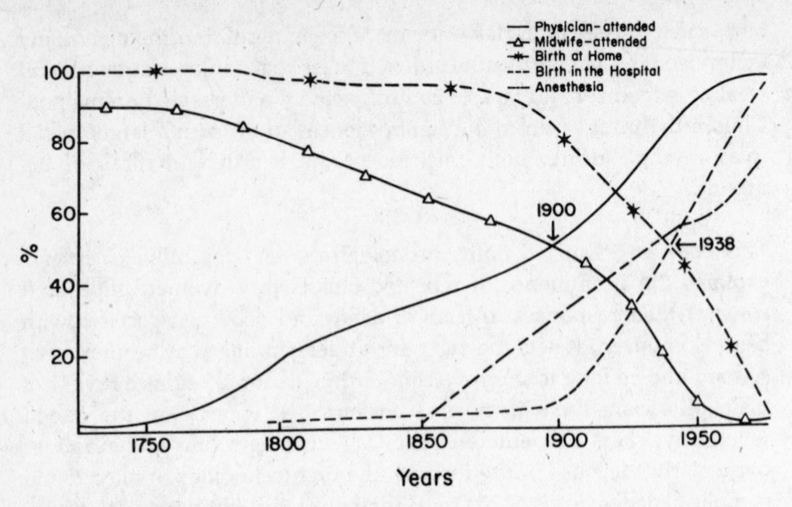

Graph illustrating trends in U.S. childbirth practices, based on estimates.
Source: Judith Walzer Leavitt, University of Wisconsin.

change in childbirth procedures and practices. A short epilogue, bringing the story into the 1980s, concludes the book.

Because of the topical organization, which sometimes requires some chronological overlap between the chapters, I have provided a graph of the trends in the major events in childbirth history and a brief chronology for readers to consult whenever necessary. A glossary of medical terms can be found (pages 271–76) preceding the Index.

1

"Under the Shadow of Maternity"

Childbirth and Women's Lives in America

In 1846 a young woman in Warren, Pennsylvania, gave birth to a son and soon after was taken with "sinking spells." Her female friends and relatives were there to help her; they took encouragement when she appeared better and consoled each other when she fell into a stupor. A woman who was with her during these days wrote to a mutual friend describing the scene around Mary Ann Ditmar's bed:

> Oh my beloved Girl—You may imagine our sorrow, for you too must weep with us—How can I tell you: I cannot realize myself—Mary Ann will soon cease to be among the living—and numbered with the dead . . . Elizabeth, it was such a scene that is hard to be described—L and I remained until the afternoon. Mrs. Mersel came and relieved us, also Mrs. Whalen came. We took a few hours sleep and returned—She had requested us to remain as long as she lived—there was every indication of a speedy termination of her suffering—Mary had come over—Mrs. N. remained to watch . . . all thought she was dying—She was very desirous of living till day light—She thought she might have some hope if she could stand it until morning—She retained her sense perfectly—She begged us to be active and not be discouraged that she might live yet—that life was so sweet—how she clung to it—Elizabeth I would wish you might be spared such a sight—we surrounded her dying bed—Each one diligent to keep life and animation in the form of one they so much loved and who at that very time was kept alive with stimulating medicines and wine—I cannot describe it for o my God the horrors of that night will ever

remain in the minds of those who witnessed it—our hearts swelled at the sight.[1]

Mary Ann lingered a few days, during which time she bestowed rings and locks of hair upon her friends so they might remember her; she made her peace with God and provided for her child. Then she died.

Mary Ann's story represents a reality visited upon countless American women in the eighteenth and nineteenth centuries, and it is a reality with supreme significance for understanding women's lives. During most of American history, an important part of women's experience of childbirth was their anticipation of dying or of being permanently injured during the event. This chapter will examine how potential dangers of childbirth influenced women's life expectations and experiences; and it will set the stage for understanding why and how women worked so hard to overcome these risks.

The physical dangers associated with childbearing—the "shadow of maternity"[2]—helped provide the justification for limiting women's lives to the domestic duties of homemaking and child-rearing. Most married women, and some unmarried women, had to face the physical and psychological effects of recurring pregnancies, confinements, and postpartum recoveries, which all took their toll on their time, their energy, their dreams, and on their bodies. The biological act of maternity, with all its risks, thus significantly marked women's lives as they made their way from birth to death.

Maternity's shadow had many dimensions. Most significant were high fertility rates. At the beginning of the nineteenth century, white American women bore an average of more than seven live children. This implies considerably more than seven pregnancies, because many terminated in miscarriage or stillbirths. For many groups in the expanding American population, fertility rates remained close to this high level throughout the nineteenth century.[3] Pregnancy, birth, and postpartum recovery occupied a significant portion of most women's adult lives, and motherhood defined a major part of their identity.

The life of Mary Vial Holyoke, who married into a prominent New England family in 1759, illustrates the strong grip that frequent pregnancies could hold over women's lives. In 1760, after ten months of marriage, Mary gave birth to her first baby. Two years later, her second was born. In 1765 she was again "brought to bed" of a child. Pregnant immediately again, she bore another child in 1766. The following year she delivered her fifth, and in one more year her sixth. Free from pregnancy and childbirth in 1769, she gave birth again in 1770. During

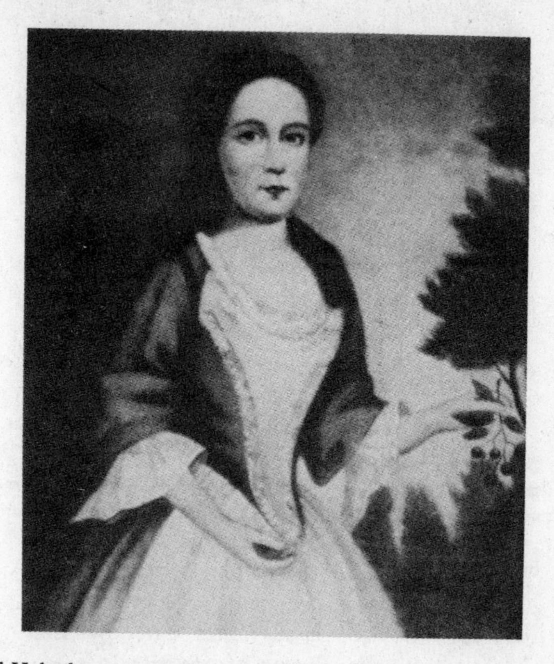

Mary Vial Holyoke, portrait painted in 1753.
Source: *Holyoke Diaries,* p. 46.

the next twelve years, she bore five more children. Mary Vial Holyoke spent the majority of the first 23 years of her married life, the years of her youth and vigor, pregnant, nursing her infants, and recovering from childbirth. (See Figure 1.) Because only three of her twelve children lived to adulthood, she also withstood frequent tragedies. She devoted her body and her life to procreation throughout her reproductive years. Mary Holyoke had more pregnancies and suffered more child deaths than her average contemporary, but her story presents a poignant example of the extreme physical trials some women endured. Her life reveals how the biological capacity of women to bear children has translated historically into life's destiny for individual women.[4]

Mary Vial Holyoke and two of her daughters kept diaries, portions of which have since been published, and these journals meticulously record the family's birth and death experiences. Entered frequently amidst the notations of family occasions, visiting schedules, and daily housework were the citations of confinements in the family and friendship circle. In 1765, for example, one third of the entries in Mary Vial

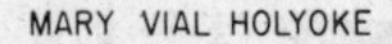

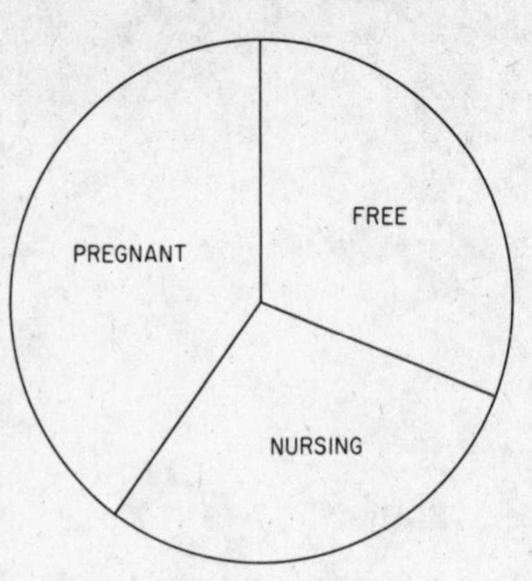

Figure 1. Chart dividing the first 23 years of Mary Vial Holyoke's married life into three parts. She had 12 pregnancies, nursed her infants an estimated 12 months if they lived, otherwise calculated by months of life, and was free from bodily reproductive duties the remainder.

Holyoke's diary contained references either to her own confinement or to those of her close friends. Eleven of her friends were "brought to bed" that year, and three others in the months of December and January immediately surrounding the calendar year. Historian Mary Beth Norton concluded from such accounts that married fertile colonial women accepted a child every two or three years as a "rhythmic part of . . . everyday existence."[5] Women chose to document childbirth frequently in their diaries and letters in part because it happened so often, but they found it a worthy topic also because of the significant physical risks it held for almost all women. Both the frequency of the event and its physical dangers created the burdens that women of the past carried with them through life.

A closer look at the obstetrical histories of the women in the Holyoke family reveals how commonly childbirth affected the course of women's adult lives. Before marrying Mary Vial in 1759, Edward Augustus Holyoke had been married to Judith Pickman. Judith became pregnant within the first six months of her marriage. She carried to term an infant daughter, but both mother and daughter died within months. This woman's life was snuffed out from childbirth-related causes eighteen months after her wedding. Edward and Mary Vial's daughter Susanna Holyoke Ward bore six live children and endured one still birth (thus putting her closer to the average white American woman of the period, who bore seven live babies). Susanna's obstetrical history, shown in Figure 2, illustrates that even if a woman produced below the average number of children, childbirth and the ensuing lactation could dominate her adult life. Judith Holyoke Turner, Susanna's sister, bore eight children during the first 18 years of her married life; four of her children died in infancy.

Of the other women in the Holyoke family whose obstetrical histories can be reconstructed through the family diaries, Mary Elliot Holyoke bore ten children between 1677 and 1697; Elizabeth Holyoke bore two infants in 1718 and 1719 and died herself before her second wedding anniversary; (another) Elizabeth Holyoke bore nine children between 1725 and 1739; Margaret Holyoke bore eight children between 1726 and 1739; Susannah Holyoke bore eight children in the years 1731 to 1746; Mary Holyoke bore five children with her first husband and one with her second between the years 1724 and 1742; Hannah Holyoke bore eight children in the twenty years between 1761 and 1781; Anna Holyoke Cults gave birth to eight children between 1763 and 1777; and Sarah Holyoke bore ten children during her first twenty years of marriage from 1775 and 1795. For all of these women childbearing and childrearing consumed a major portion of their adult lives.

The obstetrical history of Sarah Everett Hale, wife of Nathan Hale and mother of Edward Everett Hale, provides an early nineteenth-century example of childbirth's domination over women's time and

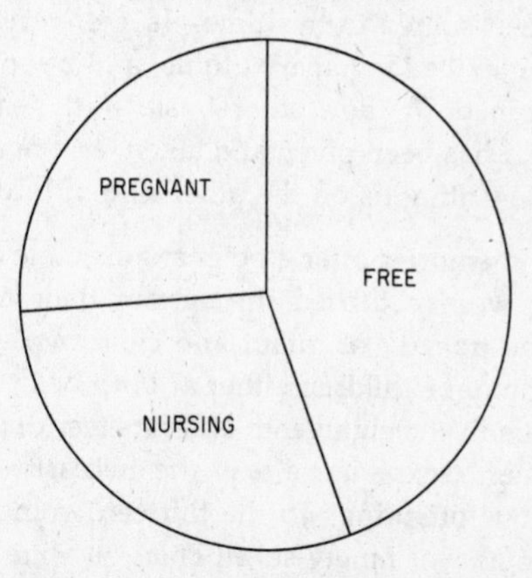

Figure 2. Chart dividing the first 20 years of Susanna Holyoke Ward's married life into three parts. She had seven pregnancies, nursed six live children, and was free from bodily reproductive duties the remainder.

energy. She experienced eleven confinements during the first twenty years of her marriage. (See Figure 3.) Sarah Everett married Nathan Hale on the morning of her twentieth birthday on September 5, 1816. One month later she was pregnant, and nine months later she delivered her first child. In another eight months Sarah again conceived, bearing her second child after a little more than two years of marriage; her next nine children followed in rapid succession. Sarah's diary reveals the centrality of childbearing and rearing to her life, and it illustrates the dimensions of the experience that women could share with one another. Looking back on her married life on her twenty-fifth wedding anniversary, in 1841, Sarah Hale wrote:

> I have borne eleven children, and have been permitted to keep until this day seven—One blossom of hope, just dawned upon this world, lived but a brief hour, and was transplanted by the all knowing Creator to his gardens of joy.—Another remained with us for seven months, learned to return smile for smile, and was just beginning to show the germs of intelligence when a short space of suffering and anxiety was closed by our laying him away in the dark chamber, which then was but a few paces from the nursery where we had cherished and nourished him—Then came another bright cherub—our darling "other Susie"—bright and hopeful and promising with her earnest and deep glance, and her thoughtful spirit, and in her seventh year, it pleased God to take her from us. . . . Three weeks had past away after her death, when another little girl was given us—She has been spared to this time—Is like, very like her sister,—God grant she may be long spared to us, and be so trained here that she may be joined to the "other Susie"—in heaven—Since then another little girl has been given and taken, and now there are seven here, and four awaiting us on the other side of Jordan.[6]

Sarah Hale's memories offer a poignant example of another part of the shadow that women carried throughout their married lives, the frequency and the tragedy of infant and child mortality. The woman who did not lose any of children either at birth or in the early years of their lives was rare in the eighteenth and nineteenth century. Far more common to women's experience was the necessity of accepting the deaths of numerous offspring. To the thirteen women in the Holyoke family mentioned above, ninety-seven children were born, and thirty-eight of them died as infants or small children. Statistics of course do not tell the whole story; a woman might lose just one child and carry the grief forever. But coming to terms with the deaths of numerous

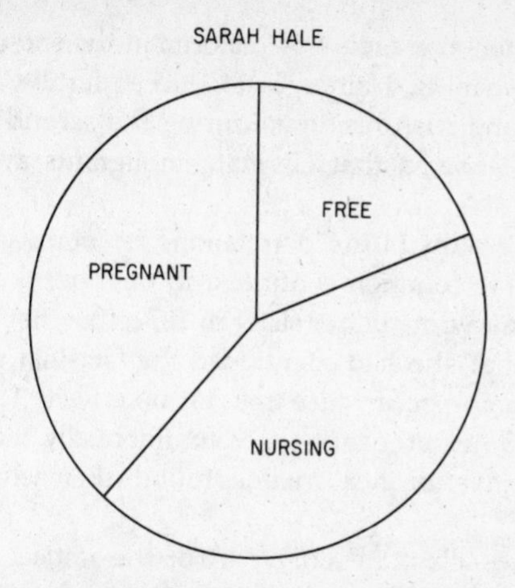

Figure 3. Chart dividing the first 22 years of Sarah Hale's married life into three parts. She had eleven pregnancies—ten live births, and one infant died at six months—and was free from bodily reproductive duties the remainder.

small children added a particular burden to women, especially during the time they were pregnant and had to anticipate the possibilities of disaster. For women, birth and death, life and loss, were intimately entwined in their daily existence.

Experiences with frequent pregnancies like Sarah Hale's and Mary Holyoke's became less common in nineteenth-century America as fertility rates declined. By 1900, white women, showing the ability to cut their fertility in half over the century, averaged 3.56 children. Historians and demographers trying to understand this decline have suggested that as much as 75 percent of the dropping fertility can be explained by active fertility control, including abortion and birth-control techniques.[7] Some people seem to have succeeded in beginning to assert control over the size of their families, but it is important to keep in mind, also, that the fertility decline that demographers have identified in nineteenth-century America applies mostly to white native-born women; immigrant and black women continued to have babies in larger numbers. Significant differences even among white native-born women suggest that fertility control was exceedingly variable. Southern white farm women, for example, continued to bear an average of almost six children at the end of the nineteenth century. Black women bore an average of more than five children.[8] Demographers have noted significant variations in fertility according to ethnic group. Foreign-born white women averaged 4.54 children at the end of the nineteenth century; but Michael R. Haines, who studied fertility among Philadelphia's German and Irish residents during the second half of the nineteenth century, showed that German immigrants averaged 7.22 and Irish 7.34.[9]

Among all groups in the population, the popular perception that large families were common continued throughout the nineteenth century. One woman wrote to her sister in 1872: "Mother said that she did not know whether she had mentioned the fact that we have another son. Such a common occurrence that it is no novelty." Ellen Whitehead wrote in 1877 to her pregnant sister confidentially that she was pregnant and that five of her friends found themselves in the same condition.[10]

Fertility rates illustrate only part of the impact of childbirth on women's lives. Maternity cast a shadow greater than its frequent repetition alone could have caused. Maternity, the creation of new life, carried with it the ever-present possibility of death. The shadow that followed women through their childbearing years was the fear of the physical risks of bearing children. Young women perceived that their bodies, even when healthy and vigorous, could yield up a dead infant or could carry the seeds of their own destruction. As Cotton Mather had warned at the beginning of the eighteenth century, and as many American women continued to believe, conception meant "your *Death* has Entered into you." Nine months of gestation could mean nine months to prepare for death. A possible death sentence came with every pregnancy.[11]

Women spent considerable time worrying and preparing for the probability of not surviving their confinements. During Nannie Stillwell Jackson's pregnancy in 1890, she wrote in her diary: "I have not felt well today am afraid I am going to be sick I went up to Fannies a little while late this evening & was talking to her, & I told her to see after Lizzie & Sue [other children] if I was to die & not to let me be buried here . . . & I want Lizzie & Sue to have *everything that is mine*, for no one has as good a rite [sic] to what I have as they have."[12] A pregnant Clara Clough Lenroot confided in her diary in 1891, "It occurs to me that *possibly* I may not live. . . . I wonder if I should die, and leave a little daughter *behind* me, they would name her 'Clara.' I should like to have them." Three days later she again was worrying: "If I shouldn't live I wonder what they will do with the baby! I should want Mamma and Bertha [sister] to have the bringing up of it, but I should want Irvine [husband] to see it every day and love it so much, and I should want it taught to love him better than anyone else in the world." With the successful termination of the birth, Clara's husband wrote in his wife's diary, "Dear Clara, 'mamma and Bertha' won't have to take care of your baby, thank God." He continued, "Everything is all right, but at what a cost. My poor wife, how you have suffered, and you have been so brave. . . . I have seen the greatest suffering this day that I have ever known or ever imagined."[13]

When her sister Emma experienced a difficult pregnancy in 1872, Ellen Regal went to be with her and found her "so patient and resigned." Ellen wrote to her brother, "it is not strange that she should tremble and shrink at the thought of that Valley of the Shadow of Death which she must so soon enter." Another woman wrote to her parents late in her pregnancy, "If I live and regain my health I will surely write to [all the people to whom she owed letters]." Lizzie Cabot in the middle of the nineteenth century wrote to her sister when she was pregnant with her first child, "I have made my will and divided off all my little things and don't mean to leave undone what I ought to do if I can help it." Sarah Ripley Stearns, returning from church near her time of confinement, wrote in her diary: "perhaps this is the last time I shall be permitted to join with my earthly friends."[14] Writing to her friend in 1821, another pregnant woman confided, "Could I have you . . . with me I should enjoy it much . . . for this life may soon be closed. I feel my dear friend that there may be but a step between me and eternity." Young Nettie Fowler McCormick confided in her diary, "I am feeling quite well but the time is *near at hand*—O God preserve my life to my husband & children."[15] Young, vigorous, healthy women who should have been anticipating a long life instead faced the very real possibility that in creating a life they would pay with their own.

Death fears remained central to women's perceptions of their birth experiences throughout the nineteenth and early twentieth centuries. Georgiana Kirby began to keep a journal when she learned she was pregnant in 1852 because, she wrote, "I think that perhaps I may die and my babe live." She was afraid she might not survive "this great trial of my physical powers" and wanted the child to have a remembrance of its mother.[16] Bessie Rudd, whose tuberculosis compounded her worries just a few years later, wrote to her husband that preparatory to her confinement she was arranging her household accounts so that he could understand them. "I have everything in order & fixed to my mind, should any unforeseen Sorrow come to me. You know we must think of all things, Edward & have everything in readiness . . . I sometimes think I am ready to [die] . . . though Life was never dearer to me than now, with *you* to *live for* & help along life's *pathway.*" Another day she wrote, "What record have I left for you, dear Edward, should I be taken away?" Even more melancholic, she wrote again, "if a Separation comes you *will* believe that I *loved you devotedly* dear Edward and I shall wait for you in the better home to which I know you will have an entrance and be blessed."[17]

Women like Bessie Rudd, whose illnesses portended especially dangerous labors and deliveries, had particular reason to fear death as their pregnancies advanced. Similarly, women whose mothers or other relatives had died during childbirth carried strong fears for their own possible demise. Sarah Jane Stevens, for example, whose mother had died in confinement, became acutely apprehensive during her own first pregnancy in 1880. She confided her fears to her doctor, who wrote to assure her that her labor "probably will be slow and tedious, as first labors almost always are, but with a strong will and resolution, such as I know you to have, no such abnormal conditions as you apprehend, will mar the normality of your confinement." Despite a successful first delivery, Sarah's fears did not diminish during her second pregnancy in 1885. Her brother, a physician, wrote to her that she should "look forward to confinement with less apprehension than to the last. The circumstances of our mother's unfortunate death were altogether abnormal," he concluded. "The immediate cause of her death was nervous shock at the *brutal* and *brutally ignorant* preparations for a surgical operation. . . . The lack of a skilful physician with good sense and humane instincts. . . . You have nothing of that sort to fear." Despite constant reassurances from her family, friends, and medical adviser, Sarah Stevens continued to feel anxious throughout both of her pregnancies.[18]

The extent to which these fears of death spread beyond the parturients to other family members is evident in the diary of Albina Wight, whose sister was pregnant and near confinement in another state. In 1870 Albina wrote, "I am so affraid [sic] she won't live through it." Three days later, she continued to think of her sister: "I could not keep Tilda out of my thoughts[.] It has seemed like a funeral all day . . . I fear she is not living." With relief Mary E. Cooley wrote her daughter-in-law: "I am very thankful that you are safely and comfortably through your trial."[19]

Women and family members were not the only ones who anticipated maternal death. Physicians who attended parturients through the fearful hours of labor and delivery also brooded over mortality. Dr. James S. Bailey of Albany, New York, in the 1870s, pondered the sometimes sudden and unexplained deaths of women following childbirth. He wrote, "To see a female, apparently in vigorous health until the period of accouchement, suddenly expire from some unforeseen accident, which is beyond the control of the attending physician, is well calculated to fill the mind with alarm and gloomy forebodings" and make it impossible "while attending a case of confinement, to banish the feeling of uncertainty and dread as to the result of cases which seemingly are terminating favorably."[20] Similarly, Dr. William Lusk, after relating the tragic story of a 23-year-old "very beautiful young woman" who died after delivery, warned his fellow physicians, "the exhausted condition in which the woman is left after childbirth render[s] her an easy prey to the perils of the puerperal state."[21] Fort Wayne, Indiana, physician H. V. Sweringen agreed that "Parturition under the most favorable circumstances is attended with great risk."[22] Physicians and families were well aware of the possibility of death: fears of the dangers of childbirth permeated society.

The extent to which society's fears reflected a reality of high death rates is almost impossible for historians to determine with any degree of confidence. The graphs that can be constructed from the available evidence illustrate that deaths from causes associated with maternity seem to have been declining toward the last part of the nineteenth century. But the statistics also show that the death rate leveled out toward the end of the century and continued at a high (and even increasing) level in the twentieth century. The statistics show that deaths from maternity-related causes at the turn of the twentieth century were approximately 65 times greater than they are in the 1980s, a comparison that helps us to understand the dangers women faced.

The best available evidence for the maternal mortality calculation comes from the statistics from New York City. Although New York is not necessarily representative of the rest of the country, health officials there collected information about maternal deaths for a longer time and in a more reliable way than elsewhere. Graph 2, based on health officer Haven Emerson's relatively complete recording of births and deaths in New York City, illustrates these trends in maternal mortality.[23]

These data are of limited value in determining the actual dangers women faced from childbirth-related causes before the middle of the twentieth century. The graph illustrates maternal death rates—that is, the number of maternal deaths per number of live births, which is calculated by dividing the number of deaths by the number of births. But the number of live births represents only part of the total pregnancy and delivery experiences. The figure omits from the denomina-

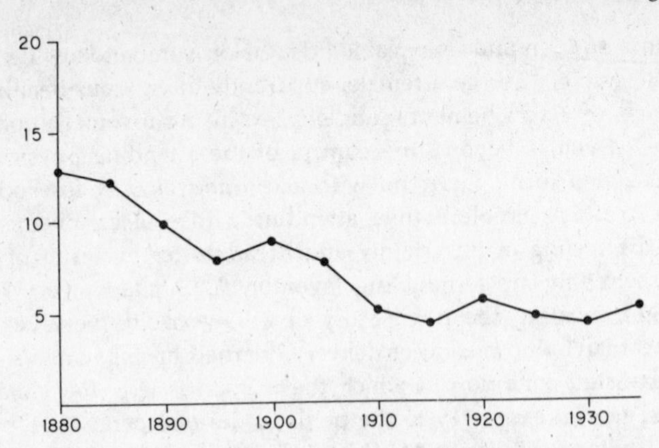

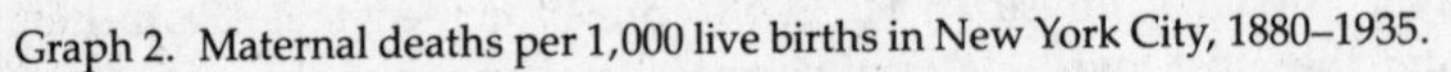
Graph 2. Maternal deaths per 1,000 live births in New York City, 1880–1935.

Source: Haven Emerson and Harriet Hughes, *Populations, Notifiable Diseases and Deaths Assembled for New York City*, New York (New York: Dehamar Institute of Public Health/College of Physicians and Surgeons, 1941). My thanks to Eve Fine for constructing this graph.

tor stillbirths, abortions, miscarriages, and other accidents that terminate a pregnancy prematurely or unsuccessfully. If we are interested in determining the actual dangers a woman faced when she became pregnant, we need to base our calculations on the total number of pregnancies women experienced, not just the ones that resulted in live births. But this tabulation is unavailable: we simply do not know how often women in the past found themselves pregnant or even how frequently women labored to give birth. It is only in the twentieth century that the recording of births (live and still) began to be noted reliably by local and state health departments, and even today we cannot calculate precisely the risks women face each time they become pregnant. Because we can not be sure about the number of labors or pregnancies, our statistical conclusions have limited meaning.

Even more frustrating for the historian trying to reconstruct the actual degree of danger associated with maternity is the fact that the recording of puerperal deaths itself (the numerator in our equation) is frequently incomplete and may bear little relationship to actual causes of death. Officials might have recorded that women who died while pregnant or within a month of childbirth died from other than puerperal causes. They might instead have implicated tuberculosis or any number of other diseases. Attributing the death to tuberculosis masked a large percentage of deaths that were actually childbirth-related. Physicians knew that an active case of tuberculosis could be exacerbated by pregnancy and especially by a difficult labor and delivery, but they attributed the death the woman suffered to the disease of tuberculosis rather than to the "disease" of childbirth. Their assumption that the women in fact died from tuberculosis may have been technically correct; but the result of their labeling hampers our ability to determine the actual risks parturient women faced. Tuberculosis in the nineteenth century disproportionately attacked young women between the ages of 15 to 45, and frequent pregnancies in these same women put them at a greater risk of early death. Because women suffered extensively from tuberculosis, their often repeated pregnancies were more dangerous to them.[24]

Further complicating our reading of the mortality data is the practice of some physicians of knowingly reporting a childbirth-related death as due to another cause to cover their own reputations in the community. One doctor wrote of this tendency in fellow physicians who wanted to pretend that they never had a case of puerperal infection: "he may have avoided signing a death certificate for a patient recently delivered, the certificate bearing the words, 'peritonitis,' 'blood-poisoning,' 'inflammation of the bowels,' or 'puerperal fever'; but cases occasionally perish some weeks after labor, with 'jaundice,' 'pneumonia,' 'congestion of the liver,' or 'malaria,' that, on closer study will be found to be the results of puerperal septic infection."[25]

The further frustration historians face with historical mortality statistics is that even the imperfectly reported maternal deaths and live births are available in the nineteenth century only for certain parts of the country for certain years. Much of women's experience, therefore, is unavailable through the statistical records. Those numbers we do have must be used with extreme caution.

Despite the inability of the statistics to speak adequately to our question of just how dangerous childbirth was, we can interpret the data that do exist to underscore society's perceptions of the dangers of childbirth for young women. Early in the twentieth century, by which time statistics had improved considerably over nineteenth century standards, approximately one mother died for each 154 living births (compared to 1980 standards of one maternal death for each 10,000 live births). If women delivered, let us estimate, five live babies during their childbearing years (the fertility rate for white women was 3.56, but an estimate that includes black and immigrant women would increase the rate to around five), then one of every thirty women might have been expected to die in childbirth over the course of her fertile years. That is, her risk during each pregnancy may have been one in

150, but her risk over her five pregnancies compounds to one in 30. Put this way, it is possible to understand women's fears for themselves in a more dramatic and realistic way.[26]

One of every 17 men who applied for life insurance in an early twentieth-century study said they had a mother or sister who had died as the immediate result of childbirth.[27] This figure included the women whose deaths might have been medically attributable to tuberculosis or other diseases, but which family members attributed to childbirth because of its proximity to the woman's confinement. If the figure one in seventeen represents family experiences, as this particular tabulation indicates was the case for many families in the early twentieth century, women's and family's fears of maternal death were based in reality.

Certainly the perception of childbirth's dangers, as we have already noted, was a constant in the minds of pregnant women and their families. Ellen Regal wrote to her brother in 1872 that their sister had survived her confinement: "It was a hard day for her in every respect; but she has escaped the fever we feared and is, apparently, doing well in every respect." A. G. Chatfield wrote to his brother in 1837 expressing relief that his brother's wife "got over the worst of all human Perils, that of giving birth to a child," and he reported that his own wife had just "had a fearful time" delivering a baby.[28]

Over and over again, the fears of death in childbirth were confirmed. A daughter wrote: "My mother died suddenly, giving premature birth, when I was seventeen (in 1879). She herself was only thirty-eight." A husband wrote: "In June [1875] my wife gave birth to my youngest daughter. From this sickness she never recovered. She suffered terribly . . . and finally died . . . leaving three boys and two girls to mourn her loss." A neighbor wrote of a mission wife in Oregon who, while her husband was away, "went down into the valley of the shadow of death" after delivering her first baby. A New England woman wrote: "My friend, Mrs. John Howard, of Springfield, has died as she has expected to,—under the most aggravated circumstances that a woman can leave the world. She never gave birth to her child; but died in the effort. In this dreadful manner have six of my youthful contemporaries departed this life." A desolate husband turned from his wife's death in childbirth in 1830: "I am undone forever." Another husband wrote to his mother-in-law in the 1860s:

> My dear wife is no more, you dear daughter is gone, Melissa is dead. In our deep and mutual affliction let us weep scalding tears of sorrow and anguish, my pen will not describe the depth of my woe.

> The world that so lately seemed so bright and lovely before me with happiness, is suddenly but a dark and dreary wilderness before me . . . . She was confined on the 28th of Nov. and after extreme suffering brought us a little girl . . . a fever set in, with inflamation, known as child bed Fever . . . She has suffered on until this morning at 10 minutes past 4 Oclock death came to her relief . . . our dear little baby . . . will never know a mothers love.

These were not isolated incidents. The U. S. Children's Bureau studies in the early twentieth century catalogued the intimate knowledge of death that pregnant women, especially in isolated rural areas, carried with them along with their swollen bellies. Childbed deaths were so familiar to Americans, from the eighteenth to the twentieth century, that fearful anticipation characterized the common and realistic attitudes toward pregnancy.[29]

Despite the decline in number of births women endured, and somewhat of a decline in the rate of maternal deaths, women remained fearful of maternity.[30] Women might have been at risk of puerperal death fewer times during their lifetimes, but for them the fear of dying during childbirth continued to define the shape of their lives. In the early twentieth century part of this fear was related to the fact that maternal deaths continued at higher than expected levels. Women and physicians saw that deaths from various infectious diseases were dropping rapidly at the turn of the twentieth century, but that deaths from childbirth-related causes remained high. Since many of those deaths could be attributed to infection, and since physicians supposedly understood how to prevent infection after the 1880s, both the medical and lay communities agreed that much of maternal mortality should be preventable. Furthermore, maternal mortality statistics from other countries showed that women in several nations fared better than they did in the United States. In 1910, when the United States recorded that one mother died for every 154 babies born alive, Sweden's record showed that one mother was lost to every 430 live births.[31]

Another reason birth anxieties continued, despite declining fertility and mortality, was that first births contained the largest actual risk (i.e. maternal deaths were higher for primiparas than for multiparas),[32] and women continued to have first babies at the same rate throughout the nineteenth century. That is, between 1800 and 1900 when the size of families declined, the percentage of families in the population remained the same; women had smaller families, but they still had families. Married women continued to bear first children as their grandmothers had, but the total size of their families diminished. Their fears continued to be related to the experiences of their first pregnancies, when, young and vulnerable, they faced the possibility of their own death. Dr. Beatrice Tucker, Director of the Chicago Maternity Center, realized as late as 1948, "There are all kinds of women who come into a doctor's office to seek care during pregnancy. Some are educated and well-bred; some ignorant; some well adjusted; some phlegmatic, and some neurotic and high-strung. But most of them have this in common—fear."[33]

Death fears were promoted, too, in the culture at large. Religion taught that childbirth was God's punishment to women, and this perspective of women's fate was strong in women's private writings. Countless women, either explicitly or implicitly, related their fears and their pregnancy-related trials to God's will and accepted it as such. Nineteenth-century fiction writing also shaped women's perceptions of what to expect during their confinements and led them to anticipate suffering.

Women today continue to think about mortality for themselves or their offspring, even when their own experience and the experiences of their friends and relations contradict the probability of death. Whether dangers are reported as one in every 150 births or one in 10,000, women find themselves thinking about death as soon as they discover they are pregnant. Part of this represents a lag time in perceptions catching up with improving statistics. But, in addition, the few cases of women dying in childbirth reported in the United States today are enough to force pregnant women to face their own mortality. Because they are young and because the possibility of death, even though remote, occurs to them perhaps for the first time in their lives, its emotional impact is beyond its actual danger. The centrality of childbearing to women's lives emphasizes the seriousness of the dangers it holds.

In the past, the shadow of maternity extended beyond the possibility and fear of death. Women knew that if procreation did not kill them, it could maim them for life. Postpartum gynecological problems, some great enough to force women to bed for the rest of their lives, others causing milder disabilities, hounded many of the women who survived childbirth. For some women, the fears of future debility were more disturbing than fears of death. The worse problems were the vesicovaginal and rectovaginal fistulas (holes between the vagina and either the bladder or the rectum caused by the violence of childbirth or by instrument damage), which brought incontinence and constant irritation to sufferers. Women knew also that unsutured perineal tears were likely to cause slow postpartum recovery and significant daily discomfort. Postpartum infections similarly threatened young women's health and life during their prime. Newly married women looking forward to life found themselves almost immediately faced with the prospect of permanent physical limitations that could follow their early and repeated confinements.

Chicago physician Henry Newman believed that the "normal process of reproduction [is] a formidable menace to the after-health of the parous woman."[34] Lacerations—tears in the perineal tissues or in the walls of the vagina, bladder, or rectum—probably caused the greatest postpartum trouble for women. The worse of these, the fistulas, which led to either urine or feces constantly leaking through the vaginal opening without the possibility of control was, in the words of one sympathetic doctor, "the saddest of calamities, entailing . . . endless suffering upon the poor patient . . . death would be a welcome visitor."[35] Women who had to live with this condition sat alone and invalided as long as they lived unless they were one of the beneficiaries of Dr. J. Marion Sims' repair operation after the middle of the century. Their incontinence made them unpleasant companions, and even their friends and relatives found it hard to keep them constant company.[36]

More frequent and less debilitating, but still causing major problems for many women, were tears in the vaginal wall, cervix, and perineal tissues that might have led to prolapsed uterus, uncomfortable sexual intercourse, or difficulties with future deliveries.[37] One physician noted, "the wide-spread mutilation . . . is so common, indeed, that we scarcely find a normal perineum after childbirth."[38] Most perineal lacerations were probably minor and harmless; but if severe ones were not adequately repaired, women might suffer from significant postpartum discomfort. Women complained most frequently of prolapsed uteri. This displacement of the womb downwards, sometimes even through the vaginal opening, usually resulted from childbirth-related perineal lacerations and relaxation of the ligaments. The practice of keeping women in bed for ten days to two weeks postpartum and the corset women donned soon after childbirth exacerbated this problem. One doctor noted that fallen womb was often a temporary condition; but he also found it recurrent: "Any woman subject to ill turns, lassitude, and general debility, will tell you that not unfrequently upon these occasions she is sensible of a falling of the womb."[39]

The condition caused misery for women. Albina Wight's sister Eliza, to give just one example from the 1870s, had a difficult delivery that was followed by prolapsus. Six weeks after one of her sister's confinements, Albina recorded, "Eliza is sick yet can only walk across the room and that overdoes her. She has falling of the Womb. poor girl." Eliza's medical treatment by "a calomel doctor" who gave her "blue pills" did not help. Five months following the delivery she could only "walk a few steps at a time and cannot sit up all day." A second doctor predicted, "it will be a long time before she will get around again."[40]

The typical treatment for this common female ailment was the use of a pessary, a mechanical support for the uterus inserted into the vagina and left there as long as necessary. (See illustration.) Pessaries, of which there were literally hundreds of types, themselves often led to pelvic inflammations and pain for the women whose conditions they were meant to alleviate. In the opinion of one doctor, "I think it is indisputable that a pessary allowed to remain for a very short period will invariably produce irritation, and if continued longer, will produce almost as certainly, ulceration. I have removed many pessaries that have produced ulceration; one in particular, hollow and of silver gilt, was completely honey-combed by corrosion, its interior filled with exuviae of the most horrible offensiveness, the vagina ulcerated through into the bladder, producing a vesico-vaginal fistula, and into the rectum, producing a recto-vaginal fistula; the vagina in some portion obliterated by adhesive inflammation and numerous fistulae made through the labia and around the mons veneris for the exit of the various discharges."[41]

Uterine displacements puzzled doctors and pained women throughout the nineteenth century. A midcentury physician noted that uterus-related problems were "the dread of almost every physician, and the constant, painful perplexity of many a patient." He told of his recent case:

> In the winter of 1863, I was consulted by a young lady from a distant part of the State, on account of a disease from which she had suffered for nearly four years. She had received the advice of many a physician of high and low degree—had worn the ring pessary—the globe pessary—the horseshoe pessary—the double S pessary and the intra-uterine stem pessary—and the common sponge . . . . The patient gave a history of frequent inflammation of the uterus and ovaries, and there appeared to be quite strong adhesions binding the womb in its assumed place. She had had too frequent menstruation—profuse and intolerably painful—frequent and painful micturition [urination].

The physician inserted his "modified" ring pessary and happily reported that "the patient went to her home after a few weeks entirely relieved from all bad symptoms."[42]

In the last half of the nineteenth century physicians reported in-

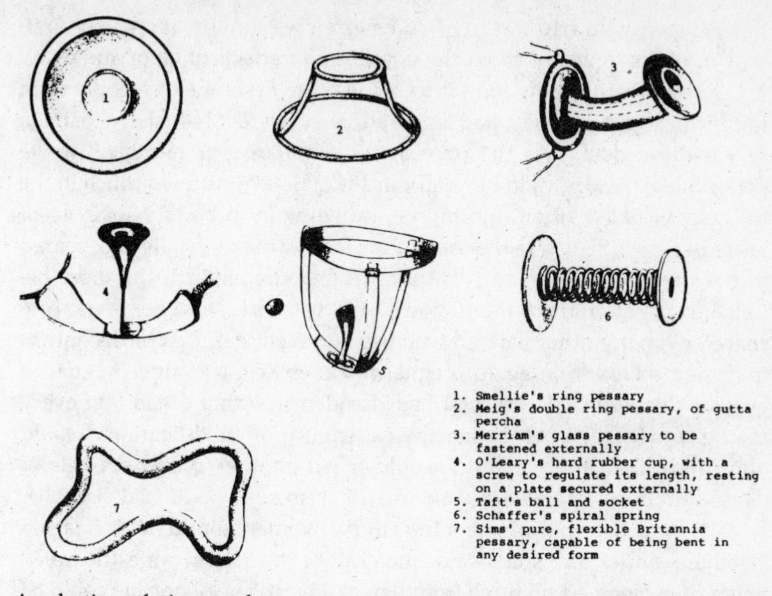

A selection of nineteenth-century pessaries, used internally to support a prolapsed uterus. Hundreds of varieties existed.

Source: Augustus K. Gardner, "On the Use of Pessaries," *Transactions of the American Medical Association* 15 (1865): 109–22.

creased numbers of perineal and cervical lacerations and their accompanying gynecological problems, attributed by many observers to increased use of forceps in physician-directed deliveries. If it is true that physicians' interventions caused increasing problems for women in this period (a question explored in Chapters 2 and 6), it is also the case that physicians became increasingly adept at repairing the problems. The medical journals were filled with case studies of women whose badly managed delivery had caused them problems, which could then be resolved by superior medical care. For example, an Iowa physician, Dr. Nicholas Hard, reported in 1850 a case he salvaged: a 35-year-old woman "with her first child, having had the forceps applied at an improper time during her labour, suffered from inflammation of the vulva, vagina, and contiguous soft parts, and had a tardy convalescence . . . . The vaginal orifice was perfectly closed . . . she suffered exceedingly from retained catamenial [menstrual] fluid." The doctor instrumentally reopened the vagina and reported that his patient now "walks to church, visits, and does house-work."[43]

Women who had already had children were more likely than first-time mothers to worry about the possible aftereffects of labor and delivery. Remembering how long it took them the first time to recover from the birth and how they had suffered, they were particularly loath to repeat the ordeal. "As the time draws near I fear & tremble," wrote Persis Sibley Andrews in her diary in 1847, "I have suffered much in the last four weeks & often find myself indulging in forbodings of evil—of years of ill health as was the case before & all & the worst ills to be feared in the case. God help me."[44] Andrews feared childbirth the more because of the invalidism that followed her first birth, and her fears were shared by many other women who had survived their first births only to find themselves soon again pregnant. Agnes Reid's second pregnancy evoked this letter: "I confess I had dreaded it with a dread that every mother must feel in repeating the experience of child-bearing. I could only think that another birth would mean another pitiful struggle of days' duration, followed by months of weakness, as it had been before."[45] Another mid-nineteenth-century woman found herself again "walking under the shadow of maternity . . . . Then came the week when there seemed no hope from day to day that even one life could be given for the other, but that both would perish together."[46] Mary Kincaid resigned herself to her coming trials when she found herself again pregnant in 1896. She wrote this poignant message to her cousin:

> Mamie I got two hard months before me yet that if I count right, I just dread the time coming. . . . O Mamie I wish there was no such thing as having babies. I wish I took George Willard's receit [for abortion?] and left the nasty thing alone. I will next time you bet I will not have any more if I live through this time what I hope I will. Well, Mamie it is there and it has to come out where it sent in. Sumner [husband] says that I could cough all I am [she had a cold] and I couldn't cough it up. Well might as well laugh as cry it be just the same.[47]

Apart from their fears of resulting death or debility, women feared pain and agony and "suffering beyond bearing" during the confinement itself. They worried about how they would bear up under the pain and stress, how long the confinement might last, and whether trusted people would accompany them through the ordeal. The short hours between being a pregnant woman and becoming a mother seemed, in anticipation, to be interminably long, and they occupied the thoughts and defined the worries of multitudes of women. Women's descriptions of their confinement experiences foretold the horrors of the ordeal.

"Between oceans of pain," wrote one woman of her third birth in 1885, "there stretched continents of fear; fear of death and dread of suffering beyond bearing."[48] Surviving a childbirth did not allow women to forget its horrors. Lillie M. Jackson, recalling her 1905 confinement, wrote "While carrying my baby, I was so miserable. . . . I went down to death's door to bring my son into the world, and I've never forgotten. Some folks say one forgets, and can have them right over again, but today I've not forgotten, and that baby is 36 years old."[49] Too many women shared Hallie Nelson's feelings upon her first delivery: "I began to look forward to the event with dread—if not actual horror." Even after Nelson's successful birth, she "did not forget those awful hours spent in labor."[50]

Women recounted their trials with wrenching repetitiveness. One wrote that her child "nearly killed me as he tore his way into life." Another: "My body and spirits were so extremely weak, I could only just bear to look at those I loved." Another: "The two of us were close to death. . . . The strain of having him had exhausted me." Another: "The angels of life and death wrestled over my baby's life and over mine in that little pioneer fort." Another: "I lay at the point of death. And out of that hour in which I touched the hand of death, two months before her time, came my daughter." Women suffered in the anticipation and in the reality of childbirth.[51]

Most women managed to find joy or purpose in the experience despite their hard times. Mary Foote recounted her 1877 childbirth as a "long dreadful day and night . . . a dim bewildering Hall of pain all day—growing worse & worse and then came Heaven at last. . . . I am weak and happy." In another letter to her friend she admitted that motherhood was "a sort of pendulum . . . between joy & dread."[52] Josephine Preston Peabody wrote in her diary of the "most terrible day of [her] life" when she delivered her firstborn, the "almost inconceivable agony" she lived through during her "day-long battle with a thousand tortures and thunders and ruins." Her second confinement brought "great bodily suffering," and her third, "the nethermost hell of bodily pain and mental blankness. . . . the *will-to-live* had been massacred out of me, and I couldn't see why I *had* to." But, she concluded in her diary, "Now that it is over—I would not for anything—give up the awfulness of it. For I am wiser in the height and the depth, for this knowledge of the almost inconceivable agony . . . I can never forget—or explain—that apocalyptic hugeness of the thing. . . . I have crossed the abyss now. . . . That anything so wonder-small and wonder-soft and helpless and exquisite should come of anything so cruel and unimaginable as Birth," she marveled.[53] And yet another new mother rejoiced that out of her "time of great difficulty and distress" she had emerged "the living mother of a living and perfect child."[54]

Regardless of the particular fear that women carried along with their swelling uterus, the prospect of often repeated motherhood promised hardship and anxiety, even at the same time as it might have promised wonderment and hope. Hannah Whitall Smith understood this and wrote in her diary in 1852:

> I am very unhappy now. That trial of my womanhood which to me is so very bitter has come upon me again. When my little Ellie is 2 years old she will have a little sister or brother. And this is the end of all my hopes, my pleasing anticipations, my returning youthful joyousness. Well, it is a woman's lot and I must try to become resigned and bear it in patience and *silence* and not make my home unhappy because I am so. But oh, how hard it is.[55]

Hannah Smith wrote in this short diary passage, which has strong religious overtones, how unhappy she was when she found herself pregnant, because pregnancy meant that she had to give up the parts of her life that she enjoyed—the youthful happiness and the hopeful days. But she accepted what was coming with her pregnancy, she determined not to complain about it, and she knew it was what her position demanded. The diary entry is all the more poignant because it voiced meaning for two generations in this family. Hannah Whitall Smith's niece, M. Carey Thomas, found her aunt's journal and was so moved by this notation that she copied it into her own diary in 1878. For Hannah Smith, as well as for Carey Thomas, marriage meant having children. Unable to prevent conception, Hannah Smith accepted its demands even while expressing to her diary how much against her wishes it was. Her lot—woman's lot—was to be Mother.[56]

Many women walked with Hannah Smith under the shadow of maternity, experiencing repeated and agonizing births in unrelenting succession with no relief throughout their fertile years. Many women suffered physical complications through their confinements that stayed with them the rest of their lives. For many women the physical hardships of childbearing determined the parameters of their lives and defined their social destiny. Mathilde Shillock, a German immigrant who settled on the Minnesota frontier in the 1850s, wrote to her sister how childbearing compounded her already difficult settler life:

> God has entrusted us with a son, a blooming healthy child. He was born on the 1st of December. It seems that his father is happy over it; I myself do not wish for any more children, as I look upon life as a heavy burden. The three years of western life have so thoroughly exhausted me that I am no longer capable of joy or hope or love. I am speaking the naked truth so that I may in a measure at least write quietly without exertion of dissumalation [sic]. What a cleft there is between the outpourings of my heart over our first children and this little stranger! pity is all that I can offer him. Pitty [sic] and a feeling of duty towards him to lighten his blameless fate.[57]

Although childbearing and the ensuing motherhood held many rewarding times for women, the hardships and the dangers created the boundaries within which most women had to construct their lives. The childbirth experience was, of course, heavily influenced by cultural and economic conditions, the particular time and place in which women lived, and their socioeconomic class or ethnic group. But much of the meaning of childbirth for women was determined not by the particulars of the event but by what women shared with each other by virtue of their common biological experience.

The biological capacity to bear children itself was not what determined the course of women's lives, but rather the cultural use to which that capacity was put during most of American history. Because women found themselves repeatedly pregnant and because this condition involved certain physical risks, women found themselves bound by what appeared to be their biology. In fact, they were bound equally by ideology, an ideology of domesticity and nurturance, which the women as well as the men in society accepted as the proper order of things. The ideology affected all women, although the difficulty of raising large families under conditions of poverty meant that it became particularly burdensome for poor women.

In the following chapters I shall examine how women coped with their lives led under the shadow of maternity. The analysis centers on the event of childbirth itself, and it looks at how birthing women participated in changing the event, particularly after the middle of the eighteenth century when physicians first began attending normal labors and deliveries. The next chapter examines the initial impact of physician obstetrics by focusing on the introduction of the forceps, the instrument that worked particularly to the advantage of doctors as they began to participate in the traditional women's event of childbirth.

2

"Science" Enters the Birthing Room

The Impact of Physician Obstetrics

At the end of the eighteenth century, Dr. William Shippen, Jr., of Philadelphia attended all the childbearing women in the well-established Drinker family. The family members chose Shippen instead of a woman midwife, in spite of their ambivalence about having a man in the traditionally all-female birthing room, because they believed the physician offered the best hope for a successful outcome. The Drinkers, and many others like them, considered themselves fortunate to be living at a time when male physicians began replacing female midwives in the birthing rooms of the American urban elite. The families expected—and believed that they received—better care at the hands of physicians than they thought possible with traditional female attendants. This chapter examines the promises of the new physician-directed obstetrics—beginning in the 1760s, when American physicians first entered the practice of normal obstetrics, and ending in the early twentieth century, when physicians delivered most of America's babies—and evaluates the extent to which those promises were kept.[1] The chapter focuses on the forceps; other physician-based interventions will be examined in Chapters 5 and 6.

Before 1760 birth was a women's affair in the British colonies of North America. When a woman went into labor, she "called her women together" and left her husband and other male family members outside. "I went to bed about 10 o'clock," wrote William Byrd of Virginia, "and left the women full of expectation with my wife." Only in cases where women were not available did men participate in labor and delivery, and only in cases where labor did not progress normally did physicians

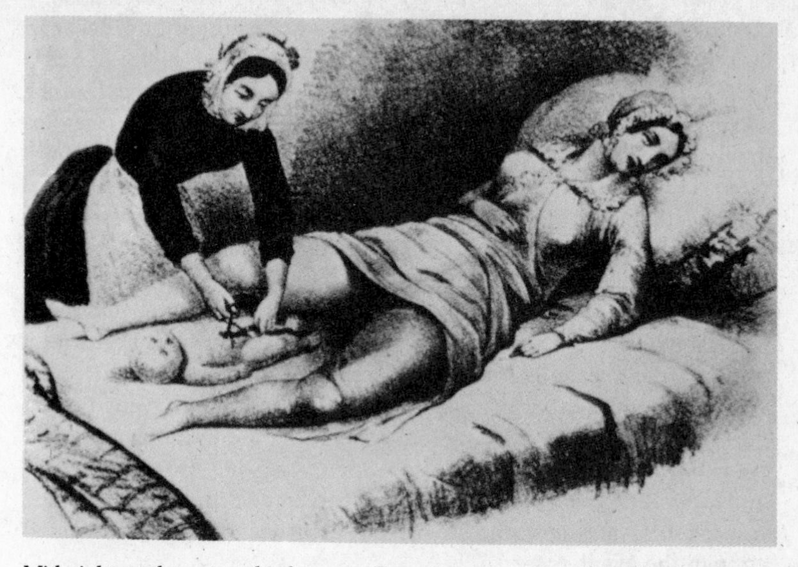

Mid-eighteenth-century birth scene. Parturient woman attended by a midwife. Source: W. Beach, *Improved System of Midwifery* (New York: Baker and Scribner, 1848).

intervene and perhaps extricate a dead fetus. The midwife orchestrated the events of labor and delivery, and the women neighbors and relatives comforted and shared advice with the parturient.[2]

When Mrs. Ebenezer Parkman was brought to bed in 1738, she called her midwife and six other women to help. Seventeen women attended Mrs. Samuel Sewall during her lying-in period. Midwife Martha Ballard attended hundreds of women in childbirth and recorded in her diary the presence of numerous other neighbor women. The common pattern of American childbirth was that women attended other women in their confinements. Trained midwives or experienced friends and relatives came to help before or when women began labor, and many of them stayed for days or weeks afterward, participating in the transition to motherhood. Women suffered through the agonies and dangers of birth together, sought each other's support, and shared the relief of successful deliveries and the grief of unsuccessful ones. This "social childbirth" experience united women and provided, as Carroll Smith-Rosenberg has argued, one of the functional bonds that formed the basis of women's domestic culture.[3]

Within their own homes, birthing women controlled much of the experience of childbirth. They determined the physical setting for their confinements, the people to attend them during labor and delivery, and the aids or comforts to be employed. Midwives traditionally played a noninterventionist, supportive role in the home birthing rooms. As much as possible they let nature take its course: they examined the cervix or encouraged women to walk around; they lubricated the perineal tissues to aid stretching; they delivered the child and tied the umbilical cord; and sometimes they manually expressed the placenta. In cases of protracted labor, midwives might have turned the fetus—"version"—or fortified women with hard liquor or mulled wine. They may have manually stretched the cervix or, rarely, administered ergot, a drug that stimulated contractions. Midwives spent most of their time, as the written record reveals, comforting the parturient and waiting. The other women attendants supported the midwife and the birthing woman, and the atmosphere in the birthing rooms—if everything proceeded normally—was congenial and cooperative. Parturient women, who felt vulnerable at the time of their confinements, armed themselves with the strength of other women who had passed through the event successfully.[4]

Despite the very positive aspects of social childbirth, a romantic image of childbirth in this early period would be misleading. Women garnered suppport from their networks of companions, but they continued to fear childbirth because of the possibilties of death or debility. It was precisely these fears that led women away from traditional birthing patterns to a long search for safer and less painful childbirths. Some women, especially those who were economically advantaged, tried to modify traditional births by incorporating new possibilities as they became available. Like the Drinkers, these eighteenth-century women readily invited physicians to attend them, despite their worries about the propriety of having men participate in intimate female events, in hopes that the "man-midwives" could provide easier and safer births.

The entrance of physician-accoucheurs into the practice of obstetrics in America during the second half of the eighteenth century marked the first significant break with tradition. The story of this new midwifery, familiar to historians of medicine, centers on William Shippen, who in 1762 returned from his studies in London and Edinburgh to establish the first systematic series of lectures on midwifery in America. Shippen initially trained both female midwives and male physicians in anatomy, including the gravid (pregnant) uterus, but he soon limited his lectures to male students. He established a private practice of midwifery and became a favorite of Philadelphia's established families. The Drinkers found him "very kind and attentive" during labor and delivery and noted that he remained with his patients even during protracted labors and "sleep't very little."[5]

Shippen was the most famous of late-eighteenth-century physicians who practiced midwifery, but he was not alone. Numerous doctors expanded their practice of medicine and began to attend women in labor. The transition to male attendants occurred so easily among advantaged urban women in the northeast that it can only be explained by understanding the women's impression that physicians knew more than midwives about the birth process and what to do if things went wrong. Women overturned millennia of all-female tradition and invited men into their birthing rooms because they believed that male physicians offered additional security against the potential dangers of childbirth. By their acknowledgement of physician superiority, women changed the fashions of childbearing and made it desirable to be attended by physicians.[6]

Women had good reason to believe that physicians could provide services that midwives could not. Many of the physicians who practiced obstetrics at the turn of the nineteenth century had trained in Great Britain, where a tradition of male accoucheurs had already developed. The men had access to education then denied to women, and this medical education provided theoretical understanding of female anatomy and the process of parturition. Whereas women midwives relied on practical experience and an appeal to female traditions—factors to some extent taken for granted and unappreciated—men physicians had the extra advantage and prestige associated with formal learning. Even though most American practitioners had not attended medical school and were themselves apprentice-trained, physicians carried with them the status advantages of their gender and of the popular image of superior education. Furthermore, birthing women perceived that the male presence had already contributed opium and forceps to obstetrics and promised even greater benefits in the future. The appeal to overturn tradition was strong.[7]

When Shippen attended Sally Drinker Downing's 1795 birth, which was complicated by a footling presentation, he administered opium to relieve her suffering. Two years later, faced with another of Downing's difficult labors, Shippen "was oblig'd to force her mouth open to give some thing with a view of reviving her." In 1799 Downing again suffered a protracted labor, and Shippen took fourteen ounces of blood and then gave her eighty to ninety drops of liquid laudanum, an opiate. According to Downing's mother, when labor still did not progress, Shippen gave "an Opium pill three grains he said, in order to ease her pain, or to bring it on more violently." When this still did not produce the desired result, Shippen threatened to use his instruments, but finally Downing delivered without them.[8]

Shippen's practice of allaying painful and lengthy labors by bleeding, giving opium, and occasionally using forceps illustrates why women wanted physicians to attend them. The prospect of a difficult birth, which all women fearfully anticipated, and the knowledge that physicians' remedies could provide relief and successful outcomes led women to seek out practitioners whose obstetric armamentarium included drugs and instruments. In the eighteenth and nineteenth centuries the option of calling in physicians was limited to those women who could afford to pay the extra fee physicians commanded over the midwife's charge. In the second half of the nineteenth century extremely poor women, whose birth options at home were limited by their resources, and single women, who likewise could not garner the family-centered support needed, delivered their babies in hospitals and maternity centers where they, too, had access to physician attendants (see Chapter 3).[9]

The promise of the new obstetrics developed in part through formal physician education in midwifery. Shippen's first lectures covered pelvic anatomy, the gravid uterus, the placenta, fetal circulation and nutrition, natural and unnatural labor, and the use of obstetrical instruments. He demonstrated on manikins and on patients—poor women for whom he provided accommodation—and used drawings and textbooks. Other physicians followed his example, and courses in midwifery became available in Boston and New York as well as in Philadelphia.[10]

During the first half of the nineteenth century medical education in obstetrics took root and expanded. Schooled in the values of their culture, many professors and students found the subject embarrassing, and students generally did not observe women in labor but received only a theoretical education. Samuel D. Gross, a student who observed Thomas Chalkley James teaching obstetrics at the University of Pennsylvania early in the nineteenth century, noticed that "it was seldom that he raised his eyes from his manuscript, or looked squarely at his audience. His cheeks would be mantled with blushes while engaging in demonstrating some pelvic viscus, or discussing topics not mentionable in ordinary conversation. It was often painful to witness his embarrassment."[11]

Although the embarrassment of physicians about their role in obstetrics disappeared as their experience with the subject increased, the question of a man's proper behavior in a woman's birthing room continued to influence the teaching and the practice of obstetrics. Of William Potts Dewees, who succeeded James at the University of Pennsylvania, Gross observed, "he did not hesitate to call things by their proper names. No blush suffused his cheek in the lecture-room."[12] But Dewees, whose influential text, *A Compendious System of Midwifery,* went through twelve editions, remained as horrified by the idea of visual inspection of women's genitals as his most modest patients. Using manikins, he taught his students how to perform unsighted digital explorations of parturient women. As the illustrations show, students learned to examine women's genital tracts without looking at what they were doing. Even when applying forceps, Dewees taught, "every attention should be paid to delicacy . . . the patient should not be exposed . . . even for the drawing off of the urine. . . . The operator must become familiar with the introduction of the instruments without the aid of sight."[13]

Walter Channing, who was the first professor to teach obstetrics at

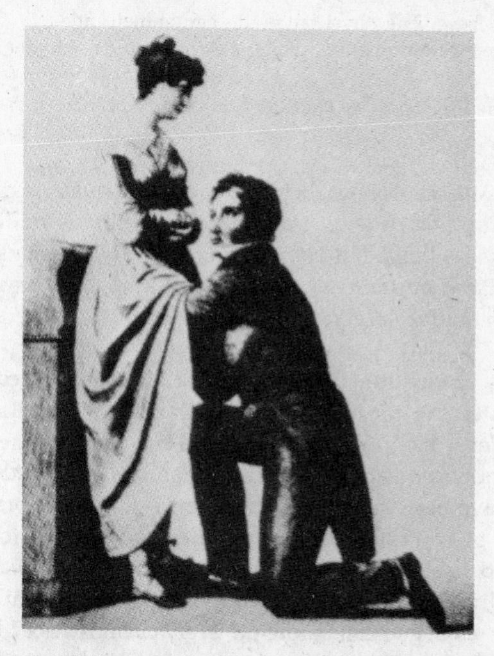

Vertical touching. This illustration, from an 1834 text, shows a physician doing a pelvic examination without looking at the woman's genitals.
Source: J. P. MayGrier, *Midwifery Illustrated* (New York: Harper Bros., 1834).

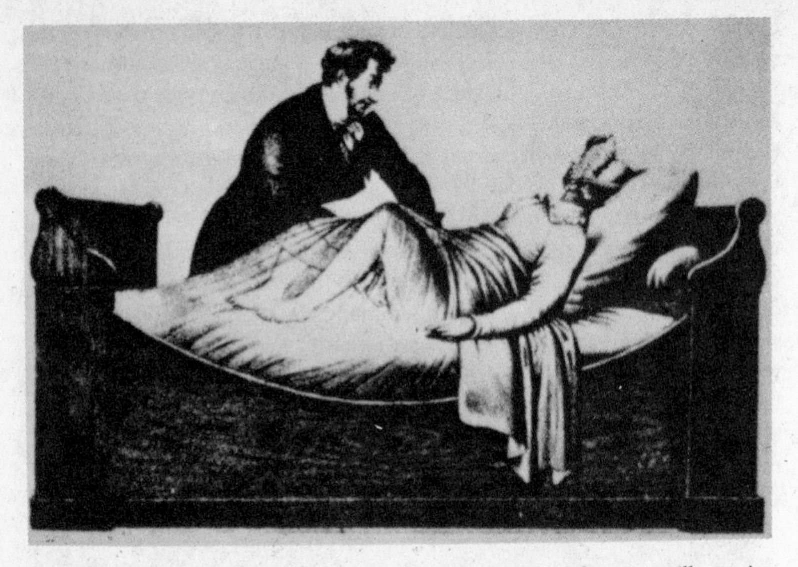

Horizontal touching. The physician in this early-nineteenth-century illustration performs a pelvic examination while looking directly into the eyes of the woman.

Source: J. P. MayGrier, *Midwifery Illustrated* (New York: Harper Bros., 1834).

the Harvard Medical School, beginning in 1815, similarly did not teach his students on live patients. According to one of his students, practical obstetrics was limited at Harvard to one or two sessions: "A female pelvis was placed on the table. The head of a rag baby was thrust into it. It was our duty to ascertain the presentations, and to deliver with forceps."[14]

Students graduating from such didactic obstetrics courses were forced to enter the birthing rooms of their first patients in relative ignorance. Never having witnessed actual births, and armed with only theoretical knowledge about how parturition was supposed to proceed, they must have been somewhat apprehensive. Yet doctors knew that they had to be confident to gain confidence, and they forged ahead and delivered babies. One medical graduate wrote: "I was left alone with a poor Irish woman and one crony, to deliver her child . . . and I thought it necessary to call before me every circumstance I had learned from books—I must examine, and I did—But whether it was head or breech, hand or foot, man or monkey, that was defended from my uninstructed finger by the distended membranes, I was as uncomfortably ignorant, with all my learning, as the foetus itself that was making all this fuss."[15] Those physicians who had formal medical education, still a minority in the early nineteenth century, tried to raise the practice of obstetrics to a higher level by emphasizing anatomy and physiology, but they suffered some difficulties early in their practices.

The physician elite armed with theoretical training believed that they could expand the practice of obstetrics beyond individual experience and that apprentice-trained midwives and physicians remained limited by their particular mentors'—or their own—experiences. The study of the anatomy and physiology of parturition removed knowledge from its anchor in individual experience and brought it to a more abstract and generalizable level. Learning what was possible and probable in labor and delivery, what was normal and abnormal, provided these birth attendants with general knowledge that they hoped would allow them to make educated judgments on the individual cases they examined.

While the potential for this increased enlightenment may have existed, the question remains whether or not individual medical graduates related their theoretical knowledge to the actual cases they faced in their practices, and whether their didactic training made them better accoucheurs. Did male physicians enhance or improve childbirth, as women believed they would? Did "science," the symbol of the promises of physician-directed obstetrics, come to the aid of birthing women?

Either because of their training or because of families' expectations, male physicians, the apprentice-trained and medical-school graduates alike, intervened in the birth process more than midwives. Whereas midwives followed a noninterventionist pattern, the physicians' model was just the opposite. As Walter Channing put it, a doctor, when called to attend laboring women, "must do something. He cannot remain a spectator merely, where there are many witnesses, and where interest in what is going on is too deep to allow of his inaction. Let him be collected and calm, and he will probably do little he will afterwards look upon with regret."[16]

Physicians' favorite interventions during the first half of the nineteenth century were bloodletting (venesection), drugs (typically opium or one of its derivatives), and forceps, frequently all used together. Dewees advocated substantial bloodletting. In one of his difficult cases, for example, with the woman standing on her feet, he took "upwards of two quarts" until she fainted. Dewees remarked that "every thing appeared better . . . I introduced the forceps, and delivered a living and healthy child." In another case:

> We placed the patient on her feet, taking care to have the perinaeum guarded, during the operation. Upon taking away about ten ounces of blood, (a small amount because the patient was delicate) she became very faint; she was immediately laid upon the bed; and the most complete relaxation had taken place; the forceps were applied, and our patient was delivered in a few minutes of a fine healthy girl.[17]

Physicians believed that venesection could relieve pain, accelerate labor, soften a rigid cervix, ease podalic version, and reduce inflammation. They even bled patients who were hemorrhaging, using the logic that further reducing circulation would produce blood clotting and stop the hemorrhage. They also relieved puerperal convulsions by bloodletting. In fact, as one historian has concluded, "bloodletting . . . was uncritically accepted as the fashion in early American obstetric practice."[18]

The use of opium or laudanum (tincture of opium) seems to have been equally popular among physician-accoucheurs in the nineteenth century. In cases of protracted labor, as in the Shippen/Downing cases cited above, physicians tried opium to accelerate cervical dilatation and ease suffering. They also employed cathartics to open the bowels, ergot to stimulate contractions, tobacco infusions to encourage the cervix to dilate, and techniques of manually breaking the waters to accelerate labor. In cases of extreme need physicians could surgically separate the pubic bones to facilitate passage of the fetus's head or they could introduce the crochet, the instrument used for fetal dismemberment and extraction.[19]

The forceps were the favorite instrument of physician intervention, and women both feared and respected the "hands of iron." When Shippen referred obliquely to forceps in front of Sally Downing's mother, she "was afraid to ask him, least he should answer in the affermative [sic]" that he needed to use it. Her confidence in its benefits, however, remained intact. Women were grateful for the tool that could extricate a fetus in difficult labors.[20]

In 1812 a medical graduate of the University of Pennsylvania entered practice in a town where two aging physicians already practiced. These physicians "had never used forceps, and were in the habit of resorting to Smellie's scissors and the crotchet [to dismember and remove a dead fetus] in all cases where the fetal head became obstructed in the pelvis." (See illustration.) The young doctor soon established himself among the women in the community by successfully using forceps to deliver healthy babies who might otherwise have been

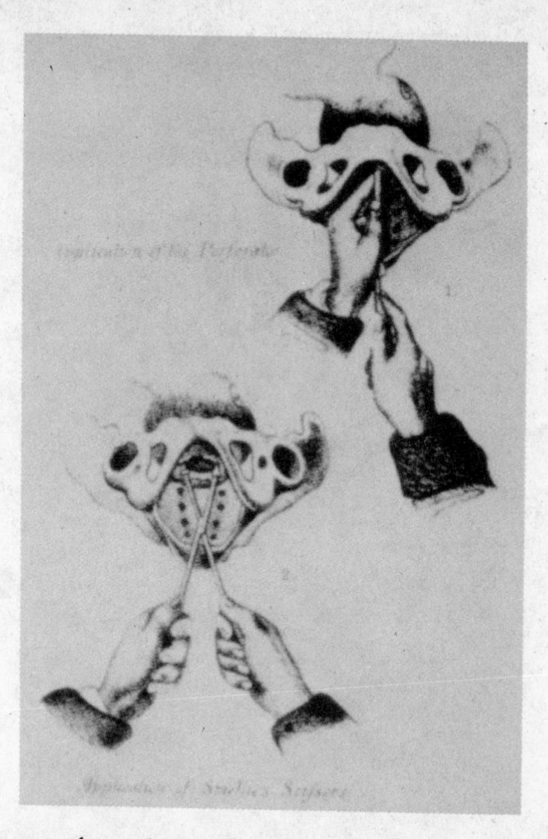

The performance of a craniotomy. First the skull of the fetus is perforated and then the cranial contents are removed.
Source: J. P. MayGrier, *Midwifery Illustrated* (New York: Harper Brothers, 1834).

destroyed. This sort of success story achieved a legendary quality in the nineteenth century as physicians expanded the use of forceps at the same time as they developed their practices.[21]

When well used, forceps could save lives; when misused, they could increase women's perineal lacerations and cause head injuries to the fetus. Dewees repeatedly called attention to the "mischief" that forceps could cause, and he believed that their dangers were enhanced because physicians used them too often and unnecessarily. He cautioned:

> The greatest care must be taken, before we begin our traction, that no portion of the mother is included in the locking of the blades—

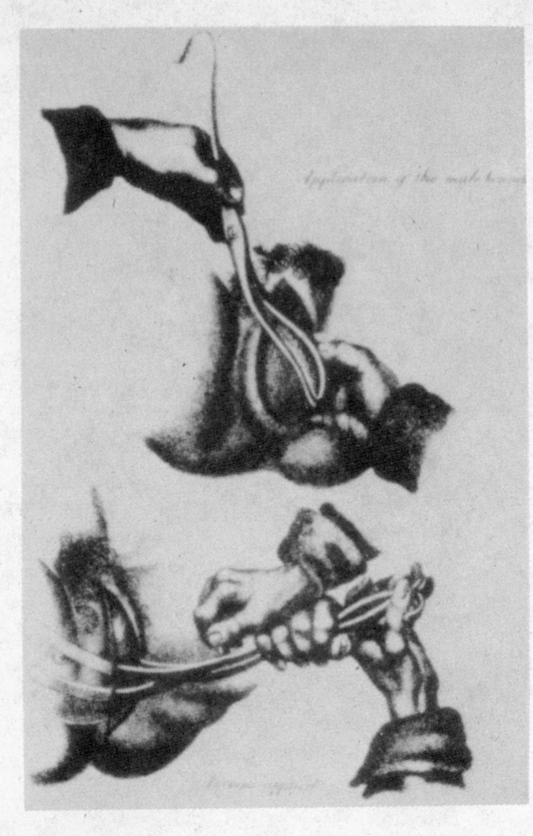

Application of the forceps.
Source: J. P. MayGrier, *Midwifery Illustrated* (New York: Harper Bros., 1834).

> this must be done by passing a finger entirely round the place of union. . . . I was once called to a poor woman who had had a considerable portion of the internal face of the right labium [the fold of skin on the side of the opening of the vagina] removed, by having been included in the joint of the short forceps.[22]

Physicians who had been trained to use forceps only on manikins and who were required by custom to perform the forceps operation without the benefit of sight ran considerable risk of creating new problems for the women whose obstructed labors they tried to ameliorate.

Countless stories testify to the severe perineal lacerations—tears in the perineal tissues—nineteenth-century women suffered in childbirth, and they suggest an increase in the problem as the century progressed. The accusation of "meddlesome midwifery" followed physician-accoucheurs, and textbooks cautioned against forceps misuse often enough to suggest that a significant problem existed. Dewees, for example, wrote: "The frequency with which [forceps] have been employed in some instances is really alarming, and I had like to have said, must have been to [sic] often unnecessary."[23] It is impossible to count women's perineal lacerations or other obstetric complications or to determine whether the incidence of laceration increased in direct relation to forceps use. Many contemporary observers believed this to be true. As one physician concluded, writing in the 1880s, "grave perineal lesions were more common now than formerly, and this increase has been coincident with the increased use of forceps and of anaesthetics in labor."[24]

Certainly the leaders of academic obstetrics—Shippen, Dewees, Channing, and others—were not the perpetrators of forceps excessiveness. Professors of midwifery repeatedly warned against unnecessary use of forceps. But their students or apprentice-trained physicians practicing in America's communities found forceps a very valuable tool, and because of their eagerness or their limited practical experience, they may have overused and misused them. Forceps, after all, gave the male physicians a significant advantage over traditional female midwives as they tried to establish themselves in practice. Dewees observed so many cases of misused forceps that he concluded, "The forceps, therefore, in the hands of those who consider them as a means by which a difficult labor may be terminated, but who apply them without rule, or without a knowledge of their mode of action, are nearly as fatal as the crochet itself."[25]

If forceps were at fault in the "meddlesome midwifery" of the early nineteenth century, they were not the only problem. Almost any intervention by the physician created a potential for harm. If a birth could not proceed without help, the physician provided a life-saving service not available elsewhere. If, however, as was statistically more probable, labor was proceeding normally and physicians intervened anyway, their actions introduced dangers not otherwise present. Dewees's caution about careful use of forceps inadvertently informs us about the concurrent dangers of infection. He taught his students to check that no part of the mother was caught in the blades of the forceps by "passing a finger entirely round the place of union." Yet an unwashed and ungloved finger could have carried a higher risk to women's lives than a perineal laceration. (Infection is examined in greater detail in Chapter 6.)

H. B. Willard, a medical graduate who practiced obstetrics in Wisconsin beginning in 1849, rarely used forceps because "the idea of instruments is *horrible* to *friend & patient* beside there is much liability to injure the parts." But Willard had no reservations about using opium and ergot, internally manipulating the fetus to change its presenting part, and routinely rupturing the waters with his fingernails. Willard chose his therapeutic activities by weighing the effects they would have on his reputation in the community. He tried not to use emetics, for example, because he knew "the idea of being vomited at such a time is exceedingly repugnant to the patient & to friends." By the same reasoning, Willard, when called to attend a laboring woman, followed Channing's dictum to do something. He knew his patients expected action. The only cases in which Willard did not interfere at all were those in which the baby had been born before his arrival. In those cases he might still have had opportunity to extract the placenta manually.[26]

The mental state of the birthing women helped Willard decide on the necessity of intervention. His assessment of a woman suffering from "nervous temperament" justified his playing a more active role in birth management. Just what Willard meant by nervous temperament, however, is unclear. Many physicians who attended labor and delivery, including Willard, saw parturient patients for the first time when they arrived during active labor. To judge a woman's temperament from her behavior at this stressful time was at best difficult. Thus interventions planned on this basis were susceptible to miscalculation.

Physicians' obstetrics courses taught them the theoretical basis of their craft, and their apprenticeships gave them tools with which to effect a successful birth, but nowhere did they receive clear guidelines for the practical application of their knowledge. Doctors had numerous techniques at their command and complete leeway in their use. If physicians used forceps too often, or if they intervened in the birth process too eagerly, it was because they were more persuaded by the faces of women in agony than by the cautions of their elders. The instrument provided one important differentiation between the skills of doctors and the skills of midwives, and doctors needed to remind their patients of this distinction. Medical decisions about interventions were made on the spot and in relative isolation. Even the professors at the medical schools and the leading textbooks taught by anecdotal example, making generalizations or patterns hard if not impossible to construct. Physicians could convince themselves easily and in good conscience that their judgment to intervene in labor was in the best interests of the patient. The majority of successful outcomes in each individual's practice justified these conclusions. Early obstetric "science" provided some knowledge and technique, but the practical application remained at the bedside in the hands of individual, isolated doctors such as Willard.[27]

Throughout the nineteenth century, the decision of whether or not to employ the skills of the physician remained with women, where it had been traditionally. The parturient, her midwife, and her assistants might have decided to call a doctor after labor had begun, and then they gave or withheld permission for each procedure suggested. The nineteenth-century home birthing room (as Chapter 4 will examine more closely) frequently contained the traditional female attendants right alongside the newer medical attendant, and these people all decided what procedures might be employed during the labor and delivery. William Dewees, for example, after one successful forceps operation, was called to other cases because "the influence of this case upon many of the midwives of this city, procured me many opportunities of applying the forceps." In another instance, Dewees wanted to take blood from a laboring woman: "I represented to the friends of the patient, the danger of her case. . . . They agreed to the trial." Similarly the young Pennsylvania doctor's success in delivering babies using forceps led women to refuse to let other doctors use the crochet. "The women in attendance put their veto upon [the crochet] procedure and demanded that 'the boy,' as they sneeringly styled him (for he was but twenty years old), should be called in consultation [to use the forceps]." Although physicians had broken the gender barrier and birth was no longer exclusively a women's event, women, by making their own choices about attendant and procedure, continued to hold the power to shape events in the birthing room.[28]

Despite the strength of tradition, however, birth had changed for the women who invited physicians to attend them in their homes. These women formed a minority of all birthing women at the middle of the nineteenth century, and they probably were limited geographically to the major cities and economically to the advantaged classes. Most Americans still could not afford doctors and employed midwives and delivered their babies in the same ways as had their mothers and grandmothers. But for those women who chose physicians instead of or in addition to midwives, birth became less a natural, immutable process and more an event that could be altered and influenced by a wide selection of interventions. Middle-class birthing women and their physicians realized that fate no longer held women in such a tight grip and that decisions could be made and actions could be taken that would determine what kind of birth a woman would have and perhaps whether she and her baby lived or died. This mental perception of the ability to shape the birth experience became even more important in the second half of the nineteenth century, when anesthesia emerged as the newest birthing panacea and physician interventions became more routine.

Most physicians continued to manage the birth process in the second half of the nineteenth century as they had earlier. The introduction of anesthesia to obstetrics at midcentury, discussed in Chapter 5, contributed to this trend. Other interventions, such as drug use and procedures for suturing perineal tears, became increasingly routine in the second half of the nineteenth century, as Chapter 6 will explore. In addition, physicians continued to use the methods that had served them well already, most particularly the forceps.

Reports of new types of forceps were legion in the nineteenth century. One physician, in introducing his own favorite variation, remarked that "there seems as many forceps as there are individual obstetricians."[29] There were long forceps and short forceps, curved forceps and straight forceps, mechanical forceps and axis-traction forceps. "This lack of uniformity proves the non-existence of a scientific basis," complained one physician, who tried to introduce "precise and absolute" laws for forceps use even while introducing his own favorite forceps variation in 1889.[30] To use the forceps effectively, physicians had to become familiar with at least a few different types for the different presentations they would encounter and to learn which sort fit each circumstance.

Skill in applying forceps varied widely in the second half of the nineteenth century, as it had earlier. Physicians estimated that 75 percent of the problems that gynecologists saw had been "from errors or incidents occurring during the parturition state," and one doctor thought that "seven-eighths of the women coming under his observation (about 1600 confinement cases) for treatment have been delivered by forceps." He feared that physicians were driven to using drugs and forceps because women preferred to call a doctor who had "the reputation of not allowing his patients to suffer."[31] But, he noted, these tendencies caused the suffering upon which gynecologists built their practices.

A California doctor also saw widescale forceps abuse. She wrote about her experiences and reservations about forceps use in unskilled hands:

> I have asked people to assist me in delivery (not me, my patients in delivery), and they put on a pair of forceps, and with great strong muscles that could lift probably two hundred pound dumb-bells, they pull. They seem to think that the only thing to be done is to deliver the child; if they cut off its circulation or bruise the mother, that is a matter of minor importance. That to me is all wrong. It is not brute force that we want. . . . I am not a strong woman, but I am strong enough for all the child or woman can bear. It seems to me that it is a lack of anatomic knowledge that destroys so many and makes so many failures.[32]

Commenting on four cases of uterine traumatism, the editors of the *Woman's Medical Journal* similarly concluded that "the fatality in each [was] clearly due to the wrong and improper application of the forceps by inexperienced or unskilled men." Although these two examples come from female physicians and contain elements of a specific female point of view, there is no evidence that women were any more avid than men in calling attention to the dangers of excessive and misdirected forceps interventions. Male critics such as William Dewees, whose objections to forceps abuse was widely known and publicized, were just as vociferous. Dr. W. P. Manton of Detroit estimated in 1910 that "not one in ten of those who are now employing [forceps] do so intelligently. . . . In the hands of the bungler, they become weapons of danger, leaving destruction and sometimes death in their wake."[33] Forceps could be an instrument of salvation for birthing women; it could also be—and was—the means by which women were reduced to postpartum invalidism.

Not only did physicians' skill in manipulating forceps vary, but the extent of their forceps use in the second half of the nineteenth century differed widely. As forceps became "fashionable," in the words of one physician, young doctors were pressured to use the instrument without waiting "sufficiently long to know what nature can accomplish, because of the vivid picture of impaction, sloughing, death of child, etc., which will rise before his excited fancy. It will be long, if ever, before he learns that such dangers are very much overstated."[34] Dr. H. H. Whitcomb of Philadelphia proudly reported in 1887 that in 616 obstetrical cases, he had used forceps only twice: "My success I ascribe to patient waiting and conservatism. I do as little meddling as possible. . . . I see so many doctors who, in almost every case of obstetrics they get, if they arrive before the child is born, put on the forceps to 'hasten delivery and shorten the woman's suffering.' I am very positive that this frequent use of the forceps is abuse."[35] When Dr. Hiram Corson of Pennsylvania made a similar point that "forceps are used very often," and attributed their overuse to the fact that "the physician has never hurt *himself* by using the instrument and wished to get away speedily, as he had other patients who needed attention," he incurred the ire of the editor of the *Journal of the American Medical Association*, who objected to the implication that obstetrics "advanced backwards." The editor accused Corson of imagining forceps misuse.[36]

Some observers perceived excessive forceps use; others believed that most physicians used the instrument prudently. All agreed at least on the potential danger of forceps use. The medical journals repeatedly urged caution. One doctor recommended "the final resort is the forceps." He said the more experience he had the less he resorted to forceps:

> I recall a case some years ago where I had spent the night at a case of lingering labor and at five o'clock in the morning I told the patient that she must be delivered with instruments. I went across the street to ask my friend Dr. Porter for his forceps and found he had left them at his office. Returning to the house to send a messenger for my own case, I was most agreeably surprised to find good labor pains had set in, and before the forceps arrived the case was terminated without mechanical aid. The moral effect on the patient's mind had evidently been sufficient to assist her.

This doctor believed, as did so many others, that "many practitioners . . . put on the forceps early in labor," without waiting for serious indications. Dr. Charles Budd advised his students to leave the forceps at home when they travelled to attend laboring women, so that if they were tempted to use them, they would have to travel back to their homes first, thus giving the parturient more time to achieve the delivery without them.[37] Dr. Joseph Hoffman of Philadelphia urged his fellow practitioners: "The forceps are to be applied, neither because the mother demands them nor because they are a time-saving convenience for the obstetrician."[38] Logic, he said, should govern the use of the instrument. In the words of another physician, "The forceps should never be used simply to gratify nervous patients, interfering nurses or meddlesome women, nor to save the time of a practitioner, busy or otherwise."[39]

Nineteenth-century physicians were remarkably candid in the medical journals in their descriptions of the labors and deliveries they attended, and their case reports help us understand some of the difficulties physicians faced in private practice. Dr. Dan Millikin, of Hamilton, Ohio, for example, told of a woman he attended in labor:

> Finding a head of moderate size above the brim of the pelvis . . . I was sure that I could deliver it with forceps in spite of a slight asymmetry . . . In this opinion I was all amiss, for it was afterwards demonstrated that the child could not be delivered in that position. . . . Because the woman's general condition was excellent, the effort to deliver by forceps was much prolonged. When, finally, it was determined to essay delivery by podalic version . . . The upper blade of the forceps—the one which passed to the right side of the woman's pelvis—would not come out! . . . Then my hand, passed into the uterus, revealed the fact that the child's right hand had passed through the fenestrum of the blade and that, in fact, the blade hung on the bend of the elbow, as a basket hangs on one's arm. . . . Presently, when the child had been delivered by the feet, it was seen that violence had been done to the forearm.

The physician tried to draw a lesson about the shape of the ideal forceps from his "error of judgment" and his "sorry job." The story gives us insight into the dilemmas physicians faced in the midst of labor and away from other help. They made decisions and took actions that had grave implications for the health of women and babies, and they did this under the severe pressures of progressing labor. They encountered situations of which they had no experience or teaching, and their judgments might have been faulty or wise just as their manipulative skill might have been excellent or deficient. Sometimes the results showed that the risks taken were justified; other times avoidable mistakes resulted from the physician's action.[40]

Part of the confusion for nineteenth-century physicians about when and whether to use forceps can be attributed to the difficulty in recognizing those cases in which immediate forceps application was indicated and in differentiating them from cases in which caution and watchfulness indicated forceps use only as a last resort. Dr. Coe of New York reported numerous cases in which he believed immediate application of forceps was necessary even before complete cervical dilatation to save the life of the baby: "The application of the forceps . . . did not present special difficulties. The perineum might be badly torn, or the cervix lacerated, in consequence of the rapid delivery; but patients would gladly overlook such accidents if the child's life was saved by the physician's prompt action, especially if former children had not survived."[41] This doctor recommended superseding the common practice of using forceps only when the first stage, the part of labor up to the point of complete cervical dilatation, was complete, and substituting in its place physicians' on-the-spot judgment about the state of labor.

A controversy in the pages of the *Journal of the American Medical Association* in the mid-1880s indicated some of the difficulties doctors had in judging the proper time for forceps application and called into question the very rule that forceps should be applied only to a fully dilated cervix. One "original thinker of prominence" wrote: "I regard the rule (not to apply the forceps till the os is completely dilated), long held by the ablest men, to be entirely erroneous, and capable of doing much harm to womankind and to the obstetric art." Instead, said this physician, "though my experience with the forceps is very limited. . . . I take pride in stating that, as far as my recollection goes, in no case of my own was a woman ever allowed to lie in suffering and danger till the os was 'completely dilated.' " The editors of the *Journal* suggested that this writer's " 'limited experience' with the forceps disqualifies an operator for the expression of opinion upon the subject" and concluded: "We are very decidedly of the opinion that a serious study of the nature of the case, and a careful weighing of the opinions of those obstetricians whose views are entitled to distinguished consideration, will furnish evidence sufficient to establish the proposition that *complete dilatation of the cervix uteri is an essential condition to the typical forceps operation.*" The editors admitted that there were unusual cases when forceps might be introduced prior to full dilatation, but only with extreme caution: "The dangers of injury to mother and child are obvious. It is a very easy matter to grasp a portion of the cervical walls between the blade and the head. A case in point has recently come under our observation. The forceps was applied to the head, resting in the mid-plane of the pelvis, through an undilated os, by an able and experienced practitioner. Together with the head, a shred of tissue, six inches long by two broad, was extracted. . . . The danger of injury to the foetus is frequently not less than that to the mother."[42]

Another physician entered his opinion: "It is as unwise as inhuman to allow women to suffer the pains of the first stage of labor [before full dilatation] when protracted for hours beyond physiological limits. The loss of sleep, the want of nourishment, the anxiety of protracted labor, and above all the nervous depression produced by pain; all of these tend to exhaust the patient and prepare the way for uterine inertia [the slowing and stopping of labor]. Postpartum shock and haemorrhage, septic infection, and least of all, a slow convalescence, are some of the *sequelae* of protracted first stage." This physician believed that early forceps use constituted "timely interference exercised in the first stage as well as in the later ones."[43]

To decide whether to intervene early or late was truly a dilemma for nineteenth-century physicians, who had to judge each case on its own merits and make their decisions without recourse to clear guidelines. "Is it not more perfectly fulfilling the purpose of our professional attendance, promptly to respond to the first intimations of evil and not wait to be driven to a last resort?" asked one Cincinnati doctor. "Is it not true conservatism to *avert* danger and difficulties by economizing our patient's powers, by not allowing pain to continue unmitigated for hours?"[44] Similarly, Dr. J. M. Fassig insisted that usually "physicians delay too long. . . . The skilled accoucheur does not sit by for hours without some reason."[45] Dr. Agnes Eichelberger sounded the medical confusion in her advice to fellow physicians: "I would like to make a plea for early use of forceps, when we know they must be used. Also, decidedly against their use when a little patience will not only save the child, but lacerations, hemorrhage, or sepsis."[46] How could physicians with limited obstetric practice, isolated from other doctors and sometimes alone in the birthing rooms of patients, decide whether early or late or no forceps use was indicated? Doctors responded to the confusion along a spectrum from waiting until all else failed to intervening before dilatation.

Our understanding of forceps use and abuse needs to be developed within the context of the degrees of difficulty in applying the instrument. Nineteenth-century physicians made use of low forceps when they lifted the fetus, whose head already rested on the perineal floor, across the perineum, still a common procedure at the end of the twentieth century. But perhaps just as often as this relatively easy application, physicians used mid forceps (when the fetal head reached the midpoint in the pelvis) or high forceps (when the fetal head was above the midpoint) or even "floating" forceps (when the fetal head had not yet entered the pelvis) to pull the baby from deeper within the pelvis. Dr. Charles Jewett, for example, explained to the New York Academy of Medicine that "he sometimes used the forceps when the head was above the brim provided he could readily crowd it into the brim and hold it there while applying the axis traction forceps."[47] It was this high or floating forceps procedure with the associated dangers of severe lacerations, infection, and fetal damage that led physicians to try to develop alternative interventions for aiding protracted labors.

Symphysiotomy, the surgical separation of the pubic bones, frequently seemed preferable; and Cesarean section became an increasingly safe procedure in the twentieth century, preferable to the high forceps operation. Physicians themselves believed that the high forceps procedure was too commonly used in the nineteenth century and that it usually was associated with extreme risk for the mother and the child.

Nineteenth-century physicians' forceps use and skill varied and was imprecise and unscientific, but it would not be correct to conclude that it was uniformly bad. Most individual physicians conducted their practices, including their obstetric practices, by trying as best they knew how to help their patients. The written record reveals their efforts and their sincerity. But the circumstances under which physicians practiced sometimes took the upper hand. Their limited practical training may have led them to develop certain skill areas and by necessity leave others underdeveloped. Delivering babies within women's homes, with inadequate light and minimal equipment, with no trained helpers, and with interested friends and relatives contributing their opinions must have made it difficult for physicians to form their own obstetric styles and to master them. The long miles that many of them had to travel between patients, sometimes delayed by bad weather or a disabled horse, may have made them anxious about getting on to their next patient. The timing of forceps use and the skill with which the instrument was manipulated must have been affected by all these other concerns. When we add the further consideration that many of the operations that physicians carried out while leaning over the beds of the parturient women were high forceps procedures, requiring the insertion of the forceps well into the pelvis, we can understand the scope of the problem. Perineal lacerations and other postpartum gynecological problems were almost inevitable, given the circumstances under which the forceps operation took place. Moreover, forceps frequently appeared as the lesser of the possible evils attendant to a difficult childbirth.

Physicians' safety record when measured by mortality statistics matched or was worse than the record of midwives, who continued to follow a basically noninterventionist birth policy. Dr. Dorothy Reed Mendenhall studied births in Wisconsin at the beginning of the twentieth century and concluded that for both physicians and midwives maternal mortality was higher than it needed to be, but that "we must admit that the midwife is, on the whole, probably less culpable in regard to the deaths of parturient women than physicians in this state."[48] Similar maternal mortality rates for midwife- and physician-attended births indicate that physicians, with all their expertise and intervention techniques, did not, as they had promised, enhance the safety of the birth experience for women. Medicine may have improved comfort levels and may have rescued some women from complicated labors, but it did not, on the whole, increase women's chances of survival in the nineteenth century. The variation in skill, the difficult circumstances under which physicians carried out complicated interventions, and the frequent misuse of forceps all negated the benefits of the physicians' techniques.

In fact, it is probable that physicians' techniques created new problems for birthing women and actually increased the dangers of childbirth. Inappropriate forceps use and the careless administration of ether and chloroform (see Chapter 5) introduced serious maternal lacerations and infant breathing disorders that otherwise might not have developed. Perhaps even more significant, physicians often carried puerperal fever, which was potentially disastrous to birthing women. Because their medical practices included patients with communicable diseases, doctors were more likely than midwives to bring into the birthing room the agents of infection on their hands and their clothing. Epidemics of puerperal fever developed even in the practices of physicians like H. H. Whitcomb of Norristown, Pennsylvania, who did "as little meddling as possible" in normal labor and delivery. In 1886 one of Whitcomb's parturient patients developed childbed fever because Whitcomb brought the infection from a previous patient who had scarlet fever. That winter and spring, Whitcomb, by his own admission, transmitted the fever to thirty-two more birthing women. Although he understood and accepted the role of microorganisms in transmitting infection, he was unable to cleanse himself thoroughly enough to prevent its spread. Puerperal sepsis still caused the largest proportion of maternal deaths at the beginning of the twentieth century.[49]

Historians still debate the extent to which puerperal fever was exacerbated by physicians' attendance at normal confinements, especially in the late nineteenth-century period when bacteriological discoveries were revealed in the public press with wide acclaim and the public and the medical profession increasingly understood and accepted the germ theory of disease causation. Because the issue is so important both to assessing the impact of physicians' obstetrical practice and to understanding some of the pressures doctors and birthing women felt when deciding on birth procedures, Chapter 6 will further explore the issue of infection in childbirth. Meanwhile it is sufficient to note that physicians became increasingly sensitive to the question of puerperal infection and worried about their own role in its propagation. Beginning in the 1880s, many of them worked consciously and energetically to expunge the disease from the birthing rooms,[50] as we will see in Chapter 6.

Physicians offered some women relief from suffering and aided others through difficult labors, but because of the variations in ability and practices of birth attendants, most women continued to experience extreme pain and discomfort and to fear childbirth. One woman described her physician-attended confinement as "hell. . . . It bursts your brain, and tears out your heart, and crushes your nerves to bits. It's just hell."[51] Despite their continued suffering, those middle-class women who had chosen physicians to attend them did not want to return to midwives as their sole birth attendants. They believed that if birth dangers and pains were to be eased, improvements would come from progress in medicine. Instead of returning to traditional practices, which were still available to them, these women demanded more of their physicians and continued to hope that safe and comfortable deliveries would come to them from the medical world.

The presence of men and modern technology in the birthing rooms altered some parts of the women's birth experience, but the confinements of late nineteenth-century middle- and upper-class women retained many important elements of traditional births. Anita McCormick Blaine's first childbirth in 1890 illustrates how the old and the new came together in the turn-of-the-century birthing rooms. During her pregnancy Blaine corresponded with her mother, who was in Europe seeking a cure for a hearing loss, and she sought the traditional female support network to help her through the impending crisis. "If you could but be with me now, what wouldn't I give," wrote Anita to her mother Nettie Fowler McCormick. Despite all of Blaine's preparations and the doctor and nurse who would attend her, McCormick yearned to be with her daughter. She wrote detailed instructions about her care, advising, for example, rubbing olive oil over the abdomen and perineal area to ease delivery. She worried that only a mother could rightfully do such an intimate job. "I don't know if you have a person you could let do it," she wrote, "but I wish I were there to do it." Blaine sequestered herself in her childhood Chicago home, where "every chair and table speaks to me of dear familiar times . . . nothing is so sweet as to feel the presence of all it reminds me of." She surrounded herself with helpers, including her old friend Harriot ("Missy") Hammond, who traveled from Virginia to be with her. She wrote her mother:

> I never can be able to tell you what peace comes to me from being in this home of all my girlhood now. I know I should feel very differently in any other place. I did not realize what a blessing it would be but I feel it every minute—& I am so grateful that my sweet baby can come to me here—Dearest mother mine—all would be complete if you were here.

Strengthened by these traditional comforts, Anita delivered her baby while under the influence of chloroform. She was supported by her nurse and by Hammond and attended by a male physician. Her husband waited outside. She united the old traditional female-centered practices and the new medical obstetrical procedures and planned the whole event to meet her expectations. The doctor managed the birth in the context that the woman created.[52]

The decision-making process in Anita Blaine's confinement reveals how the old and the new intermingled in late nineteenth-century birthing rooms. Doctors, who may have had only minimal practical experience, were invited to attend women in their own homes in the presence of other women, many of whom had had considerable birth experience and had developed strong opinions about birth procedures. Within the birthing rooms, these attendants talked to each other and negotiated. There were desires and expectations on both sides. Women retained a lot of power in their own homes, and physicians bowed to it or risked losing patients and damaging their reputations among a whole community of women. As the new obstetrical techniques—from forceps to anesthesia—became available, they worked to the advantage of physicians, who held the monopoly over their use, while centuries of female traditions and the domestic environment in which these traditions operated worked to the advantage of women.

Inexperienced physicians sometimes welcomed the knowledge of other attendants. One doctor gratefully recorded that, while attending one of his first deliveries, early in the twentieth century, his confusion about what to do with a footling presentation was relieved when "a breezy nurse came whistling in. She took charge, and with her optimistic attitude, aided by nature's magnificent resourcefulness . . . the little fellow arrived." Morris Fishbein, a Chicago physician with a wide national reputation, admitted that when he was a student in the second decade of the twentieth century he "received better instruction" from a poor Irish woman whose eighth birth he attended than he ever had in any classroom: "She was thoroughly familiar with every step of the process." Other physicians found attending a birth in the presence of well-informed women intimidating. One physician recalled, "A young doctor, fresh from medical college, can pass many embarrassing moments in the presence of the neighborhood midwife." Another recalled that a mother's instructions to him "rattled me so that I hardly knew what I was doing."[53]

Women invited physicians to attend them in order to benefit from their expertise and technology, yet they would not give doctors approval for all the procedures they might suggest. Dr. William B. Dewees of Salina, Kansas, wrote in 1889 of one of his confinement cases, a 37-year-old German woman in labor with her first child. He was called to attend, but "it was probably an hour later before the patient would consent to an examination. . . . I advised blood-letting as a means of giving speedy relief and an easy delivery. The patient not only seriously objecting to this, but to anything what ever to be done to her person, saying most emphatically: 'I want to be left alone entirely,' consequently no attempts to give aid were made." When labor still did not progress after twelve hours the woman requested a second examination. The physician found a rigid cervix and "Bleeding was again proposed but likewise rejected by her. I then suggested a hot water enema, which was consented to." This eased the perineum slightly, but the fetus gave signs of distress: "I listened for its heart sounds, and failing to hear them, I kindly informed the patient of the fact, urging the use of the forceps, to which I soon received her consent." The baby died soon after delivery. The doctor concluded: "Here we have a clear case that, had blood-letting been consented to early, when first proposed, the child would have been saved."[54] This physician told of another patient, a woman in labor with her fifteenth child, who was opposed to bloodletting but agreed to chloroform to get her through a difficult labor.[55] Women's ideas about acceptable procedures often set the limits under which physicians' interventions had to be planned and executed.

Physicians' struggles to achieve a sterile environment to prevent postpartum infection from developing in their patients reveal the tensions that could arise as women, midwives, and physicians, present together in the birthing rooms, tried to work out acceptable settlements. A Long Island doctor in the 1890s, when public understanding of germ transmission was still new, tried to demand that his patient's helpers boil his instruments and make up a clean bed for the delivery. One woman told him: "No doctor I ever worked with had such foolish notions."[56] An Oklahoma physician explained why he could never try to shave a patient's pubic hair even though he thought it would help prevent infection:

The lack of a systematic approach to the practice of obstetrics in the early twentieth century can be traced in part to the quality and emphasis of obstetric education, which had not changed substantially during the nineteenth century. After the middle of that century some medical schools initiated "demonstrative midwifery," teaching students by having them observe actual laboring women, but many medical schools ignored this innovation and continued their didactic teaching from textbooks and manikins. In 1910, although most practitioners now received a formal medical education, many still graduated having witnessed few or no live deliveries. One 1904 graduate described her education: "My obstetrical training . . . consisted in reading my textbooks, listening to lectures dealing chiefly with abnormalities, delivery of a manikin put into presumably abnormal positions, and the witnessing from the ampitheatre of the delivery of a few cases."[62] Such training, largely theoretical and lacking clinical experience, at best prepared students to understand in principle birth pathology and the rudiments of how to intervene to rescue a woman in trouble, but it did not prepare physicians to attend women under the various conditions of normal labor. An Iowa physician remembered that when he began practice a husband of one of his patients asked if he had had any obstetrical experience. "I had schooled myself for just such a question," reminisced the doctor, "and unhesitatingly, but shamefully, replied, 'Oh, yes!' (My total college experience was with a manikin, you remember). Luckily for me, the child was born about ten minutes after my arrival, else I might have fallen into grave disrepute."[63]

J. Whitridge Williams, professor of obstetrics at the Johns Hopkins Medical School, surveyed obstetrics education in 1912 and concluded that the "average practitioner, through his lack of preparation for the practice of obstetrics, may do his patients as much harm as the much-maligned midwife." Williams found that most medical students had the opportunity during their training to watch only one woman deliver, and one quarter of the medical schools admitted that their graduates were not competent to practice obstetrics. Yet most physicians did deliver babies as part of their medical practices, and they spent on the average approximately 30 percent of their time attending childbirth.[64] In the era when scientific investigations began to permeate the medical world, when medical schools increasingly built laboratories and trained their students in research methods and findings, when specialization and hospital expansion transformed medical practice, obstetrical practices were still characterized by wide individual variation and unsystematic application of general principles. The science of obstetrics had not yet fulfilled its promise.

3

"Overcivilization and Maternity"

Differences in Women's Childbirth Experiences

At the turn of the century, Dr. Franklin Newell of Harvard Medical School observed "two distinct classes of patients" in obstetrics practice: "the one seen in hospital practice being largely composed of women of foreign birth, who have not been subjected to the action of the influences brought to bear by the high requirements of modern civilization," and the second seen in private practice among middle- or upper-class women whose nervous systems suffered because of the high stimulation of their urban environment. Newell believed, and much of the medical community agreed with him, that affluent women suffered in childbirth more than other women and needed special treatment from physicians to survive the experience without nervous breakdowns. "It seems to me," he wrote, "that this overdevelopment of the nervous organization is responsible for the increased morbidity of pregnancy and labor which is apparent among these women of the overcivilized class." The doctor went on to suggest that women whose nervous temperament could not withstand labor might be good subjects for Cesarean section. "The advocacy of an elective Cesarean section for patients who have no pelvic obstruction will undoubtedly come as a shock to many members of the profession," he admitted, but to his mind the nervous disability of the affluent urban women in his practice warranted such extreme measures.[1]

Newell's observations about the bad state of health among middle- and upper-class American women, which merely echoed the sentiments of many in the medical profession during the last part of the nineteenth century, bear scrutiny. What was the state of women's health in the nineteenth century? To what extent were health differences among women observable, and how did these affect their childbearing experiences? Were working-class women healthier and better able to bear children than middle-class women? Did socioeconomic class directly determine women's ability to withstand difficulties in labor and delivery? Perhaps most pertinent to this book's analysis of change in childbirth procedures: did differences attributed to socioeconomic class, perceived or real, influence the particular direction of obstetric developments?

This chapter will examine the nineteenth-century medical perceptions of class differences among women and the limitations of their dichotomous thinking about women's health and childbirth experiences. It will then go on to suggest a four-part differentiation in childbirth experiences during the prehospital era, a categorization scheme that may be more useful than the nineteenth-century interpretation for understanding women's actual experiences. This categorization itself, however, cannot define all the determinants for understanding the childbirth experiences of American women. As this chapter will conclude, some of the similarities among all women's experiences are more revealing than the identifiable differences.

The general state of women's health provides a very important context for understanding women's birth complications and thus for understanding women's experiences. Because of the connection between general health and childbearing health, the question of whether rich women were on the whole less healthy than poor women in the nineteenth century becomes particularly important. Many observers of nineteenth-century society noted that American women were sickly; in fact, women themselves agreed on the low state of their health. Catherine Beecher at mid-century reported her own survey of her friends and their friends across the country. Very few of this select group described themselves as healthy individuals. Beecher's informant in Milwaukee, Wisconsin, for example, described her ten friends: "Mrs. A. frequent sick headaches. Mrs. B. very feeble. Mrs. S. well, except chills. Mrs. L. poor health constantly. Mrs. D. subject to frequent headaches. Mrs. B. very poor health. Mrs. C. consumption. Mrs. A. pelvic displacements and weakness. Mrs. H. pelvic disorders and a cough. Mrs. B. always sick. Do not know one perfectly healthy woman in the place."[2] Mrs. S. M. Estee told her female readers of the *Water Cure Journal:* "You are sick and have been for months, years, and some of you your whole lives."[3]

Physicians accused "female invalidism" of potentially undermining the American race. Dr. Edward Clarke of Harvard warned in the 1870s that if things continued as they were American men would have to cross the Atlantic to find healthy wives.[4] Clarke blamed particularly the education of young girls at puberty for women's adult health problems, claiming that girls could not develop their brains at the same time their reproductive systems were forming. He favored separate schools for girls, with a curriculum that allowed for rest one week out of the month. While Clarke's interpretation that women were sickly because of their education was widely challenged, his perception that women were sickly was not. All around them, nineteenth-century social critics saw languishing women who kept to their beds in their weakness. These women seemed unable to carry out the duties assigned to them and particularly incapable of bearing healthy offspring.

The feeble state of American womanhood worried the medical community, and physicians tried to explain this seemingly national problem. To many doctors, the cause of female weakness was menstruation. They believed women, weakened by this periodic attack on the system, could not carry out vigorous mental or physical tasks. In fact, the president of the American Gynecological Society claimed in 1900, "Many a young life is battered and forever crippled in the breakers of puberty; if it crosses these unharmed and is not dashed to pieces on the rock of childbirth, it may still ground on the ever-recurring shadows of menstruation, and lastly, upon the final bar of the menopause ere protection is found in the unruffled waters of the harbor beyond the reach of sexual storms."[5] Because of their biology, women were not safe from puberty to menopause.

Dr. Cyrus Edson, the health commissioner of New York, in 1893 confirmed this view of the "physical deterioration" of American women. "Let me briefly state facts as they are," wrote Dr. Edson in the popular *North American Review:*

> An American girl, educated as it is our pride to educate her, marries the man of her choice amid the warm good wishes of all her friends. She is clever, bright, beautiful, and looks forward to years of happiness and of usefulness. One or, at most, two children are born, and if we meet her we can scarcely recognize her. She looks dragged and worn, she is fretful and peevish, she has become a burden on her husband instead of help to him, she feels as if she were a nuisance to herself and to others; worse than all, because it is the cause of all, she is a confirmed invalid, doomed to suffer more or less during the coming years.[6]

He blamed education, abortion practices, and the pressures of modern life for women's problems, and he called for a return to more healthful customs for American women.

Edson's observations on the state of health among American women became the subject of controversy in the 1890s in the pages of the *Journal of the American Medical Association*. The editors asserted that Edson's "charges against American women were based on mere assertion."[7] To evaluate the charge, Dr. Edmund Andrews of Chicago surveyed his patients and those of his close associates. Andrews concluded, in opposition to Edson, that of 163 families he identified, in which the women had produced 545 children, only five women were "confirmed invalids." "On the whole," wrote Andrews, "we finished our extempore study with a cheerful conviction that the women are for the most part all right, and can be depended on to replenish the earth."[8] Dr. James Morgan of Washington, D.C., however, agreed with Edson on the basis of his own survey of 48 mothers. "I find there are but twenty who may be said to enjoy as good health as before they were married. Of the remaining twenty-eight, seven died, incident to or following childbirth, five are bedridden, and the remaining sixteen have never regained their former good looks and health."[9] Despite the medical disagreements about Edson's assertions, many medical journal articles corroborated the precarious nature of women's health, the dangers of puberty for future health, the adverse effects of childbirth, and the physical weakness of women.[10]

Most of the medical discussion about women's health concerned middle- and upper-class women, who, physicians believed, were particularly at risk for poor health because of their attempts at education, their tight-lacing corsets, and the social activities of balls and parties with which they occupied their time. Physicians claimed that the women they saw in their private practices experienced significantly greater difficulties in general health and particularly in childbearing than the poor women they treated in the hospitals and dispensaries. Newell observed that his typical hospital patient, "in spite of the unfavorable conditions of her bringing up, poor food, privations, and hard work, comes to maturity a strong healthy woman. . . . The working woman goes through her pregnancy with little or no trouble . . . she ordinarily comes to labor in good physical condition to endure the strain, and goes through perhaps a hard labor without reacting unduly either to the pain or the muscular effort which she undergoes, and usually without aid of anesthetics delivers herself safely."[11]

Working-class women were less frequently the subject of medical discussion. However, the poverty that governed their daily activities, the environment in which they lived, and the physical labors they endured created additional risks to their health. In answer to Edward

Clarke's study of the effects of education on young women's physical development, Dr. Azel Ames wrote about the effects of industrial labor on women in early puberty, concluding that these produced equally harmful results on growing women: "large numbers of [young female workers] are of an age at which unfavorable conditions of employ act with dire results against her especial sexual attributes."[12] Dr. Elizabeth Brown studied industrial workers in New York and believed similarly that the manufacturing trades were particularly damaging to the future reproductive health of working women.[13] In fact, those doctors who analyzed the health situation of their working-class patients concluded that these women, too, carried special health burdens through their adult lives.

Newell's perceptions that the robust health of working women contrasted to the frailty of affluent women is more evident rhetorically in the medical literature of the turn of the century than it is in the case reports. It seems to have informed the ideology behind many physicians' treatment of their female patients. But when the medical literature is examined more fully, it becomes evident that physicians believed that all women suffered significant health problems by virtue of their femaleness rather than by virtue of their class. Medical observers in general agreed that women who worked outside the home, women who studied, women who menstruated, and women who had babies all faced the potential of living an adult life without their full capacities. Different problems affected the health of the various classes of women, but according to nineteenth-century observers, women, by virtue of being women, were a high-risk population.

Tuberculosis, the incidence of which was significantly higher among young women than among young men in the nineteenth century, produced particular problems for women in their childbearing years.[14] Although exacerbated by the crowded tenement conditions of the poor population, this was a health problem that affected all groups of women. In the nineteenth century, physicians posited that pregnancy might improve the physical condition of women suffering from pulmonary tuberculosis, but by the first decade of the twentieth century, they realized that the opposite was true. Women who had active tuberculosis could put themselves at increased risk for ill health or death if they continued their pregnancies, and many doctors believed the risk was great enough to justify abortion in these women. Because they believed hygienic conditions were nearly impossible to achieve in the crowded urban tenement dwellings, some doctors felt that poor tubercular women who found themselves pregnant should be aborted.[15]

Dr. Charles Sumner Bacon of Chicago estimated at the beginning of the twentieth century that approximately 1.5 percent of all pregnant women suffered from clinical, diagnosable tuberculosis. He further estimated that significant numbers suffered from subclinical, undiagnosable tuberculosis and that "nearly every individual has a little tuberculosis." The health of women suffering from the disease was endangered by their pregnancy, increasing as the uterus pushed against the diaphragm, according to Bacon. "The detrimental influence of the latter part of pregnancy and of labor is revealed during the puerperium [the period following delivery], which is characterized by a rapid progress of the disease," he wrote. "The puerperium itself, with its usually enforced confinement in imperfectly ventilated and overheated rooms, is injurious and its influence is added to that of labor. As a result, this period is always a critical one, even for milder cases and for those more advanced it is very dangerous."[16] Dr. Alice Tallant of Philadelphia agreed that "tuberculosis can progress to a fatal issue in a woman who was but slightly affected by the disease before her delivery."[17] Bessie Huntting Rudd's fear of dying as a result of her childbearing experiences (noted in Chapter 1) was heightened by her knowledge that she was tubercular. She removed herself from city life when she became pregnant, which meant separation from her husband, in order to let the fresh country air improve her chances for survival.[18]

For women who had suffered from rickets during childhood, or who had manifested its adult form, osteomalacia, childbirth also held specific dangers. Dr. J. Whitridge Williams of Johns Hopkins University Medical School observed at the turn of the twentieth century that rachitic pelves were not unusual, afflicting 0.8 percent of white and 10.8 percent of the black women delivered at Johns Hopkins Hospital.[19] Giving vaginal birth through a distorted pelvic canal caused labor complications that were difficult for most birth attendants, both midwives and physicians, to handle. The inability of the fetus to fit through a deformed pelvis could be blamed for the deaths of significant numbers of mothers and babies. Unfortunately for our understanding of this problem historically, adequate statistics do not exist about rickets, and it is impossible to determine the class or racial distribution of the disease. A vitamin D deficiency disease, rickets especially affected children with inadequate diets and low exposure to sunlight, most likely the poor and urban dwellers.[20]

The effects of gonorrhea and syphilis on the health of childbearing women have yet to be explored adequately by historians. Phillips Cutright and Edward Shorter believe that the reproductive functions of non-white women particularly were adversely affected by sexually transmitted diseases during the late nineteenth and early twentieth century. They suffered from increased incidence of miscarriage, from infertility, and from earlier deaths. Contemporary observers did not limit their worries about venereal diseases to any specific racial or ethnic group, but noticed the too common occurrence of these diseases among all races and classes. In 1904, for example, a group of New York physicians estimated that 60 percent of the male population in the United States contracted syphilis or gonorrhea during their adult lives; others believed 35 percent a more realistic figure. With either estimation, it is evident that these diseases were harmful to women's reproductive health.[21]

But childbirth menaced the health of all women, not just the ones who had tuberculosis, rickets, or sexually transmitted diseases. Chapter 1 discussed all women's fears about dying during or immediately following their confinements and the high mortality associated with childbirth. Dr. Charlotte Brown of San Francisco painted a typical scenario in 1895: "A healthy girl of 20 years marries, becomes pregnant and is delivered in the first year, she has a bad laceration of the cervix and perineum. Neither is repaired at the time nor does she nurse the child. Her youth and good constitution help her. She makes a fair recovery, resumes the care of her family and calls herself well." But then follows quickly the second and third children, and, perhaps, economic hardship. "Pregnancy at this stage is unfortunate as her mental force is not quite equal to it," observed Dr. Brown: "in a short time she is a physical wreck."[22] Dr. Joseph DeLee as late as 1934 called attention to the "immense army of women suffering, if I may coin a phrase, subinvalidism and who say they have never felt well since their first baby was born." Women perceived that the physical stresses of delivering children, especially when added to other pressures, quickly made them invalids. As one woman told her cousin, "I have had such poor health since the baby is born I have taken medicine for a month now . . . I haven't done a bit of housecleaning . . . I don't think I will be able to do any this spring." Similarly, a patient told her doctor, "I had one child ten months after marriage, and the seven years since have been years of sickness and misery."[23]

In light of the evidence about the health risks of all groups of women, the medical and lay observation that middle- and upper-class women were more sickly and suffered more in childbirth than did their working-class sisters needs amplification. By physicians' own accounts, poor women, too, suffered major health problems, leading to difficulty in bearing children and sometimes infertility. The medical evidence reveals that women, rich and poor, suffered in childbirth, died in childbirth, and were at risk for a multitude of health problems that potentially affected their childbearing and may have shortened their lives.

Part of the medical perception of robust health among poorer women can be explained by the fact that physicians did not see many of the women in this group. Many women did not consult physicians when they delivered their babies or at any other time during their lives. Paul Starr has concluded that for much of American history regular use of medical help was outside the financial reach of many people. These people, when sick or about to deliver their babies, turned instead to midwives, family networks, old family remedies, and domestic practice; they did not show themselves to the physicians who have left the medical records. Physicians saw, in their private practices, the more affluent women who could afford their services, and in their charity and hospital work, the poorest women whose social networks could not provide aid. It was not until the late nineteenth or early twentieth century, according to Starr, that all groups of Americans gained access to routine medical care through the growth of hospitals, the use of the automobile and telephone, and the development of financial aid and insurance programs.[24] Many working-class and poor women did not consult physicians; because the doctors did not see them suffer in childbirth, they concluded that these women must be healthier than the women they did see in their practices. Edward Clarke's conclusions that women suffered reproductive problems because of their education grew out of his own private practice among affluent Bostonians and reflect his lack of such experience with working and poor women. Historical interpretation of the observations doctors made about women's health must be tempered by the fact that they applied mainly to the women they saw in their practices.

In addition, physicians' actual contact with the middle- and upper-class women who consulted them only occurred when those women were ailing. Healthy women did not consult physicians—except during their confinements, when evaluation of their health might have been difficult and distorted—and thus physicians were not well acquainted with many physically thriving women in this class. Medical observations should not be discounted because of these factors, but the possible exaggeration of the class-related problems associated with women's health must be considered.

Another factor usually absent from the nineteenth-century analyses about the healthy poor was that higher fertility rates among poor and immigrant women in the nineteenth century put these women at risk more often for childbirth-related health problems. As we noted in Chapter 1, immigrant and black women were likely to experience two or more times the number of pregnancies and childbirths as native-born American women, especially as the nineteenth century progressed. Sociologist Margaret Jarman Hagood, who studied Southern tenant farm women in the 1930s, found that these women had on the average 6.4 children, or "one child for each period of a little less than three years." Her figures did not include stillbirths or abortions. Larger families entailed hard domestic labor for these women, adding to their already difficult life of poverty and privation.[25]

In fact, working-class women appear to have been at greater risk of poor childbearing health than middle- and upper-class women. The poorer the woman was, the likelier she was to have more children, to be exposed to debilitating infectious diseases, to need to contribute her strenuous daily labor to provide food and shelter for her family, to live in ill-ventilated housing, to have access to fewer fresh foods, especially milk products and clean water, and to encounter more general daily hardships. All of these daily realities of life contributed to the health risks of poor women.

Poor and working-class women's risks, however, might not have been evident outside their own groups. Poor childbearing women, despite their physical trials, would have had to return to work early after their confinements and would have had to continue their household or workplace duties whether or not they felt well. Reformer Michael Davis believed that poor women could not take the time for any postpartum recovery because of their busy lives. He quoted a Polish woman from Johnstown, Pennsylvania, who described the delivery of her last child in the early twentieth century: "At five o'clock Monday evening went to sister's to return washboard, having just finished day's washing. Baby born while there; sister too young to assist in any way . . . washed baby at sister's house; walked home, cooked supper for boarders, and was in bed by eight o'clock. Got up and ironed next day and day following." Observers of this quick resumption of normal activities would have been likely to conclude that the woman was robust and healthy; in fact, it represented the lack of choice in the woman's life.

There is ample evidence that the poor population suffered higher general mortality and morbidity rates than other groups in the population. Poor women, whose fertility rates were above average, were not immune to physical debility. Newell's characterization of the women of this class as robust and healthy was a misrepresentation of their actual health conditions. His observation that upper-class women were more sickly than lower-class women seems to have been born within a particular medical and social setting that did not allow Newell or many of his associates to see the obvious contradictions. Their lack of knowledge about the lives of this class of women and their class-based ideology that fostered the image of robust uncivilized peoples precluded their ability to understand the bias of their statements.[26]

On the other hand, the women Newell observed as sickly—the middle- and upper-class women seen in private practices—also were at high risk for ill health in the nineteenth century. Tight corsets, fashionable low-protein diets, and lack of exercise have adversely affected affluent women and their childbearing. Physicians who noticed that this population of women exhibited sickly natures were not incorrect. The social norms governing the behavior of fashionable women led just as inexorably to ill health as the physical realities of the lives of their poorer sisters. A historian looking back at the lives of the nineteenth-century women must conclude that all women were at risk for physical problems and for difficulties related to their childbearing, but that different groups were led to that point by the particular causes and consequences of their specific lives.

Challenging Newell's observations on the dichotomous and solely class-based nature of female health during the nineteenth century does not lead to the conclusion that all women, suffering ill health, had the same childbirth experiences. Very important differences among women remain evident through the study of their confinements, and the most important variant among them is the degree of choice the women themselves had in determining the situations in which they found themselves.

The various childbearing experiences of American women during the prehospital era fall, in my analysis, into four kinds, and the divisions that define them are, in part, as Newell's, class-related. But in addition to socioeconomic factors, this categorization includes time period, rural or urban location, and cultural group to help define the differences in the kinds of birth experiences. The four categories are: (1) the "institutionals," the poorest of urban women, frequently unmarried, who had literally no financial or social options available to them during their pregnancies and confinements, and who turned to the charity and public institutions as their last resort; (2) the "traditionalists," a diverse group of working-class, lower-middle class, and some middle-class women, immigrant and native-born, some urban but increasingly rural as the nineteenth century progressed, who had limited choices available during their pregnancies and deliveries and who remained within the traditional female-centered network for their confinements until childbirth moved to the hospital in the twentieth century; (3) the "integrationists," largely the urban middle class, who had financial options and social networks that allowed them wide-ranging options during their pregnancies and confinements and who included physicians in their birthing plans; and (4) the "privileged," the wealthy upper-middle- and upper-class women, living in major urban centers, who had access to medical services of highest repute.

The first group, the so-called "institutionals," represents the poorest and most desperate women living in or near the urban centers. These women, often unmarried and frequently with no family support or employment, turned in their pregnant despair to public or private charity institutions. Many impoverished women, married and single, found refuge in hospitals and almshouses that provided shelter and medical aid for them through their deliveries. These institutionalized women were either unmarried and could not admit their pregnancies to their families or they did not have access to any home support to help them through their confinements. They could not afford to pay for midwife or physician assistance, and they might not have had the space at home or friends available to help them manage a confinement. These women sought the institution because it was their only choice. Within the small number of maternity hospitals, almshouses, or medical school-affiliated dispensaries and clinics, these most desperate women were joined by a number of other women who sought institutional care because they needed special medical attention and could not afford a private doctor. Perhaps because of their particularly complicated labors, some women who would not otherwise have utilized medical facilities found themselves referred to these public institutions in their time of extreme need.

Some of the women who used institutional services were able to do so within their own homes; this subgroup of the institutionalized women probably had greater options than the most desperate. These women at least had homes, as crowded and impoverished as they might have been, into which medical attendants could come. Medical students in training rotated through home delivery, called "outdoor" services because doctors travelled outside the institution, for perhaps a few weeks of their medical training, and they were supervised by their professors, as were their colleagues who delivered poor women in the hospital. Unless the students found themselves in trouble in managing the delivery, the professors themselves rarely appeared in the women's homes.

Those poor urban women who went to hospitals to deliver their babies or who used outpatient institutional services within their own homes usually received medical aid in exchange for the clinical experience they provided for medical students.[27] Some of the finest obstetricians of the nineteenth and early twentieth century attended these poorest and most desperate of women. The historical evidence about the confinement experiences of this group of women, in fact, comes mostly from the accounts doctors wrote either when they were students in training or when they themselves trained new generations of medical students in obstetrics.

The autobiographies of many physicians include descriptions of their training adventures in obstetrics, and from these it is possible to glean something about the women "institutionals." Morris Fishbein, for example, related his clumsiness around the birthing beds of his first patients as he tried to learn how to handle the laboring woman and new baby. One particular experience stood out in his mind: "I wish that either I or my accompanying student on that trip, Aaron Arkin, had known as much as did our patient. We forgot to make sure that the bowel was empty before delivering the child. Most of our time during this delivery was spent removing the excreta from the newspapers which we had spread widely over the bed to constitute something resembling a sterile covering. The patient was kind enough to compliment us on our assistance as soon as the procedure was ended." Another noteworthy physician, Charles Mayo, also wrote graphically about the logistical problems of the first delivery he attended in the 1920s: "The woman was having a slow and difficult labor, which added to my alarm. The bed on which she lay didn't have a footboard [to help her push] so I stood at the end of it with a sheet in a tight grip, gave her the other end of the sheet and begged her to pull. She cooperated at once, with which her membrane ruptured and I was drenched in her water. With practice I improved, at least so far as positioning myself."

Franklin Martin attended numerous confinements during his training at Mercy Hospital in Chicago in the 1870s. He learned obstetrics while his patients were at the mercy of his developing talents. Mary Bennett Ritter, when a student at the Cooper Medical College of San Francisco in the 1880s, received her practical experience not in a hospital but out in the community: "Anyone desiring student care in a confinement could apply to the [medical] college. . . . My memory of this angle of our preparation lies chiefly in our prowling around dark streets in the middle of the night searching for the number of the house, usually a tenement."[28] Kate Pelham Newcomb, when a student at the University of Buffalo in the early twentieth century, followed her preceptor on home rounds, and sometimes found herself left in charge of confinement cases. When she received her clinical training at the New York Infirmary for Women and Children, she delivered the children of immigrant Armenian and Italian women in New York; she gained her experience by bringing medicine into the tenements.[29] Similarly, Margaret Stewart, while a student at the Woman's Medical College of Pennsylvania in Philadelphia, delivered babies in the Lying-In Charity Hospital. She wrote about the process: "Prospective mothers were not eligible for admission there until they were actually in labor. One of the duties of the police department was to furnish free and prompt transportation to these women." Picking up the resident physician first, the patrol wagon raced to the laboring woman and transported both back to the hospital, sometimes necessitating birth in the wagon en route.[30] Leon Herman remembered his training at Johns Hopkins in the first decade of the twentieth century when he was "required to spend several weeks of our junior year in an obstetrical clinic which was located in a very poor section of the city, and to officiate at six or more deliveries."[31]

Before actually delivering the babies of the poor who sought medical aid, medical students had received some classroom education in the process of parturition. Many of them had watched their professor or other physicians attend laboring women. But physicians' accounts of their training reveal many mistakes and awkwardnesses of these first deliveries. Students did not have the experience that many of the birthing women or the neighbor women also in attendance might have had; they did not yet comprehend the range of labor and delivery patterns, and they often panicked in the face of breech presentations, hemorrhaging, or convulsions. But in difficult cases, students could and did call their teachers, and the birthing woman could then receive the benefit of more experienced medical care.

In the nineteenth century the hospitals to which these poor women went for their confinements varied enormously in quality of care. In some training centers, there was adequate staff to serve the needs of the women; in others extreme neglect characterized their treatment. At Bellevue Hospital, for example, in 1860, a *Harper's Weekly* reporter observed that one woman gave birth entirely unattended, after which rats attacked her baby before anyone noticed.[32] (See illustration.) The women employing these medical services, probably never

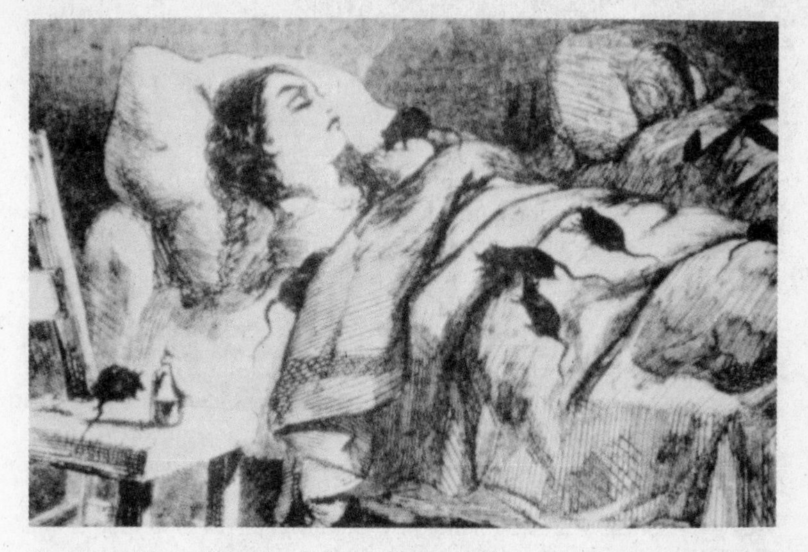

Illustration of conditions at Bellevue Hospital. The accompanying story claims this woman delivered her baby, who was attacked by rats, unattended in 1860. Source: *Harper's Weekly* 4 (1860): 273.

more than five percent of the nation's birthing women, did so for the most part because they did not have other options. The care they received sometimes was among the best available; it might also have been extremely marginal.

The poor urban women who had no choice in seeking attendance, as well as those who were able to find minimal support in their own families or communities but who also wanted or needed to include medical aid, constitute this first group of "institutionalized" birthing women. Unable to afford a private physician, and usually unable to maintain a traditional birth within their homes, they called upon the services of student physicians in training at nearby medical centers. These women represent in one sense the bottom of the opportunity scale, because their options were extremely constricted by their poverty, by their unmarried status, or by the particular medical complications they encountered during their labor. But the services that became available to them after the middle of the nineteenth century allowed them to utilize medicine within or outside of medical institutions as did women with wider birth choices.

The second category of birthing women, the "traditionalists," represents a more diverse group. Working-class, lower-middle, and some middle-class women—immigrant and native-born, urban, but as the nineteenth century progressed, increasingly rural—shared birthing experiences that were characterized by traditional female-centered practices. These women had some options available to them when they planned their confinements, but the options were limited in part by finances and also by the particulars of their local situation. Many of the immigrant women in this group chose midwives because they did not approve of the American custom of male birth attendants. Other women in this second, "traditional," grouping found themselves isolated from medical institutions and perhaps even from physicians; and they could not have chosen any but the most traditional helpers available in their community and among their friends. For most of the nineteenth century, these women called midwives to attend them along with numerous friends and relatives. Their confinements incorporated varied practices according to their cultural group; traditionalists' experiences were augmented by gradual changes in technique and procedures. Cultural rituals connected with confinement differed widely. Michael Davis recorded some of the variations, including Polish women's tradition of "scrubbing," perhaps for exercise during pregnancy, Jewish women's insistence on a pan of water under the birthing bed to draw away poisons, and Italian women's fear of bathing.[33]

The specific training of the midwife, the experience of the friends, and the course of the labor and delivery helped determine the particular practices the women in the traditionalist group chose. If all proceeded according to expectation, the birthing woman and her friends could participate in the process within a comfortable environment of shared experiences and close feelings. If the labor did not progress as expected, the women in attendance discussed calling in medical help. If they felt they could not handle the situation and if finances permitted and medical aid was available, the women called for a physician on short notice. They consulted with the doctor about specific procedures, often gave or withheld permission for suggested medical interventions and continued to serve their friend's interests. For this group of women, medical attention was a last resort only, and most often they planned and executed their deliveries within the traditional female mode. For some women in this group traditional practices were a conscious choice made because they believed birth was a natural event, not a medical one. For others the traditional nature of their confinements represented instead the limitations of their options, imposed because of limited family resources or because medical care was not available in their community.

There were significant variations within this group. Rural and frontier women, for example, remained limited in their options by the lack of birth attendants, trained or untrained. Some communities might have had only midwives available for birthing women; others might have offered more choice. Significant numbers of women, however, reported that they delivered their babies alone or only with the help of their husbands. These women might have planned to have midwives and their mothers, sisters, cousins, or friends with them, but labor caught them unprepared. It was necessary for rural women, because of their physical isolation, to make considerable preparations ahead of time. In their advanced pregnancy they may have taken rooms in the nearest town to be near a midwife or physician. Urban women might unexpectedly have had to seek the help of their close neighbors if their special friends or midwives or physicians did not have time to get to the labor.

This traditionalist group, despite their diversity, shared the common expectation, enforced or chosen, that birth only rarely needed the outside consultation of the medical profession. One doctor in a rural community served mostly by midwives noted that "Farmers' wives, who have acquired more or less experience in such cases, attend most of the confinements. They may be called neighborhood midwives, though all are unregistered, most are without training, and none make any charge for their services. Their patients give them a present of $2.00 or $3.00 for their help."[34] Partly because of limited financial resources and partly because of traditional expectations, this group of women continued the birth practices of their ancestors and incorporated new medicalized techniques significantly later than their more affluent sisters.

The third category of birthing women, identified as "integrationists," formed the bulk of the middle-class population, especially urban, during the late eighteenth and nineteenth century. This group had both social and financial options; it was possible for these women to plan their confinements. After the initial introduction of male physicians into the normal practice of obstetrics, the choices of many middle-class urban women integrated medical practices into traditional practices to create the ideal confinement. Women in this category, beginning in the middle of the eighteenth century, but more commonly during the nineteenth century, planned to incorporate physicians as attendants at their confinements to insure against physical difficulty.

They believed that medicine could offer increased safety, and they were willing to spend the extra money necessary to get the benefits of that promise. After anesthesia became available in the middle of the nineteenth century, (which will be discussed in Chapter 5) these women wanted the relief it provided and called in physicians for this purpose specifically. Many of these women continued to ask midwives to help out as well; others relied solely on medicine. Most women in this category, regardless of their preference for doctors alone or midwives with doctors, continued to ask women friends and relatives to be with them and provide the domestic help and the emotional support they needed at the stressful time of their confinements.

The variations in how this integrationist group of women used medical services depended in large part on the configuration of the medical people available to them. American medicine in the nineteenth century was a pluralistic system, and the people practicing it differed significantly from one another in training, theory, and skill. Middle-class women had the financial ability to pick and choose among these groups, and their choices represent the wide diversity within medicine and within their local areas. So-called "sectarian" practitioners practiced in most American communities, and these physicians offered services according to their particular medical system.

Hydropathy, or the water cure, incorporated warm-water baths for mother and baby. Many middle-class women found this noninvasive treatment, sometimes administered in home treatments and otherwise at water-cure establishments, most appealing. The water-cure advocates stressed natural therapies, including fresh air and exercise regimens during pregnancy, vegetarian diets, and the liberal use of water internally and externally for maintaining physical health. Many women chose this system for their confinement, even if they did not use hydropathy routinely as their usual health care method.

Homeopaths, who eschewed drugs except in infinitesimal doses, also offered women an option in health care delivery during pregnancy and confinement. Many women sought out these followers of Samuel Hahnemann, who believed that the smaller the dosage of a medicine the greater its effectiveness, because of the mildness of its treatments. The sect established itself in America in 1825, and it grew in strength through the century. Women made up an estimated two-thirds of homeopathic patients, who were located mainly throughout New England, New York, Pennsylvania, and the Midwest.[35]

Within the part of the profession labelled "allopathic" or regular, enormous differences also existed. As noted in Chapter 2, regular physicians trained before the middle of the nineteenth century received virtually no practical obstetric training in medical school. Most regular practitioners probably did not even attend medical school until well into the nineteenth century. Even those educated in the second half of the century, under the system of "demonstrative midwifery," which allowed medical students to witness live deliveries, had extremely limited hands-on experience before they started their own medical practices. General practitioners, for whom obstetrics was only one among many services offered to patients, may never have acquired systematic practical experience delivering babies.

The skill that all of these practitioners wielded within the confinement rooms probably could not be predicted or known by the women who sought their services. While women might have made their choices among the different medical systems with an understanding of the theoretical ideas that governed each, most could not evaluate ahead of time the actual prowess of the doctors they invited to attend them. Birthing women merely sought medical aid with the faith that "medicine," and all it symbolized, attended them in the person of their own physician.[36]

The fourth group of American birthing women, the "privileged," were urban upper-middle- and upper-class women who had complete opportunity to include whatever and whomever they wanted at their confinements. Because finances were not a consideration, these women could make choices limited only by their own knowledge of the available options. Although not guaranteed safe or comfortable confinements, the women in this group had the optimum chances of receiving the best care available. Because they lived in the major urban centers, they chose not just medical care, but medical care from the physicians with the best reputations in their community, usually the professors at the medical schools. This group of women were quickest to incorporate the newest techniques as they became available.

Beginning in the middle of the eighteenth century, these women utilized physicians' skills at the same time they continued to seek the help of friends and family (but probably not midwives). This group had optimal choice for everything except the actual physical course of labor and delivery. Physicians like Franklin Newell believed that in this respect upper-class women were more hampered than other women by their class and life style. If upper-class women were at highest risk in physicians' minds because of their education, dress style, and active social life, they were in a position to receive the best available care to get them out of their difficulties. Indeed, it can be argued that these women commanded the closest attention of the medical profession both because of their perceived increased physical difficulties and because of their ability to find and to pay for the most medicine could offer. By the end of the nineteenth century, these women had made the transition from using general practitioners to using specialists in obstetrics for their medical birth attendants, and in the twentieth century they moved into luxurious private maternity hospitals or private suites in general hospitals where they could receive their obstetricians' full attention.

The four-part division offered here applies to women's childbirth experiences before the twentieth century, and it fits only this prehospital era. The move to the hospital occurred for most women during and following the period 1910 to 1930 (as described in Chapter 7). The hospital acted in some ways as a great leveler, making women's childbirth experiences more similar than they had ever been. While class differences continued to exist in twentieth-century hospital-based childbirth, they took a different form from the ones described here.

This categorization of birthing women into four groups incorporates class differences, variations in urban or rural location for accessibility of birth attendants and institutions, and cultural values of the communities in which the women found themselves. It describes the important differences in women's birth experiences which affected their postpartum health. It also considers the relationship between the skill of the medical or midwife attendant and postpartum safety.

The enormous variations in ability among physicians allowed those women who could choose the most skilled medical attendants the best chances of not being harmed. In this respect, women at both extremes of the socioeconomic scale found themselves with similar, but not congruent, medical opportunities. Although the poorest women became the training material for medical students, they also had access to the students' professors, who represented the highest in medical skills. For example, the women who received their care from the Chicago Maternity Center, the poor and largely immigrant and black community in the inner city of Chicago at the turn of the twentieth century, probably received the best care available in the city. Their mortality was lower than any other group in the city, despite the fact that their births were overseen first by students in training.[37]

On the other hand, the middle-class women in the integrationist category, who utilized the wide variety of general practitioners, put themselves into the most unpredictable and risky situations. Their physicians exhibited a range of skills from poor to excellent and were among those most often accused of practicing "meddlesome midwifery." These doctors may have put their parturient patients in greater jeopardy for infection and iatrogenic (medically induced) complications than they might have been with traditional midwife attendants. Medical attendance by itself, therefore, did not make women's birth experiences similar or safer; rather the variations in medical practice added to the great differences.

The differences in childbirth experiences were substantial for the women who experienced them. Having little or no choice in determining who would attend them or their attendants' level of skill was very significant to birthing women. One has only to examine the care with which the pregnant women who had optimal choice planned their coming confinements to understand how much the control meant to them. With childbirth still a dangerous event, any precautions one could take were valuable and necessary to physical and psychological wellbeing. While no women could guarantee their survival or their postpartum health, all women wanted to provide as much insurance toward that end as possible. Women in the middle and upper classes believed that their best insurance rested with the incorporation of some medical attention. Probably unable to know the actual skill levels of the various medical practitioners, as we can do only partially even in hindsight, those women who could afford physicians to help them trusted their attendants, for better or worse.

Despite all the differences among women's birth experiences, it is important to note that significant factors connected all women's experiences in the prehospital era. Available to all but the poorest women who went to hospitals and dispensaries to deliver their babies was the home-based, largely female support network they all desired. This part of the birth experience will be analyzed more fully in Chapter 4. It is necessary here merely to note that in the prehospital era women held in common the desire for and achievement of this female cushion of security despite class or opportunity differences. As Margaret Hagood observed, "Lines of class distinction vanish" over "this most fundamental of realities." All women found comfort in the company of other women at the time of confinement and could share their experiences with each other.[38]

The second factor common to most women after the middle of the eighteenth century was the growing importance and acceptance of medical aids. The women with the least opportunity for choice utilized medical attendants because no others were available to them, but all of the women who had some choice incorporated physicians into their plans, even if only as a last resort. Those with choices increasingly consulted the medical profession. The lure of medicine and the progress it symbolized captured large numbers of birthing women as the nineteenth century progressed and the twentieth began. Women's increasing use of physicians and their increasing acceptance of medical solutions to their childbed problems combined to create the milieu in which the twentieth-century move to the hospital occurred.

Another similarity in the childbirth experiences of most women was their active participation in changing childbirth procedures and practices throughout this prehospital period in American childbirth history. Although middle- and upper-class women, who first invited male physicians to attend them and who first used anesthesia, paved the way for most changes, all women shared in this process. Even the "institutionalized" women who found themselves in the most powerless situation of any group of birthing women found ways to combat their powerlessness and to make their wishes felt. Through this common tradition of resistance to procedures they did not want and through combined action to achieve practices they desired, women together shaped childbirth practices.

Historian Nancy Schrom Dye has studied the New York Midwifery Dispensary, which opened in 1890 to serve impoverished pregnant women and simultaneously to train student physicians in obstetrics, and she has emphasized the women's active participation in confinement room events. Dye concluded that the medical training focus of the Dispensary's work meant that some of the most renowned obstetricians oversaw the deliveries of poor and working-class women and that these women were "central to the transformation of birth from a social to a medical phenomenon." The institutionalized women did not merely receive the ministrations of their medical attendants, despite the class differences between them, but they interacted with the students and physicians in actively determining what procedures could be applied. Dye found that many of the immigrant women who used the medical services of the Dispensary in their own homes simultaneously called in midwives and other neighbor attendants to help at the delivery. Despite their poverty, these poor women, supported by their gender and cultural peers, were able to keep their conventional birthing practices at the same time that they used parts of the medical services. If physicians insisted on procedures alien to the birthing women or their families, women sometimes asked them to leave.[39]

Hidden in the doctors' records of the births at the Philadelphia Almshouse Hospital during the 1890s is the same spunkiness evident among the charity cases. The women, poor, often single, overwhelmingly black or immigrant, who delivered at the Almshouse, were able to assert some minimal control over the procedures used during their deliveries. For example, the single Eliza Humbert, who delivered her first child at age 22 in January of 1895, had a very difficult delivery. After more than two hours at second stage (when she was fully dilated), the doctor wanted to apply forceps to extract the child, but Humbert refused. The doctor noted, "Nearly two [more] hours were consumed in waiting to obtain permission." Delivery was ultimately accomplished as the doctor wished, with the use of forceps, but not before the woman was able to exert the little power she had left in the institutional setting.[40] This pattern of self assertion, which developed among poor and upper-class women alike, had significant impact on the course of obstetric developments. Regardless of the class background of their patients, physicians had to adapt their practices to make them acceptable.[41]

All women exhibited direct or indirect influence on the specific events in their own birthing rooms. Poor women and rich women alike felt comfortable in making demands on physicians, according to their own expectations, and in removing physicians who did not comply with their wishes.

Because the upper-class women could pay for their medical services and because attendance at childbirth frequently led to complete family care and thus the promise of greater financial benefit, physicians probably felt more inclined to try to accommodate their wealthier patients than their poorest ones. Most observable changes over time in childbirth procedures, such as the introduction of male physicians to normal obstetrics or the use of anesthesia, occurred first among those groups of women who had the financial ability to choose the newest techniques. These women were influential in bringing new medical techniques into normal obstetric practice, including forceps and opium, anesthetics, and aseptic and antiseptic techniques, and, in the twentieth century, specialist-attended delivery in hospitals. In the large sweep of obstetric history, physicians' activities in the birthing room were molded most significantly by middle- and upper-class women in their private practices. The specific influences of these groups of women will be examined more closely in the next chapters.

American women suffered health problems that both led to and resulted from difficult childbirth-related events. Upper-class women might well have been at risk because of atrophied muscles caused by tight corsets, inactivity, and a low-protein diet. Working-class women carried their own burdens of insufficient diet, physical overwork, stress, poor housing, and polluted milk and water. Childbirth, especially when often repeated, exacerbated all women's health problems; the specifics of women's experiences were different, but the risks to health and some of the responses to the risks were common to all.

The socioeconomic differences in childbirth experiences, while very real and important to women, especially in terms of their options, did not affect women's attempts to set the stage for their confinements. All women had expectations, many of them based on historic and traditional women's activities, that they tried to play out during their confinements. In the next chapter we will examine the expectations held in common by birthing women—that other women could help them through their confinement crises—and analyze the degree to which the gender-based activity in the birthing rooms gave strength to the women who were able to have their friends with them during delivery.

4

"Only a Woman Can Know"

The Role of Gender in the Birthing Room

With all the dangers and worries connected with traditional childbirth, women easily could have given up hope of improving their birthing experiences or the hard domestic prospects that frequently accompanied the arrival of children. And no doubt some women did resign themselves to lives of invalidism and deprivation. But what comes through the written record much more strongly are the positive aspects of the experience that women chose to emphasize, the caring ways in which they tried to help each other, and the simple fact that women were able to change the childbirth experience for themselves in significant ways throughout the nineteenth and into the early twentieth century.

As long as birth remained a home-based event, which it did well into the twentieth century, women continued actively to participate in the determination of confinement practices. Historians have heretofore assumed that, when physicians started attending normal deliveries, beginning in the middle of the eighteenth century and increasing through the nineteenth century, the presence of this male authority figure changed the power structure in the room. Catherine Scholten concluded, for example, that when physicians attended delivery "women no longer dominated the activities in the lying-in room."[1] My research shows rather that for the entire home-birth period, until women moved to the hospital to deliver their babies in the twentieth century, women friends, neighbors, and relatives continued to offer birthing women psychological support and practical help and that these female-centered activities dominated most American births, whether or not they were attended by male physicians. This chapter will examine this essentially female nature of home-based childbirth and explore how the birthing women and their female attendants interacted with the male physicians who attended them. To complete the analysis of the role of gender in the birthing room, the chapter will also consider the role of female physicians, many of whom got their start in the practice of medicine through attending childbearing women.

Let us examine first the cooperative nature of the labor and delivery experience. Throughout American history until the twentieth century, most women gave birth at home with the help of their female friends and relatives. Birth was a women's event, and women eagerly gave their aid when it was needed. Ebenezer Parkman wrote in the middle of the eighteenth century of one of the twelve times his wife was brought to bed:

> My wife very full of pain. This Morning I sent Ebenezer for Mrs. Forbush. . . . A number of Women here. Mrs. Hephzibath Maynard and her son's wife, Mrs. How, Mr. David Maynard's wife and his Brother Ebenezer's, Captain Forbush's and Mr. Richard Barns's. My son Ebenezer went out for most of them. At night I resign my Dear Spouse to the infinite Compassions, all sufficiency and sovereign pleasure of God and under God to the good Women that are with her, waiting Humbly the Event.[2]

Mary Louise Fowler wrote to her pregnant sister Nettie in 1863 when Nettie was in Europe with her husband: "I think of you in anticipation of your coming *trial* . . . will you, can you have among strangers, in a foreign land, that tender care which we all require, at such a time. I know you will have all that can be procured under the circumstances, but it would relieve me of great anxiety if you were in *our* little best bed-room where I could nurse you as only a *mother* or a *sister* can."[3] Albina Wight, who was unable to attend her sister's confinement in the middle of the nineteenth century, wrote in her diary after the event: "Poor poor girl how I pitty [sic] her. She says the two wimen [sic] that were there were as kind and good as Sisters could be. I am glad of that . . . . Oh how I do wish I could be with her."[4] When possible, sisters and cousins and mothers came to help the parturient through the ordeal of labor and delivery, and close friends and neighbors joined them around the birthing bed. One woman who described her 1866 confinement wrote: "A woman that was expecting had to take good care that she had plenty fixed to eat for her neighbors when they got there. There was no telling how long they was in for. There wasn't no paying these friends so you had to treat them good."[5] To this women's world, husbands, brothers, or fathers could gain only temporary entrance. In an 1836 account, the new father was invited in to see his wife and daughter, but then "Mrs. Warren, who was absolute in this season of female despotism, interposed, and the happy father was compelled, with reluctant steps, to quit the spot."[6]

The woman's world around the birthing bed that is revealed in the letters women wrote to each other and in their diaries and private writings represents the existence of a specific female group identity among women. Women could write and speak to each other intimate details of confinement-related care; they could confide their innermost thoughts about their coming motherhood. While nineteenth-century conventions did not permit discourse about such private matters in public, among themselves, in private, women could and did speak freely. Here, around the confinement bed, women identified with each other's concerns, shared their wisdom, and united, as women, in the knowledge that they were not alone with their problems.

Most crucial to the support networks women tried to gather around them were their own mothers. Anita McCormick Blaine wrote to her mother, Nettie Fowler McCormick, in 1890 as she planned for the birth of her first child: "Dearest mother mine—all would be complete if you were here."[7] Anita had prepared thoroughly for her coming confinement, but she missed her mother's presence. Nettie re-

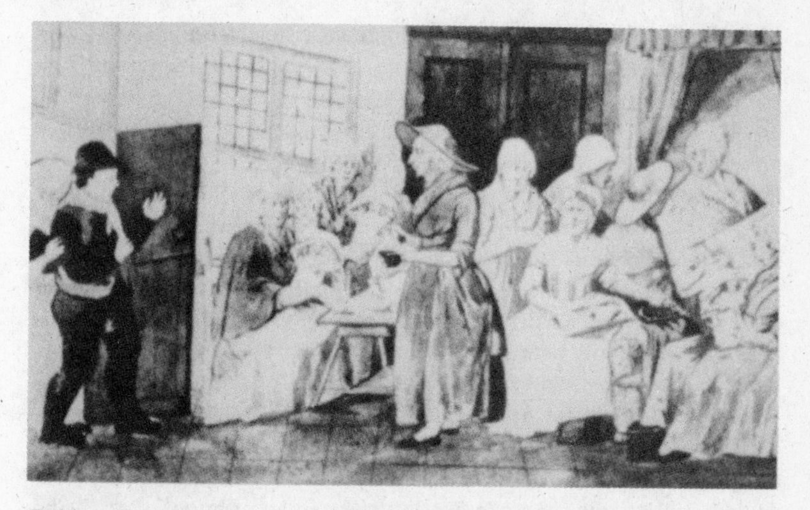

Eighteenth-century "social childbirth," illustrating women in attendance at this multiple birth ushering in the father to see the new babies.

Source: Roy P. Finney, *The Story of Motherhood* (New York: Liveright Publishing, 1937). The Bettmann Archive.

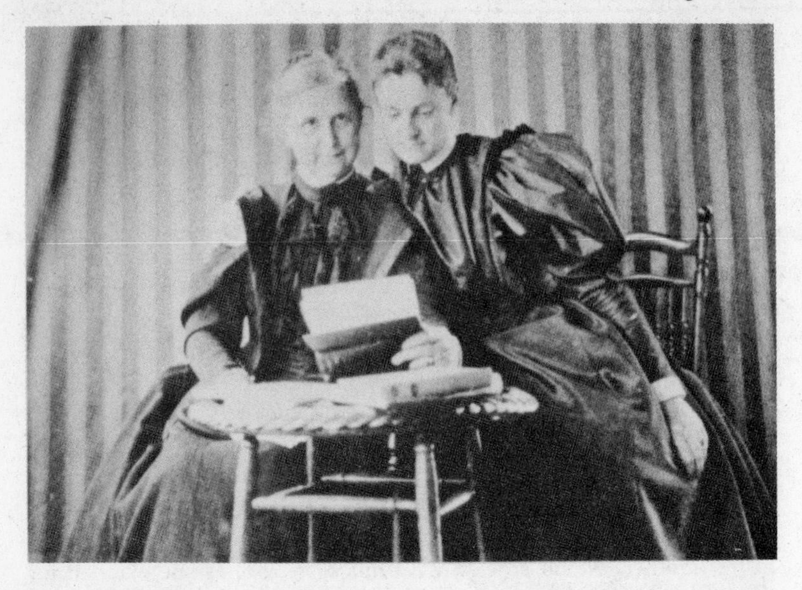

Nettie Fowler McCormick and her daughter Anita McCormick Blaine, ca. 1890.
Source: Gilbert A. Harrison, *A Timeless Affair: The Life of Anita McCormick Blaine* (Chicago: University of Chicago Press, 1979).

turned the sentiment. "Dearie," she wrote, "I wish I were there to thoroughly rub olive oil upon you hips, your groin muscles, your abdominal muscles all throughout—in short all the muscles that are to be called upon to yield, and be elastic at the proper time. See how reasonable it seems that they should be helped to yield, and to do their work if they are kneaded by the strong hand of mother, while olive oil is being *freely applied*."[8] In the highly mobile nineteenth century, many American women shared Anita Blaine's predicament of finding themselves separated from their closest relatives during their pregnancies and confinements. Georgiana Bruce Kirby followed her husband to California in 1852 and found herself both pregnant and almost completely isolated. "I have seen the face of but one woman in four months," she lamented in her diary. Mother and other relatives totally beyond reach, Kirby was ready to settle for the company of any "congenial female companion." Her husband was attentive and kind, but, Kirby concluded, "Every good woman needs a companion of her own sex." She finally spent a few days and nights visiting another pregnant woman, who, Kirby wrote, "quite made me forget myself and my ailments."

Similarly, following her labor and delivery, Martha Slayton found considerable comfort in hearing her mother-in-law's own confinement accounts. She wrote, "it was comforting to know that you had always had a hard time when your babies came. I guess that is the usual experience of mothers. Certainly the suffering is indescribable and I guess not to be comprehended by those who have not passed through it." The birth experience provided the context within which women could share their deepest feelings; out of this grew a sense of shared experiences that increased the emotional bonds among women.[9]

Letters formed a partial but usually frustrating substitute for many women whose marriages took them away from their childhood friends and relatives. Mary Hallock Foote prepared for her delivery by trying to follow the long-distance advice of her close friend Helena DeKay Gilder. "I have followed your advice in one of the two ways in which you recommended me to be anticipating the evil day that is coming—as to the hardening of the nipples—but I do not know how you mean about using oil," she wrote. "Is it the abdomen that is to be rubbed?"[10] Letters could never be as satisfying as having the people present. "I thought of my mother," wrote Leah Morton about her time of pregnancy. "I wanted her, I needed her so that I could have cried, all the way over the long miles between us." No other woman entirely met Morton's needs. "They were kind," she wrote of the women who helped her through her ordeal, "but I . . . wanted my mother with me. I did not want these strange, kind women."[11]

Trying to overcome the problem of isolation, some women traveled long distances to be with their mothers at this most family-centered time. Hannah Bingham wrote to her friend Maria Seymour in 1844, advising her to excercise during her pregnancy; she especially pressed her to leave the unhealthy environment of Detroit for her mother's more rural home for her confinement: "you know what a healthy place this is and how much better it would be to be at your own home when you should be confined." Dorothy Lawson McCall, the daughter of wealthy Massachusetts parents, went west to Oregon with her husband at the turn of the twentieth century, but returned to her parental home across the entire continent for each of her four childbirths.[12] Gladys Brooks likewise returned to the family house to have her baby in the bed where her husband had been born.[13] Despite the difficulty of travel during their advanced pregnancies, many women who could not find appropriate women to attend them went home to mother. One woman wrote about her great-grandmother's experiences in the eighteenth century:

> Before her first child was born she went to her own home in Danvers [Massachusetts] to put herself under the care of her mother, making the journey of fifty miles on horseback through what must have been at that time nearly a wilderness, where she remained until after the birth of the child, and then returned to Smithfield [Rhode Island] with her child in her arms, again on horseback. Before the birth of the second child, there still being no neighbors in the settlement of Smithfield upon whom she could depend for aid, she made the same journey in the same way, carrying the first child with her, and after the birth returning with both children.[14]

This pattern can be found in births from the eighteenth to the twentieth centuries. In Virginia at the turn of the twentieth century, Mattie Briscoe's mother came to her "rescue" for her first confinement, but after that Mattie returned to her mother's home to be confined.[15] In the antebellum South, "Grandmother Elmore" took an eighteen-mile bumpy carriage ride to her mother-in-law's house where she delivered her baby. From the North Dakota frontier in 1885, Julia Gage Carpenter traveled east to Syracuse, New York, four months before her expected confinement to spend time with her pregnant sister and to deliver at her mother's home.[16]

Emily McCorkee Fitzgerald, an army doctor's wife on the Alaskan frontier in the 1870s, could not travel home to mother, so she made elaborate plans for neighboring women to attend her during and after her delivery. She had the additional security that most women did not share of having her physician-husband at hand. Even so, after her terrible ordeal of a slow and painful labor and delivery and the difficulty of scheduling her women helpers, she wrote to her mother, "I hope I will never have any more babies where I can't have some of my relatives with me."[17]

Sarah Hale had the comfort of her family and friends with her when she was confined early in the nineteenth century. Her sister could not attend one delivery, and she wrote to Sarah how sorry she was that she could not "sit with you during your stay in your chamber." Because she understood how important women companions could be to a birthing woman, Sarah Hale wrote to her son when his wife Emily was about to be confined, offering her services. She said, "I should like very much to be with you at the time [of Emily's delivery]. . . . do not hesitate to send for me the moment [she begins labor]. . . . It is such a comfort to me if I can still be useful."[18] Emily, for her part, greatly appreciated her mother-in-law's attentions. When

Edward was out of town near the time of her confinement, Emily sent for Sarah to keep her company. Sarah wrote, "I felt quite complimented. . . . Nothing special for me to do, but Emily compliments me by saying she feels perfectly tranquil and safe now I am here."[19]

Some women could marshall only one or two women to help them, but many accounts list eight or ten women helpers in addition to the midwife or doctor who might be attending. Nannie Jackson, in rural Arkansas in 1890, gathered six women to help when she delivered her third child, and her oldest daughter noted, "Mama had a heap of company today."[20] Antebellum southerner Madge Preston gave birth to a child in 1849, which her husband, who waited in another room, reported this way: "At this birth were present Dr. J. H. Briscoe, Mrs. Margaret Carlon, Mrs. Connolly [midwife] her friend—our servant Mary Miskel, and our Negroes Lucy and Betty. They inform me that Mrs. P. bore her protracted labor, difficulty, pain and anxiety, which endured forty-eight hours, with calmness, courage and fortitude."[21]

Women went to considerable sacrifice to help their birthing relatives and friends; they interrupted their lives to travel long distances and frequently stayed months before and after delivery to do the household chores. Abbie Field wrote to her friend in 1864 that because of her sister-in-law Sue's recent confinement she was staying with her in Englishville, Michigan, although she much preferred to be in Detroit. "This seems like home now I have lived here so much," she wrote. Two weeks after the baby's birth, Sue had not yet sat up. She had had the fever, but, Abbie hoped, was finally on the mend: "If Sue is well enough so I can leave her," she wrote, "I will go to meeting next Sunday." In another family account from the early twentieth century, we learn from a ten-year-old daughter's perspective (remembered in retrospect), "Mother's younger sister Eva came from Caledonia to live at our house shortly before my kid sister arrived. . . . This aunt helped mother with the housework just before the baby came. . . . I was invited by my aunt Mary to come and stay at their home during the four days just before the baby arrived."[22] Margaret Hagood noted that among white tenant farm women in the South, "the customary practice . . . is for some female relative—mother, sister, niece, mother-in-law, sister-in-law, or cousin—to come and take charge of the housework and take care of the children."[23]

When relatives were not available, neighbors stayed for the labor and delivery and brought food and kept up with washing and other domestic duties. Agnes Reid confided to her father the difficulty she had had in 1871 in getting the right attendants. "Then at the eleventh hour my Aunt refused to be with me because of some little differences Nels [her husband] had had with her two boys. The world did not look very bright just at that point in our history. However my good Nettie [a neighbor?] offered to leave her husband to do his own housekeeping that she might help us, and three days after she came, little Jimmie was born."[24] Christiana Tillson wrote in her journal of her second confinement in 1825: "I had made the acquaintance of Mrs. Townsend, who was with me and remained until John was a week old."[25] Ann Bolton recalled with enormous fondness and gratitude a good friend: "of thirteen children which I brought into the world, she bore me company with ten of them."[26] Another woman recorded how "little Charlie" arrived "with the help of Mary Bradley, the tenant farmer's wife, Mrs. Owens and others. . . . The neighbors saw to every comfort."[27] Mathilde Shillock wrote to her sister in 1856 that during her postpartum difficulties, "Every day there were different helpers about. The ladies in the neighborhood took turns caring for me." Mary Kincaid wrote to her cousin after her second confinement in 1896: "the neighbors all was so kind to me. They brought all kinds of fruit and everything I wanted to eat and they are all good to me. Yes I am glad to have good neighbors, I don't know what I would do." Despite the support she experienced, Mary concluded, "I tell you Mamie I don't want no more babies." Recalling her own community, another woman wrote, "I remember when a baby was about to be born, all the neighbor women around living close went to be there for the borning."[28]

Women's support in the birthing room was not always easy to find nor guaranteed by virtue of previous relationships. Dr. David Kellogg related a story of a birth he attended that reveals some of the problems that might result from women's emotional ties to each other. In June of 1897 a man called on Dr. Kellogg to assist his wife in the delivery of their seventh child:

> He remarked that his wife's mother lived in the same house but that she had a mean ugly disposition and had got mad at his wife and would not speak to her. His wife was of that disposition that she would not speak to her mother unless the mother spoke first, so they had not spoken for some time. After reaching the house I found a neighbor's wife but not the mother assisting. In a few hours matters began to look serious with the sick woman, and occasionally the mother's voice was heard at the outside door asking for someone to come out. These calls became rather more frequent, until at last the

mother came in and stood by the foot of the bed and said, "Don't you want me to make you some warm tea, Mary?" This complete surrender on the mother's part doubtless helped matters on to a speedy and favorable termination.[29]

Even with the best of relationships between the women involved, the plans for gathering women together might have gone astray in the haste of an early labor or in the midst of the proverbial snowstorm. Quite often when rural women went into labor, husbands hastened to summon the nearest neighbor or to fetch the midwife or doctor only to find upon their return that the baby already had been born. Countless women found themselves unexpectedly and totally alone during their deliveries. "When mother went into labor," wrote one daughter, "she called father from the field by waving a dishtowel. He had to unhitch the team, unharness one of them, harness him again, and then drive off to fetch the woman who served as mid-wife. She lived two miles down the road from our house. But, just as father drove out of the yard, a son, large and husky, was born."[30] Another woman, finding herself in active labor three weeks before she expected, quickly turned to the chapter in her baby book, "What to do before the doctor comes." While her husband raced for the doctor, her baby was born.[31] A logger's wife recounted how her husband barely rescued her 1908 breech delivery:

> When Bill was gone once . . . I broke water and was having too much pain. Feeling that baby with my hands I knew for certain it was going to breech. I put the kids to bed to keep warm and told the older ones to keep that fire going no matter what. . . . I got . . . on a pallet under my quilts and Lordy did I pray for Bill to come back. He came blowing in that night. Said he just had a feeling. I never was so glad to see anyone. He pulled that baby out [feet first].[32]

Even in these relatively unusual events of a woman being alone for her labor and delivery, her friends usually rallied round afterwards to make sure that she got the rest she needed.[33] Women who could not summon friends were considered unfortunate: "[I] went thence to see Mrs. Ray who has been very ill in Childbed—had a little girl which died in a few hours.—She is much to be pitied having no female relation or intimate friend to be with her."[34] Another woman felt sorry for herself: "It seemed very gloomy when I found my time had come, to think that I was, as it were, destitute of earthly friends. No mother, no husband, and none of my particular friends that belong to the town; they happening to be out of town."[35]

If mothers, relatives, and friends were the preferred companions of childbirths, women settled for any women who happened to be nearby. Class, ethnic, or racial differences between women paled during this critical situation, when women as women were so needed. Susan Allison delivered her baby prematurely in 1869 before she could carry out her plan to leave her frontier home for her mother's house, forcing her to rely on the help of an Indian woman, the only woman in the area. "Suzanne was very good to me in her way," she wrote, but "she thought I ought to be as strong as an Indian woman but I was not."[36] In the same vein, Sarah Hale wrote to her daughter-in-law: "In case of failure of other assistants I dare say if needed your neighbors Mrs. Warden or Mrs. Baxter would be quite as useful as more cultivated women—But I do not believe you will need to have recourse to them."[37]

In Napa, California, in the middle of the nineteenth century, the wife of a doctor frequently found herself more in demand as a birth attendant than her husband, because of her sex. Her daughter recorded the time, apparently often repeated, when a husband sought her mother's assistance for his laboring wife, refusing the help of the doctor: "the man insisted his wife needed the help of a woman." The doctor's wife "knew all about the comfort of another woman's presence at such a time," and she went to the confinement. "Mother said she had never seen anyone so overjoyed as that woman was when she realized that help had come. While Mother could not understand her language, she said that was unnecessary, for joy and gratitude were the same in any language." Years later the grateful woman retold the story and added, "[She was] the best woman on earth. When she came in and stood beside my bed, I thought I saw an angel."[38] When Sarah Jane Stevens experienced severe anxiety about her approaching confinement in 1885, her aunt expressed her sympathy and offered a practical suggestion: "if there is an elderly woman round there of good experience you would do well to try and get her to stay with you for a time for anyone is nervous about those times especially if no woman is round."[39]

These examples are drawn from letters and diaries written over a long period of time, encompassing the eighteenth, nineteenth, and early twentieth century; they come from a variety of women, including those who were attended during their confinement by midwives and those who chose physicians. Except the most desperate poor who were forced by circumstances into institutions for their confinements all American birthing women had access to this network to varying degrees, depending on their locale and their own social acquaintances.

Women often went to help other women whom they hardly knew; when the call for help came, women responded. The women's support network that was activated when a pregnant woman found herself ready to deliver her child was impressive; and it was renewed each time a woman in the neighborhood went into labor.

Whether women chose midwives or doctors or experienced neighbors to attend them, whether they resided in the cities or in the hinterlands, whether they lived at the beginning of the nineteenth century or the beginning of the twentieth century, they sought the company of women friends and relatives to be with them through their ordeals. Scarcely any family accounts of women in childbirth fail to mention this important element of the experience. From the South, Laura Norwood wrote to her mother, "It would be a great comfort to me to have Sarah [her sister?] or some of you with me."[40] From the Wisconsin frontier in 1851, Elizabeth Atkinson Richmond wrote her mother about the gracious neighbors who came to help her, concluding "I can't tell you, dear Mother, how many times I have wished you near me to advise me."[41] From Boston, Mrs. Graves pitied her friend who delivered when "deprived of all intercourse with her kindred or friends" at a time when "the presence of a mother is so anxiously longed for and so much needed."[42] Grace Lumpkin's fictional account of a poor woman in South Carolina in the first decade of the twentieth century, who delivered her child with the sole assistance of her own father, captured the common feelings:

> As she gulped down the warm coffee she wished in herself there was a woman who would know what to do without telling. And she wished the men were where they belonged when a woman was in travail—somewhere out on the mountains or at a neighbor's.[43]

The psychological comforts women could provide for each other could not be matched. Men could not know personally the women's experience and thus could not fully empathize with women at their hour of suffering. While they might be able to provide the technical assistance necessary to aid a birth, men could not provide the psychological supports that women so eagerly sought. One man realized how important the company of women was during labor and delivery, and he formulated what he thought the reasons for this were: "His life has not been in jeopardy. Except in sympathy his nerves have not been racked, his muscles strained, his joints wrenched, his fibers torn, his blood spilled."[44] A woman physician wrote simply: "Only a woman can know what a woman has suffered or is suffering."[45]

It is necessary to document closely the importance to birthing women of the presence of women friends and relations because historians have heretofore assumed that, when male doctors began attending normal births, women's birthing network disappeared. The accounts from the birthing women and their family and friends contradict previous conceptions about the primacy of male physicians in childbirth during the home-birth period. Birthing women found trusted women companions just as important as medical attendants in planning for their confinements. Furthermore, these women played a crucial role in decision making around the birthing bed. The physicians who attended birthing women in the presence of other women shared their authority with those women. Birth in the United States remained in significant measure female and traditional in orientation until it moved to the hospital in the twentieth century.

The women's network that developed at least in part through the strong attachments formed across the childbirth bed had long-lasting effects on women's lives. When women suffered the agonies of watching their friends die, when they had helped a friend recover from a difficult delivery, or when they had participated in a successful birthing, they developed a closeness that often lasted their lifetime. Surviving life's traumas together made the crises bearable and produced important bonds that continued to sustain other parts of women's lives. "It was as if," Marilyn Clohessy wrote, "mothers were members of a sorority and the initiation was to become a mother."[46] Nannie Jackson's female support network offers one example of the importance of good friends. Her diary, which survives only for the year 1890–91, is a litany of friends helping one another. Her best friend was Fannie, who lived half a mile away; Nannie visited her daily, and sometimes two, three, and four times a day. Once, during the eighth month of her third pregnancy, she visited Fannie three times in one evening, and her husband got angry. But, Nannie noted, "I just talk to Fannie & tell her my troubles because it seems to help me to bear it better when she knows about it. I shall tell her whenever I feel like it."[47] Indeed, in this diary fragment from 1890, there is evidence of significant rebellion against her husband's wishes and her strong reliance on her relationship with Fannie. During her confinement, Fannie came and stayed for four days and nights. But Fannie was only the most important in a long list of close friends. Nannie, who was white, visited daily with many other women, both white and black, cooking special things for them, sharing the limited family resources, helping them with sewing projects, sitting up with them when they were sick, helping out at births, arranging funerals. Nannie and her friends, whose economically limited lives left nothing for outside entertainment or expense, found rich resources within their own group.

The psychological dimension of the women's network played a significant role in making women's hard lives bearable and in sustaining them during difficult times. Perhaps more significant to these women, however, was the practical assistance friends could provide during the times of crisis. During labor and delivery, when a woman might not be able to stand up for herself, she could rely on her women friends to do her talking for her. The women gathered around the birthing bed made decisions about when and if to call physicians to births that midwives were attending; they gave or withheld permission for physicians' procedures; and they created the atmosphere of female support in a room that might have contained both men and women.

In the colonial period, a birthing woman "called her women together" when she went into labor. Midwives and other attendants assessed the situation and managed the birth as long as events progressed relatively normally. If they judged the situation to be abnormal, they advised calling in a physician. In these situations, the physician entered the room as an expert, but an expert who had a nasty duty to perform. The "learned man" would use his instruments to force delivery, either by fetal manipulation and live delivery or, much to be dreaded, by fetal dismemberment and extraction. As historian Laurel Thatcher Ulrich concluded, "In a moment of extreme peril the traditional experience of the midwife gave way to the book-learning and professional aura of the minister-physician."[48] But for most of the colonial period only at the beckoning of the attending women and as a last resort would birth procedures incorporate male activity.

Not until the last half of the eighteenth century did some urban women begin calling in physicians early in normal labor as the major attendants. Yet even then, and throughout the nineteenth century, those women who asked physicians to attend them continued to call their women friends and relatives to help them and relied on the advice of the women along with the advice of the physician. Sometimes the women, usually called first, advised that no medical attendant be called. As one doctor realized, "A certain amount of inconvenience is anticipated [by the birthing woman], and so long as this supposed limit is not passed, the patient contrives, with the advice of her female friends, to dispense with a medical attendant."[49] At other times, the attending women suggested additional help. Many physicians attributed their obstetric calls to midwives or to neighbor women who were already present at a progressing labor. Dr. John Meachem, struggling to establish himself after graduating from medical school, recorded a successful first case: "Mrs. Doolittle was present, and I always thought that she had a good deal to do with engineering this call. At least I gave her the credit."[50] In Michigan, Ellen Regal, who had come to Ypsilanti to attend her sister's confinement in 1872, disapproved of her sister's choice of birth attendant. She wrote to her brother, "the more we hear of the doctors here the more we all feel as though we could not trust any of them." Ellen took it upon herself to travel home to Ann Arbor to enlist the help of a trusted family doctor.[51]

Physicians found themselves increasingly called to attend women in labor in the nineteenth century, but frequently in the company of midwives and women friends. While midwives were probably not invited into the homes of the "privileged" group described in Chapter 3, the middle-class women who asked physicians to attend them oftentimes included the neighborhood midwife in their list of birthing-room companions. These various attendants exhibited some tensions about having to work with each other, but on the whole they learned to get along together.

Physicians especially had to learn how to behave within the women's domain of the birthing room. Even in the nineteenth-century hospital deliveries among poor and unmarried women, physicians described a very female-centered scene on the wards. Dr. Franklin Martin attended obstetrics cases at Mercy Hospital in Chicago in the 1870s:

> During the long hours of the night I would sit at the bedside of these young women, many of them unwed, and endeavor to comfort them in their agonizing hours. . . . Many times several women in these small wards were awaiting the ordeal, or happily some of them, with the complacency of experience, were convalescing. There was little monotony on these occasions. Advice was exchanged, and banter ensued at the expense of the victim and the doctor.[52]

In the much more common home deliveries, physicians came into the female domestic world, and they tried to create a place for themselves. As one doctor realized, "obstetrical practice is an intimate intrusion into family affairs."[53] "Dr. Marsh stalked into the room," wrote one grateful woman, "like an easy old friend. In a few minutes he was playing with Louisa [another child] and talking to me about the new baby. . . . He did what was expected of him, ate a bite of breakfast with Kate [her friend], then made himself so much at home, he put us all at ease. He took Louisa on his lap, and soon had her speaking pieces and singing. Then, as he waited longer, he began teaching her a new one."[54] Dr. Daniel Cameron, who practiced medicine in Wisconsin in the 1850s, told of one of his obstetric calls: "Wednesday, a week ago, was called on to confine Mrs. Conklin . . . Sat up all night and talked *scandal* with some Cornish women in attendance."[55] Other physicians may not have participated in family frolic or local gossip as readily, but they too engaged in friendly conversations with the midwives and women friends who sat together in the birthing room. A typical example of midwives, physicians, and friends working together involved the confinement case of Jane B. Kelley's friend Nettie, who delivered in Wisconsin in 1886. Kelly recorded:

> I enjoyed the day at home & at night M. drove up with Sammy's rig & says, "Nett wants you." . . . They soon put the little 7 1/4 pd. babe in my arms. Mrs. Leagry was the M[id] W[ife]. Mrs. Sprague soon went home. Nettie was so faint we called Dr. Larkin & he sat with her all night. Came near having convulsions. M. & J. & F. went home at midnight. I said I always looked upon Nettie as only lent & may be she will go now. But she is all ready & to God be all the Glory. The M[id] W[ife] had helped 83 & asked the Dr. Can you bring her through & he said I hope so & It is very seldom one is like her. Did not realize her condition until most morning. She came to herself & was rational but very nervous and weak. . . . I never slept. Dr. & Mrs. Leagry slept in their Chairs.[56]

In this case, the women in attendance did not call the doctor until after the delivery, when the parturient seemed ill. Then the doctor, the midwife, and the friend continued in attendance all night together. In another instance, the physician, who arrived at the home of the birthing woman after the birth had been successfully managed by neighbor women, made a special trip later to congratulate the attending women for "having had the moral courage to do something."[57]

Often the attending women encouraged physicians' interventions and eagerly showed their gratitude. One woman wrote about her friend's confinement in 1838: "Mrs. Lee summoned Dr. White to attend her. She suffered extremely for several days; then her condition became such that the attending physician was obliged to use instruments. Between nine and ten o'clock Saturday evening, June 23, Mrs. Lee gave birth to her first-born, much to the relief of all the anxious women present."[58] One of Wisconsin's earliest physicians reported his first forceps operation "in the presence of all the old women of the neighbourhood." He was pleased to note that "all the relatives and friends expressed themselves quite satisfied with my exertions & skill."[59]

Many women, in fact, learned their birthing-room skills from the physicians who were called to attend rather than from the other women. As one recalled her early twentieth-century experience:

> I remember the first new-born baby I ever washed and dressed. The doctor was blunt and rough speaking. He told me to get water and soap and the baby's belly-band and diaper ready. . . . I supposed that was all I had to do; to my surprise, he handed me the squalling, slick baby, and said, "Here, take care of it." I said, "Oh, I have never done this—let some of the older women do it." He said, "No, this is your job. Just as well learn now, there's always a first time, you know." Well, I washed the baby with it on my lap, face up. I said, "Now, what will I do?" He said, "Turn it over and wash its back, then dress it." "Oh, no, I can't do that. I'm afraid I'll drop it, it is so slick," I told him. He grabbed it by one arm and flipped it over, and said, "You can't hurt 'em when they are newly hatched." Well, I got the job done and was proud when the mother said I could name the little baby boy. I named him Carl.[60]

Although many doctors accommodated themselves well to the female environment in the home birthing rooms, some did not feel comfortable within it. Early in their experience with normal obstetrics, in the eighteenth and early nineteenth century, many physicians tried to stay out of the confinement room except when actually needed for the delivery. Dr. William Dewees advised, for example, "When the patient is about to be placed for labour, the practitioner should withdraw, and leave this arrangement to the nurse. . . . Do not remain with the patient longer than the state of the labour may make it necessary."[61] Such physicians not only did not feel comfortable, but they realized that the birthing woman's friends could provide psychological supports that they could not. In the words of Dr. Alexander Hamilton, "Every woman in general is impressed with much apprehension at the beginning of labour, which, if indulged, may be productive of very bad effects; it is therefore important that a chearful friend or two should be present on such occasions, in order to inspire the patient with spirits and courage."[62]

By the middle of the nineteenth century, physicians tried to increase their own role in the birthing rooms by counseling that women about to deliver limit the the numbers of women friends and relatives to one or two. Dr. Edward Henry Dixon, for example, suggested in his popular advice book in 1857 that physicians "mildly, yet firmly exclud[e] from the room all who are not absolutely necessary as attendants."[63] Dr. Frederick Hollick agreed that "all useless persons should leave the room, and also those who would be likely to alarm or grieve the patient by uttering cries, or exhibiting fear," but he allowed that "no objection should be made to any one being present whom she wishes to see, unless they cannot be depended upon."[64] Another physician advised women that one "confidante be selected in some judicious and affectionate married friend, whose presence during the hour of trial, will ensure sympathy and yet encouragement." This friend, the nurse and the doctor "are all the assistants the occasion demands," wrote Dr. Thomas Bull, "The lying-in-room is not the place for a crowd."[65] He continued:

> The patient also is much disturbed by their conversation, and what is a much greater evil than this, by their imprudent remarks they frequently diminish her confidence in her own powers, or in the judgment and skill of her necessary attendants. The mind in a state of distress is easily excited and alarmed, and whispering in the lying-in-chamber, or any appearance of concealment, quickly produces an injurious impression.[66]

This medical perception of friends as impediments is in direct contrast to most birthing women's accounts of friends as necessary psychological supports. Physicians found it difficult to assert their authority in the presence of many friends, especially those who had had considerable birth experience, and it is likely that their perception of the non-usefulness of female friends in the birthing room was influenced by their own discomfort in their presence. Many physicians realized that their own effectiveness as attendants could be curtailed by these meddling friends. One physician baldly advised that the doctor be the only voice of authority in the room:

> All chatterers, croakers, and putterers ought, at these times, to be carefully excluded from the room. No conversation of a depressing character should for one moment be allowed. Nurses and friends who are in the habit of telling of bad cases that have occurred in their experience must be avoided as the plague. Boisterous conversation during the progress of child-birth ought never to be permitted; it only irritates and excites the patient. . . . The only words that should then be spoken are the few words of comfort from the doctor, announcing, from time to time, that her labor is progressing favorably, and that her pain and sorrow will soon be converted into ease and joy.[67]

The limitations of prescriptive literature, such as textbooks and advice manuals, for understanding what actually happened in America's birthing rooms is evident in these examples, for, despite their desires for exclusive attendance in the birth rooms, most doctors in fact had to submit to patients' desires to have their friends with them during labor and delivery. These women friends negotiated with the physicians about what procedures would be used and made sure that the birthing woman was represented in decision-making. Dr. John Duff of Pittsburgh unhappily recorded, "The obstetrician can not always control the general environment of his patient," and he worried about his parturients' "obstreperousness." This physician lamented the "sometimes dangerous interference of ignorant and superstitious neighbors and friends." His colleague Dr. Joseph Price of Philadelphia agreed: "Very few households will permit the practice of well-organized and disciplined maternity work."[68] Dr. Charles A. Budd advised his students in the 1860s how to gain the help of the women attendants without having to suffer their advice. When administering anesthesia, Budd said: "Three assistants are required, two to hold the limbs and one to administer the anaesthetic. . . . [They will be] generally women, those garrulous old women of whom I have spoken not a little. You choose two who seem the most intelligent. Sometimes you get stuck with those who cannot hold their tongues, and so soon as you take your position, the first thing they do is to speak up, and perhaps tell you what to do. Now to avoid this, just set them down [with] their backs to you."[69]

Dr. E. L. Larkins of Terre Haute, Indiana, believed that pressures from these other birth attendants led physicians to poor practices: "The sympathy of attending friends, coupled with the usual impatience of the woman from her suffering, will too often incite even the physician, against his better judgment, to resort to means to hasten labor, resulting in disaster which time and patience would have avoided." Similarly, Dr. L. A. Harcourt of Chicago related that, contrary to his advice, the friends of one of his parturient patients refused permission for him to suture the birthing woman's ruptured perineum.[70] Until birth moved to the hospital, however, physicians had little choice about sharing their authority with neighbor women, most of whom had had significant birth experience.

Over and over again doctors noted ruefully that they could not control events in the birthing rooms as much as they wanted. One reported a difficult presentation when the doctor was stopped from doing a procedure he thought would be helpful: "Midwife persisted in

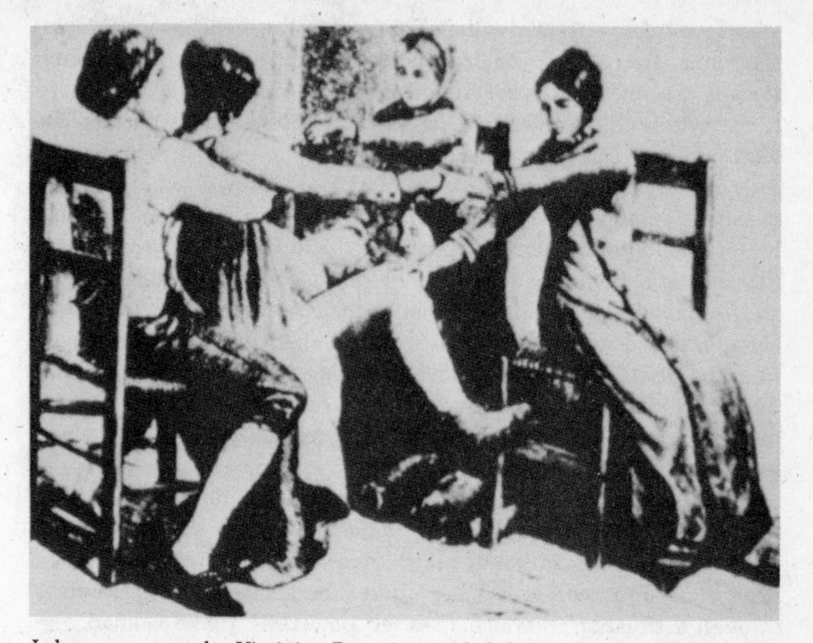

Labor scene, early Virginia. Parturient aided by husband, midwife, and friends.

Source: G. J. Engelmann, *Labor Among Primitive Peoples*, 2nd edition (St. Louis, J. H. Chambers, 1883).

interfering. . . . Midwife, husband and sisters objected to further assistance from us. Podalic version [turning the fetus in order to effect delivery] was again attempted but was forcibly interfered with by friends."[71] Another doctor disclosed early in the twentieth century that in general he "cannot be too insistent with his patients over whom, usually, he has no control."[72] In the mid-nineteenth century, a physician wrote: "The officiousness of nurses and friends very often thwarts the best-directed measure of the physician, by an overweening desire to make the patient 'comfortable' . . . all this should be strictly forbidden. Conversation should be prohibited the patient. . . . Nothing is more common than for the patient's friends to object to [bloodletting], urging as a reason, that 'she has lost blood enough.' Of this they are in no respect suitable judges."

Other physicians complained that they found it difficult to accomplish aseptic conditions because of the interference of the woman's friends. In fact, birth accounts from people actually in attendance at the labors and deliveries show that, contrary to the advice manuals' proscriptions, the parturients' friends and family made decisions about forceps use, anesthesia use, and other interventions usually considered to be within the control of the attending physician. Whether the woman was wealthy or poor, she was likely to resist procedures she thought improper or unnecessary. Dr. E. K. Brown, who practiced obstetrics among the tenements in New York City, wrote in 1908 that he repeatedly found his advice "rejected" and "persistently refused."[73] Physicians in home deliveries either persuaded the birthing women and the attending friends to agree to their suggestions or they went along with the womens' demands; the alternative was to be removed from the cases. Because of the overcrowding in the medical profession during the nineteenth century, physicians felt it necessary to find ways to modify their medical interventions and modulate their behavior to meet their patients' wishes.

The power that the friends had did not necessarily result in better care for the parturient, but it does indicate a level of support that the birthing woman could count on. Because of this network of women supporting one another, women found the ability to get themselves through a situation in which they felt powerless.[74] One woman concluded that "the most important thing is not to be left alone and to know that someone is there who cares and will help you when the going gets rough."[75] Through their social network women were able to keep considerable control over childbirth despite the presence and authority of male physicians.

It is not possible from the data left to historians to quantify women's birth experiences or to be able to say what percentages of American women found the kind of emotional and practical female support networks that Nannie Jackson and others cited here developed. Nor can it be determined to what extent these friendship groups might have worked better among the middle classes. My research uncovered them across class and ethnic lines, in the rural areas and in the cities, in the beginning of the nineteenth century and at its end. But the successful female network was not a universal experience. There were many women who underwent their severest suffering virtually alone or accompanied only by their husbands with whom they might not be able to share their deepest feelings. Unremitting poverty took its toll on many suffering women who could not develop even the outlines of a support network. These women delivered their children alone in the hospital or almshouse, without any familiar faces to comfort them or voices to speak for them. Some rich women, too, may have stood outside a meaningful collection of friends, isolated perhaps by their status or distance from family and friends.

But personal accounts of childbirth by women and birth attendants suggest that the birth experience was a crucial factor in creating the social dimensions of most women's lives. The biological gender experience of giving birth provided women with some of their worst moments and some of their best ones; the good and the bad were experiences that all women could share with each other. Regardless of the specifics of the birth procedures and practices, women shared certain fears and anxieties and suffered similar physical problems. These shared experiences created a biologically based, socially determined bond among women, which in turn influenced important common aspects of their lives. Anita McCormick Blaine, living an affluent life in Chicago at the end of the nineteenth century, shared in many respects the birth experience of Nannie Jackson, living in impoverished rural Arkansas at the same time. They both needed, sought, and received the help of their close women friends at the crucial time of their confinements. While it is certainly true that Blaine had more advantages and more choice in the particulars of the birth experience, to both women the female context in which they delivered was crucial to a successful experience.

From the eighteenth to the twentieth century women's experiences of birth changed dramatically with the major alterations of place of birth, of amount and kind of interference in the birth process, and of choice of birth attendant. Despite the very real changes in the technical and physical experience of birth, women's perceptions of its dangers and methods of dealing with those dangers within a female-centered protective environment remained very much the same during the time that birth remained in women's homes. In the twentieth century, when birth moved to the hospital for the majority of American women, women lost their domestic power base and with it lost certain controls they had traditionally held. The exclusion of attendant women friends and relatives from the hospital birthing rooms both represented a weakening of the female network and further encouraged that weakening. This is the change, discussed in Chapter 7, that caused the basic transformation in womens' birth experiences.

The silver lining in maternity's shadow that accompanied the crisis of childbirth during the home-birth period—women actively helping each other shape their childbirth experiences—enabled women to find each other and to learn to give and receive solace and support. Childbirth customs formed a cornerstone of women's group identity and sense of community. Most women thus had their network to help them when they needed help, and if successfully confined, they had the joy and toils of motherhood ahead. Childbirth and motherhood, for all the difficulties and all the dangers, were among the most rewarding parts of women's lives and led to happiness and fulfillment for many of the same women who worried and complained so much about them. Because almost all shared this experience, women were drawn to each other through the event of childbirth, and together they made decisions that influenced the course of childbirth history in this country.

It is, in fact, in the combination of shadow and light, of despair and of hope, that we can best view women's procreative experiences. While the fears and dangers of childbirth followed women, the experience itself opened up new vistas and created practical and emotional bonds beyond the family that sustained them throughout the rest of their lives. Sharing this functional bond of procreation led women to be able to share other aspects of their lives in close intimacy. This "female world of love and ritual," as Carroll Smith-Rosenberg so aptly called it, with its strong emotional and psychological supports and its ability to produce real change in women's lives, was in large part created around women's shared biological moments. The valley of the shadow of birth gave to women the possibility of a life made richer through close friendships at the same time as it provided a strict definition of that life's domestic boundaries. In uniting women, the childbirth experience ultimately provided the ability for women to stretch the boundaries of their world.[76]

Gender played an important part in the birthing experiences of American women above and beyond the domestic female context in which birth took place. It was a significant factor in the choice of birth attendant for those groups of Americans who worried about modesty and about the cost of delivery.

For millennia women attended other women during labor and delivery because birth was women's private business. Women knew how to help because they had themselves experienced the pain and anguish of delivery. They knew how to comfort because they knew what women felt and needed at their times of travail. And they knew how to intervene because they had watched others manage labor and delivery. Furthermore, many birthing women could accept only other women witnessing the intimate physical details of birth. Revealing their genitals to strange men, some women felt, might threaten their virtue. The experience women got as they witnessed and aided at the confinements of their friends and relatives helped them develop skill in coping with difficulties that commonly arose. Many midwives, only some of whom received formal training in parturition processes, learned their skills first at the bedsides of their neighbors. Through watching and helping other women in labor, these women acquired a practical excellence that allowed them to be valued attendants in part because of their developed skill and in part because of their sex. The necessity that women shield their bodies from male eyes, common to the thinking of many groups of women, led to women's expertise in the birthing room. They belonged in the birth chamber; they were part of the birth tradition.

When male physicians began attending normal labor and deliveries, and standards of excellence began to change in eighteenth- and nineteenth-century America, birthing women faced a dilemma. Women who were accustomed to female birth attendants had to decide whether to retain their traditional female attendants or to increase their chances of survival and future health, as they saw it, by inviting men into their birthing rooms. We have already seen that some urban, advantaged women made this decision quite easily and chose male attendants. Modesty being less important for them than safety, they opted for the physicians who represented science because they believed that medicine held out promises for increased safety. But even the Drinkers, the Philadelphia family who welcomed William Shippen and his colleagues into their birthing rooms, noted with relief, when a new attendant was brought in to relieve a protracted labor by bloodletting, "he is a married man."[77] Strange men witnessing intimate female events produced, at the least, a fear of loss of female modesty. Willing to accept the new ways, women were not always comfortable with them.

Indeed, some women continued to prefer female attendants even though they may have thought that male medicine provided the best birth methods. As one physician realized, "Confidence in her physician is of the greatest moment, but at once all the innate modesty of the young girl rebels against the appearance of a stranger—and male, too—in the most delicate position. A shock of startled modesty at once takes the place of all that reliance, trust and confidence that should exist." To this physician, such "adverse circumstances" threatened successful delivery.[78]

As the nineteenth century progressed and physician-directed obstetrics became increasingly acceptable among those Americans who could afford medical services, the decision for those women who were concerned about modesty remained difficult. Especially after physicians introduced anesthesia into obstetric practices and could promise relief from the worst pains of labor, women who wanted female attendants felt their choices increasingly limited. Some women rationalized that keeping birth a domestic event monitored by women made it all right to have male attendants. Most of the nineteenth-century births that physicians attended (and these were at most half of America's births) also continued to be attended by women whom the birthing women selected and trusted and to be governed at least in part by decisions those women made together. Into this still female environment many women found it possible to invite male practitioners.

But for other women in the nineteenth century, and especially for most immigrant women, who retained the traditions of the old world, delivery by a male physician remained unthinkable. Only in the most dire of circumstances would these women consider consulting a man. As Dr. Josephine Baker realized early in the twentieth century when she addressed the problem of regulating obstetrics practice in New York City, "If deprived of midwives, [immigrant] women would rather have amateur assistance from the janitor's wife or the woman across the hall than to submit to this outlandish American custom of having a male doctor for a confinement." Baker claimed that what she called "inherent racial prejudice and the even greater prejudice of their husbands" encouraged immigrant women to chose only female attendants.[79]

But these women, in order to keep their traditions, had to give up whatever promise scientific medicine held out to women. Traditional births meant only women midwife attendants, but they meant, too, birth without forceps, anesthesia, or other medical aids. The only way women could utilize what medicine had to offer and keep faith with their beliefs, in the eyes of many, was to employ female physicians. With increasing numbers of women entering medicine in the second half of the nineteenth century, this option became a possibility, especially for women in the urban centers. In 1900, women comprised 6 percent of all physicians practicing in the United States: in some cities, like Boston and Minneapolis, almost 20 percent of practitioners were female.[80]

Employing women doctors increased birthing women's options to manage their confinements at the same time that they benefitted from developments in medical science. Dr. Helen MacKnight Doyle assisted in confinement cases in San Francisco because, she wrote, "The Chinese preferred American women doctors to attend their women in confinement."[81] Numerous women doctors wrote that their entrance into medical practice was facilitated when they were invited to attend women in childbirth, who wanted them because of their sex. "Dr. Bessie," who began her practice in rural Wyoming around the turn of the twentieth century, related, "for baby cases women generally preferred a lady doctor to a man, and these cases gave me an opportunity to gain the confidence of the people for other cases."[82] Dr. Josephine Baker, setting up a practice in New York with a medical graduate friend of hers, noted that "our only asset was that we were women doctors. . . . For many years women came to us because we were women and the competition in that line was small. . . . Obstetrics," she concluded, "have been a godsend to many a young doctor just starting his [sic] career."[83] Similarly, Dr. Lilian Welsh realized, "Naturally the early cases that come to every woman in her practice are gynaecological and obstetrical."[84] As Regina Morantz-Sanchez has concluded in her study of women physicians, many women got their start in medicine through this route, finding themselves desirable attendants to a class of patients who were extremely reluctant to be examined by male physicians.[85] Many women believed that "the room of confinement is properly woman's place," and it was this belief that facilitated women doctors' entry into medical practice and allowed some women patients the advantages of medicine within the traditional all-female environment.[86]

Women doctors could offer medical techniques, and they could at the same time accommodate the needs of women who did not want strange men to intrude on their intimate moments. Perhaps even more important to some women was the special consideration they believed they could expect from women attendants. As one woman physician wrote, "By the sympathy of one woman with another, in this trying time, a relation is established between the doctor and patient that goes far to relieve the mental anxieties of the helpless sufferer."[87] Women, even those who had not themselves given birth but who had the potential to do so, provided other women with a security that came with shared experiences. Women doctors could, many women believed, "relieve the mental anxieties" with far greater success than could men.

An example of the kind of sensitivity women could provide for other women was evident in an article Dr. Margaret Colby of Clear Lake, Iowa, wrote in the *Woman's Medical Journal* in 1902 in which she looked at parturition "from a woman's point of view." Colby understood, as few male physicians seemed to in their writing on the subject, that a birthing woman was an individual with a "right to the control of her own body" and with needs that developed out her own experiences as mother and wife. "We, as physicians," Colby wrote, "must come to the rescue of this portion of our clientage with a better understanding of her [knowledge and experience] . . . and a keener sense of our own responsibility for her wellfare [sic]." Similarly, the editors of the *Medical Woman's Journal* concluded, "We need the woman 'family physician,' the wise friend and helpful counselor; the woman who can meet other women on their own basis and with a most helpful and understanding and sympathetic feeling for their problems; the woman whom other women can approach without that fear and trembling which is so often apparent when they go to a man doctor; the woman who can inspire in her woman patients the confidence that will enable them to tell all the facts and thus enable a correct diagnosis to be made."[88]

Dr. Mary Dixon-Jones, a New York physician and assistant editor of the *Woman's Medical Journal,* believed that women physicians' understanding of other women allowed them to be better birth attendants. She told of a case of tedious labor she attended in 1894 during which other (male) doctors in attendance urged a craniotomy but she held out for a live delivery: "I spoke as a woman," Dixon-Jones wrote, saying to the other attending physicians, " 'The child must not be destroyed. All the long eight years this woman has had no baby; this will be her comfort, her happiness; it may be her last; we must save it.' I insisted that it should not be destroyed. . . . The mother and child were saved." Dr. Inez Philbrick of Lincoln, Nebraska, found the educated woman physician to be the highest step on the obstetric evolutionary ladder because of her ability to understand the women's point of view at the same time she could apply science to solve women's health problems. Philbrick wrote, "the male obstetrician will someday be a vestigial remnant, and go the way of the appendix, wisdom teeth, hair, et cetera."[89]

The notion that women had something special to offer medicine was a common one in the nineteenth century, and women physicians used the argument as an important part of the justification for their place in medicine. Dr. Eliza Mosher believed, for example, that women, by heredity, had "a sympathetic understanding of the meaning of pain" and that this inborn sense when carried into medical work "bestowed always . . . that touch of the human which heals hurt souls as well as sick bodies."[90] The idea of women's distinctiveness served women well as they fought for a place within the profession, and its application to obstetrics was particularly effective.

The extent to which women physicians actually offered birthing women something different from what they could receive from male physicians is more difficult to assess. Historians have interpreted the evidence both to argue female uniqueness and to show female identification with the male profession. Certainly women doctors used the rhetoric of how they differed from their male colleagues as an entering wedge into practice; their advantages as women attendants could be beneficially called upon especially on the subject of childbirth. Although some women practitioners wanted to set themselves apart from their male colleagues, most women also sought to emphasize their connection to the male medical establishment. Their ambivalence on the subject marked their own precarious perch between the two worlds of medicine and domesticity.[91]

This living in two worlds brought women physicians into birthing rooms—sometimes not from modesty or need for feminine understanding—but from even more domestic notions of what women physicians offered. Dr. Margaret Stewart, practicing in San Francisco in the early twentieth century, remarked:

> A few patients gave reasons for selecting me which were hardly complimentary to my medical ability, but certainly amusing. One patient engaged me because when her last baby was born, the doctor put a bottle on her mahogany dining-room table, and she had never been able to remove the stain. Another woman said they had had four boys and wanted a girl so much that they decided if they had a woman doctor, the next baby would be a girl. As it turned out, it was a boy. One young chap, who arranged for me to attend his wife, told me he had decided that since I was a woman doctor I wouldn't be likely to charge as much. When I informed him my fee was the same as other doctors asked, he said, "Oh, well, I'll take you anyway, because you're a woman and probably need the money more than the men do."[92]

Economic considerations might have been far more important than the extant evidence allows us to understand. Women doctors struggling to begin their practices or establish their reputations in a traditionally male field might have eagerly sought patients regardless of the fee in order to build up their practices. Many women doctors began their medical careers in poor urban neighborhoods where they frequently treated patients for little or no money.[93]

Women physicians, although never more than six percent of all physicians, provided a bridge between the two worlds of tradition and medicine, and this proved important for many groups in the American population. The desire for women attendants seems to have been strongest among first generation immigrants. But when women physicians began to be available, their services were sought by women from all economic and cultural backgrounds. Some native-born upper-class women in the middle of the nineteenth century went to extreme lengths to procure the services of women, although many in this class usually accepted male attendants. Samuel Gregory related one such story:

> In the summer of 1851 the author was applied to by a gentleman of intelligence and influence, at the present time (1854) a member of the legislature of Vermont, from a town in that state bordering on Canada, who came to Boston expressly, as he stated, to engage a female physician to attend his wife in confinement. Several months later, in midwinter, the person engaged went on her distant professional visit, and performed her responsible duties with the highest degree of satisfaction to her employer, having carried the patient safely through her critical period. . . . In December, 1853, the same professional woman a second time performed this journey of some 300 miles to attend the same lady, and with results alike satisfactory.[94]

Immigrant women preferred or even insisted on only women attendants, usually calling on the services of midwives from their own country; but many of these women accepted the compromise of women physicians. The experience of Elizabeth Blackwell in establishing a practice among the poor of New York City and of numerous other women physicians across the country confirms that women who desired traditional birth experiences found the move to women physicians more acceptable than allowing men into the room. Their daughters, the second generation, more readily accepted male doctors, whom they associated with American ways.[95]

The experiences of women attended by women doctors reveals how much a part of the same world the professional and the patient were in these cases. Dr. Lilian Welsh wrote about her experiences in a practice of three women physicians:

> It was our obstetrical service, however, and the conditions under which we found women bearing children that stirred most deeply a feeling of medical responsibility. We early determined to use all our opportunities to instruct women in the hygiene of maternity and infancy, and to lead women to demand more enlightened care for themselves in childbirth. . . . This obstetrical service was not only a source of education to us, a source of despondency at times, but also a source of pleasure. We were admitted to share the joys as well as the distress and sorrows of our patients.[96]

Historians have argued that women's hospitals such as the New England Hospital for Women and Children also tried to provide a milieu in which traditional women's supports could be maintained within a female-centered environment for those women who had no choice but to give birth in the hospital. Regina Morantz-Sanchez and Virginia Drachman have both noted that the atmosphere at the New England Hospital for Women and Children illustrated the feminine touch in medical care.[97]

The female network drawn around the birthing bed and the importance of women physicians in bringing the two worlds of medicine and domesticity together illustrate that gender was an important factor in American obstetric history. Female tradition and female activity specifically and consciously dominated childbirth practices throughout the home birth period. To birthing women, the sex of their birth attendants remained important because women could offer support and aid that men, who moved in a separate world, could not. Male medicine, even as it expanded its technical contributions, could not intrude upon the female nature of birth significantly as long as birth remained a domestic home-centered event. When male medicine entered the birthing rooms of America in the eighteenth and nineteenth centuries, it entered on tiptoe. Men who were at ease in the sickroom and who believed they had much to offer to birthing women knew that they were attending the parturient at her beckoning and in a world very much of her making. Women, because they still felt they had options and could exercise them at any time in the birth process, retained a significant element of power in confinements. Men learned how to fit into the women's environment, knowing they might be invited to leave or not invited back in the future. They learned to be flexible in their suggestions for interventions, and they modified their actions on the basis of the desires of the attending women. Men did not make significant changes in women's birth experiences unless and until women invited them to do so. Although women gradually accepted more and more of what medicine had to offer, indeed, accepted the promises of scientific advances, they retained their ability to pick and choose among the medical options in the period before birth moved into medical institutions in the twentieth century. The next chapter will analyze further the negotiation process between birthing women and their physicians in the prehospital era through the example of the introduction and use of obstetrical anesthesia.

5

"The Greatest Blessing of This Age"

Pain Relief in Obstetrics

From the birthing women's perspective, the greatest contribution nineteenth-century obstetrics achieved was in providing pain relief during labor and delivery. Women feared their confinements in the nineteenth century and, like their grandmothers before them, eagerly sought new birth procedures, especially those that might make them more comfortable during the long hours of their travail. By the middle of the century middle-class women had become accustomed to male birth attendants, although a large segment of the population—probably growing as immigration soared in the latter part of the century—remained faithful to female midwives and traditional birth procedures. Advantaged native-born urban women sought every obstetric improvement that male physicians could offer because they continued to fear childbirth and its attendant discomforts and because they had the financial ability to alter their traditional experiences. Next to the fear of death, pain was probably the single part of birth most hated by birthing women. Fanny Longfellow's exuberant description of her childbirth under ether in 1847, the first in the United States, demonstrates just how ready women were to alleviate the pain of childbirth. "I never was better or got through a confinement so comfortably," she wrote her sister-in-law:

> Two other ladies, I know, have since followed my example successfully, and I feel proud to be the pioneer to less suffering for poor, weak womankind. This is certainly the greatest blessing of this age, and I am glad to have lived at the time of its coming and in the country which gives it to the world.[1]

Women who experienced their childbirths as the hour in which they "touched the hand of death" eagerly sought relief from the frightful event. Ether and chloroform, anesthetic agents of different chemical properties that blocked the perceptions of pain, promised such relief. At the middle of the nineteenth century, when the two drugs were introduced, women like Longfellow embraced anesthesia enthusiastically. One of Walter Channing's patients told him after her etherized birth "how wonderful it was that she should have got through without the least suffering, and how grateful she was."[2]

Women, in fact, initially were more eager than physicians to use anesthesia. Among physicians, there was some uncertainty about the safety of the new drugs for midwifery practice and about the wisdom of masking pain, the progression of which could mark labor's progress. Charles D. Meigs of Philadelphia, who rejected both chloroform and ether, carried on a well-publicized campaign against their use, claiming that he had "not yielded to several solicitations as to its exhibition addressed to me by my patients in labour." He believed that "a labour-pain [is] a most desirable, salutary, and conservative manifestation of life-force." Meigs relied upon women's painful contractions to help him determine labor's progress and believed that their inhibition would make him a less effective birth attendant. Furthermore, he worried that the drugs might not be safe: "should I exhibit the remedy for pain to a thousand patients in labour, merely to prevent the physiological pain, and for no other motive—and if I should in consequence destroy only one of them, I should feel disposed to clothe me in sack-cloth, and cast ashes on my head for the remainder of my days."[3] Meigs' melodramatic admonition reflected the views of other American physicians who likewise hesitated to use the new agents.

But many physicians went ahead and tried ether and chloroform on their laboring patients. Walter Channing, one of ether's most ardent supporters, in 1848 surveyed forty-six Boston-area physicians' use of anesthesia in natural labor and found that many of them held back on using the drugs except in cases when "patients have demanded it with an emphasis which could not be resisted . . . in many cases, and in the practice of some physicians, it has only been used when such demand has been made."[4] In the early years of obstetrical anesthesia some physicians rarely or never employed the drugs, but others responded to their patients' wishes and used anesthesia often. A. R. Thompson of Charlestown, Massachusetts, wrote Channing the following account, which was not unusual:

> This lady had informed herself fully as to the use of ether, and had made up her mind to take it. . . . When called to her, I frankly told her that I had never used the ether, nor had I ever seen it used in any case, but that I had no prejudice against it, and would consent to its administration in her case. . . . Upon careful examination I found every thing favorable for a safe and speedy termination of the labor, and told my patient I believed that the child would be born within two hours, without any interference; but she was resolute, and demanded the ether . . . I poured an ounce of ether into the sponge, and the lady held it to her mouth and nose.[5]

This example clearly illustrates the powers that women held in America's birthing rooms, the easy assertion of their decision-making authority, and physicians' acceptance of the necessity to alter their own plans in the face of women's expectations. A successful outcome and a happy patient convinced this doctor to use the drug in subsequent cases. After his second trial of ether Thompson concluded confidently; "My conviction at the time was strong, that the ether had greatly diminished the sufferings of the mother, and shortened the term of her travail for many hours."[6]

When Dr. A. K. Gardner used chloroform for the first time in New York City in 1848, his patient told him that she would "never again be confined without using the chloroform." Dr. Charles Gordon of Boston wrote to Walter Channing about his first use of ether: "the mother . . . expressed, in very enthusiastic terms, her *love* for an article that had so completely annihilated her suffering." Dr. C. H. Allen of Cambridgeport, Massachusetts, told of a woman he attended in labor who had been reluctant to call a physician at all, but finally had sent for him after twelve hours of "excruciating pains" to "save her life." Dr. Allen administered chloroform and delivered her healthy baby. "She told her female friends, that with chloroform it was nothing to have babies; that she meant to have another."[7]

With such satisfied patients, doctors were encouraged to increase their use of anesthesia. Furthermore, the early trials of ether and chloroform seemed to establish the safety of the drugs. Dr. Charles Gordon became convinced of the safety of both ether and chloroform after his first five cases:

> These agents were employed in natural labor; and also at a period when the circumstances of each case justified the expectation of speedy delivery; when the os uteri was well dilated; the pains regular and severe; every thing announcing the beginning of the expul-

sive stage. At this period these agents, cautiously administered, afforded the patients great relief; and in neither case occurred a single circumstance to the mother or child, to render their use unsafe or improper. I should not hesitate to employ them at the advanced periods of natural labor.[8]

Despite the early encouraging results, both perceptions of safety and patterns of anesthesia use varied enormously among physicians throughout the second half of the nineteenth century. The medical journals reported both safe and hazardous results of ether and chloroform in midwifery. A Massachusetts physician, for example, wrote in the *Boston Medical and Surgical Journal* that chloroform was "a dangerous and often deadly agent," and a Detroit physician who used chloroform in one-half of his 3,000 obstetrical cases over forty years of practice concluded in the *Journal of the American Medical Association*, "I have yet to see my first case of the least evil result to mother or child."[9] With such variation in the literature, individual physicians relied heavily on their own experiences and on the desires of their patients to make their own anesthesia decisions. A rural Iowa doctor, who practiced in an immigrant community where women used midwives and called him only "when nature failed," attended 500 women over a twenty-year period and wrote: "I do not use an anaesthetic of any kind, especially in forceps cases. I want the patient to know what is going on." Another physician came to the opposite conclusion and recommended anesthesia "not only in troublesome instrumental labor, but in all cases where the pains of travail fall upon women."[10]

Anesthesia use revealed wider practitioner variation than any other obstetric intervention technique. Dr. Bedford Brown from Virginia believed that chloroform should be used "in every case where the labor is at all slow, painful, and not easy. I believe that it is not only justifiable, but that it would be inhuman to withhold it." A physician from Philadelphia concurred: "for twelve years I have never refused a single patient this comfort."[11] Other physicians limited chloroform use to "tedious and protracted cases of labor where the patient's sufferings, on account of their severity and great duration, became almost intolerable." Dr. B. E. Cotting of Massachusetts believed ether should be "allowed in moderation when importunately demanded by the patient" but otherwise reserved for abnormal conditions when it should be "administered with the greatest caution, so that the safety of the patient may not be unnecessarily put at hazard."[12] The American Medical Association's Committee on Obstetrics found that "the opinions of the profession are so widely at variance," but they, too, had arguments to make on both sides of the issue. "The progress of anaesthesia has not been an unbroken triumph, its mission has not been one of unmingled good," the committee report admitted. Numerous women had died as a result of the use of ether or chloroform; many others had benefited, "substituting sweet repose for restless suffering." Very reluctant to take a position favoring either the use of anesthesia in general or the particular use of ether or chloroform, the committee concluded in 1849 that anesthesia use in American obstetrics was warranted:

> Who that has seen the etherized patient, after a severe and protracted operation, rouse from a state of unconsciousness, as from a refreshing sleep, and receive the announcement that all is over with a smile of wondering joy; who that has seen this, and compared it with the condition of her to whom this great boon has been denied, and who, after cries and screams of agony, and struggles that would not be controlled, has sunk sobbing and shuddering into a state of utter nervous exhaustion; who that has seen this, can doubt, that, under such circumstances, the chances of recovery are augmented by anaesthesia? The committee deliberately believe that they are; and that, in the more severe obstetric operations, not only may anaesthetics be rightfully given, but that they may not be rightfully withheld.[13]

With the medical journals providing anecdotal experiences that showed wide variation in use and indication, individual physicians relied on their own experiences and those of their close colleagues to make their individual policy. If patients demanded anesthesia, most doctors agreed to try it; if the outcome was successful and the women grateful, physicians were encouraged to continue its use. If they had a negative experience, they might have reserved anesthesia for those patients whose labors seemed extreme. Some doctors continued to use no anesthesia in normally progressing labors, still agreeing with Charles Meigs that labor pains were natural, and others used it almost universally.

Many physicians felt pressed, if their time was limited and other patients were waiting, to use forceps, anesthesia, or both to direct labor into patterns under their control. This inclination was reinforced by women eagerly seeking relief from their suffering. A Colorado physician related that after several hours of hard labor one of his patients "implored me to do something, and, with many misgivings, at last I decided to use instruments [and] chloroform."[14] One Wisconsin observer noted at the turn of the twentieth century that "to the rural practitioner laboring under stress of limited time, fatigue, and pressure of other work, there is a great temptation to resort to any means which to him may seem safe in expediting labor." Likewise, an Iowa doctor observed, "The country doctor who is called to go out six or eight or even twelve miles . . . has a good deal asked of him if he is expected to sit down and patiently wait. He has a terrible temptation there to use the medium for haste which he has in his bag."[15]

The rapidity with which anesthetic drugs were adopted in obstetrics produced an absence of standardization about drug dosages. Physicians learned to use anesthesia so generally in obstetrics that by 1895 one physician observed that "chloroform is given in labor often recklessly, carelessly, and copiously." As physicians delivered the babies, other attendants—"ignorant nurses, husbands, bystanders, and even . . . the patients themselves"—dripped chloroform or ether on to a sponge or cloth and held it to the woman's nose. One doctor explained, "If there is no one present to assist me in the final stages of labor, I have the expectant mother hold a drinking glass with the bottom filled with cotton and upon which the chloroform is poured, then have them hold the glass over their nose. When their hands become unsteady and the glass falls away from the nose, I know they are sufficiently asleep to give them relief and I continue to accelerate the delivery." No standard procedures guarded physicians' drug administration or dosages.[16]

Physicians' reports of their obstetric practices in the second half of the nineteenth century indicate that use of anesthesia did not necessarily lead to increased forceps use. While most doctors did come to use anesthesia routinely in forceps deliveries, the reverse was not true. Physicians did not use forceps routinely on patients to whom they gave ether and chloroform. By 1900, physicians employed forceps in approximately 8 percent of their births; whereas some used anesthesia at almost every birth they attended, and on the average about 50 percent of all physician-attended births utilized chloroform or ether.[17] Thus, despite the haphazard use of open-drop ether or chloroform and the consequent potential for overdosing, actual anesthesia use must have remained light. Profound anesthesia would have caused labor to decelerate and would have made forceps necessary to lift the baby that the woman was unable to push out. But with light analgesia physicians did not require forceps. Physicians aimed at pain relief, not total unconsciousness. One physician advised maintaining what he called a "dreamy sleep, in which the patient follows in her imagination the direction of the physician." While labor progressed, he conversed with his patients about scenes from their childhood or the Sunday school picnic. One of his patients "almost immediately after the first inhalation burst out in a beautiful song, and continued singing one after another until her babe, a large boy, first child, was born."[18]

As the symbol of what science had to offer, anesthesia enhanced the place and role of physicians in birthing rooms across America. Women who could afford physicians and their new panacea demanded the advantages of painlesssness. And physicians who early were cautious about anesthesia came to use it generously. Dr. J. Herbert Claiborne of Virginia explained his practice:

> I came into practice just when the God-given boon had been first used and commended to the world. . . . I heard it denounced by a distinguished and revered preceptor as dangerous, cruel, and a criminal contravention of the Divine curse: 'In sorrow shalt thou bring forth children.' . . . And though I used it at as early a date as any of my compeers, I used it for a time only in bad cases, and I used it hesitatingly—and as it were under protest—accepting it as an evil. . . . Since then I have learned to accept it as a boon—a benefaction beyond all computation, and now I believe that the conditions and circumstances should be very rare and very peculiar which would justify a practitioner in withholding its blessing from a woman in the agony of childbirth. Nothing gives me so much pleasure as the promise of that Lethe [oblivion; from Greek myth] to the expectant mother when the fearful hour draws nigh, except the fulfilment of that promise, and her grateful expression of returning consciousness—"Is it indeed all over, and is my baby born?"[19]

Many physicians underwent a similar change of heart and adopted anesthesia generally in the last part of the nineteenth century. Dr. H. C. Ghent of Texas told his tale in 1884: "Having been taught by Dr. Charles D. Meigs, of Philadelphia, not to use chloroform, for a number of years after I began the practice of obstetrics, I was afraid to have a bottle of it in the house. But, after many years of labor in this field, in which I had been witness of so much pain and anguish during parturition, I at last ventured on the use of this anaesthetic in some of the most painful cases of childbirth. . . . I used chloroform, at first, gradually, advancing a step at a time, until now (and for the past fifteen years) I use it in *every case* of labor, whether natural or preternatural, unless the woman positively refuses to take it."[20]

Having decided to use ether or chloroform on their obstetric patients, physicians then had to consider how to administer it safely and how much to give. The degree of safety depended on the amount of the drug used and the time during labor when it was administered. The earlier in labor the drugs were given the greater their chance to cross the placenta and affect the health of the fetus. Similarly, the drugs' ability to irritate and affect muscle function was enhanced the longer they were in use and the greater the dosage. But the actual administration and dosages of anesthetic agents varied from doctor to doctor, and the variation was great enough, especially during the early years of the obstetrical use of anesthetics from the 1840s through the 1880s, to make comparisons of their safety records or of their effects on the course of labor extremely difficult.[21]

Individual physicians' problems in figuring out drug dosages grew from the indecision of the profession at large. Recommendations about anesthesia use varied from strict regulation of dose to no recommendation about quantity at all. The American Medical Association Committee on Obstetrics recommended in 1848, very early in obstetrical use of anesthesia, that chloroform be applied by pouring one-eighth of an ounce (a drachm, or dram) onto a folded handkerchief, which was to be applied over nostrils and mouth, excluding atmospheric air. With each contraction more chloroform was to be added to the handkerchief to produce maximum benefit.[22]

But the open-drop method advocated in 1848 became less popular as the century progressed. Dr. Sayer, debating in front of the New York Academy of Medicine in the 1880s, advocated the use of an inhaler, "which by a rubber attachment can be made to fit any face perfectly: thus the patient is not allowed to breathe any air not charged with chloroform." (See illustration.) Some doctors believed the addition of atmospheric air to the drug inhalation was desirable; others thought it absolutely to be avoided. One physician reporting his anesthesia use before the Academy preferred the "choking plan" for administration of ether: "at the beginning the patient is allowed sufficient air to prevent the sensation of strangulation so often complained of," but once the effect was produced, pure ether inhalation should follow.

The editors of the *Journal of the American Medical Association*, commenting on the great variety of application methods, concluded: "It must be said that much of the trouble from anaesthetics is due to careless or faulty administration. There is a wide-spread impression that anyone can give the anaesthetic. . . . All anaesthetics are dangerous, and become more so when administered in unknown quantities

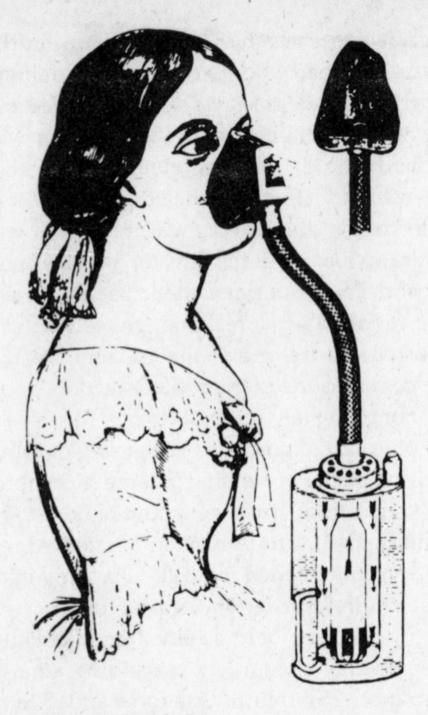

Nineteenth-century chloroform inhaler.
Source: National Library of Medicine.

and in an unsafe manner."[23] But physicians recognized "an extraordinary degree of tolerance in parturient women for chloroform" and believed it safe.[24] Chloroform is "absolutely safe when properly administered," wrote Dr. J. F. Baldwin of Columbus, Ohio, in 1890. But proper administration meant different things to different physicians in terms of dosage, administering agent, and time during labor.[25]

A Boston physician, revealing the variations that characterized obstetrical anesthesia administration in the 1890s, reported a common method of chloroform administration and pointed out why it was so popular:

> The patient rather likes it and will call for it when not given to full anesthesia, and is able to think and talk and help the physician, quite different from ether. So that the assistance of the nurse and one other woman is all the help really required. I put the chloroform on the handkerchief and keep watch on the patient. The whole appara-

> tus required is a lady's pocket-handkerchief, folded as it comes to me, and a small phial having a small neck for the chloroform. Then by placing the kerchief firmly over the mouth of the phial, the bottle is inverted so that only a few drops escape on to the kerchief. This bottle I keep within my reach and handle myself, using my left hand and removing and inserting the cork with my teeth. Thus any woman can hold the chloroform to the patient, returning the kerchief to me for renewal of the chloroform just preceding the next pain and keeping the more or less exhausted kerchief to the nose in the intervals of the pains. Thus more or less of the anesthetic can be used as the exigency requires to keep the pains bearable. . . . And even in instrumental cases, it is rare to need any extra skilled help; for by the time this is reached the woman giving the chloroform has become quite competent to follow the directions of the physician and take full charge of giving the anesthetic herself. . . . it is a most glorious blessing to this feature of suffering humanity. . . . I believe no woman should be left to suffer much without it.[26]

While most physicians insisted on physicians administering anesthetics during major surgery, many agreed that "lady friends" could be helpful in the the childbed administration of ether and chloroform: "I take a napkin large enough to fill a common tumbler about half full, when well packed in. I drop chloroform on this napkin in about drachm quantities at a time, and the irregularities of the patient's face render it impossible for my lady assistants to shut out entirely atmospheric air, should she hold the glass down close over the patient's nose and mouth."[27]

Because of the variations in the application of ether and chloroform, physicians realized that anesthesia use during normal labor and delivery could cause problems for birthing women. While most physicians favored either chloroform or ether and became adept at using their chosen agent, both of these drugs were reported to carry significant negative side effects. The medical literature indicated that either ether or chloroform could increase the danger of hemorrhage, could lead to protracted labor, could decrease uterine contractions, and could cause a newborn breathing difficulty.[28] Especially worrisome for obstetricians was the muscle-suppressing action of ether and chloroform. Labor could be prolonged rather than shortened through the use of either of these drugs.[29] Many physicians strongly decried the routine use of anesthesia in childbirth because of the problem-causing physiological actions of the painkillers.[30]

Because of these difficulties, many physicians believed that anesthesia use should be moderate during labor, and some even continued to believe that it should not be used at all. But increasing numbers of physicians voiced the opinion that some anesthetic agent was essential for American women, especially middle- and upper-class women, so many of whom, in their opinion, exhibited nervous tendencies. Dr. I. N. Love of St. Louis in 1893 described his average patients:

> We all know that the pregnant woman is prone to having her nervous system out of joint; in fact, the condition in itself is a severe test to the female nervous system. It is needless to recall to your mind how the very beginning of pregnancy is announced in many cases by peculiar nervous phenomena. During the entire term the imagination of the woman often becomes exalted or depressed. Her disposition is irritable. In many cases she is continually between two fires; upon the one side the greatest gloom, upon the other an excessive joy. Suspicion, jealousy, general sensitiveness are present, which under other conditions are never dreamed of. Nervous pains abound, migraine, facial neuralgia, toothache, itching in various parts of the body, together with smarting and other evidence of irritation of the peripheral extremities of the nerves. The most grave nerve troubles sometimes are present; eclampsia, chorea and often mania. Truly we have evidence in favor of the thought that pregnancy is a severe test to the stability of the nervous system.

Having identified—however paternalistically—such a range of troubles, this doctor developed the belief that women needed special care during labor; anesthesia was one agent that could pave the way to successful labor and delivery. "Pain long continued is dangerous, particularly to those not well endowed by nature for the bearing of pain."[31]

Dr. Bedford Brown agreed that pain was "the great terror of parturition" and that anesthesia could relieve this curse:

> For some years before I adopted anesthesia in my obstetrical practice, I have time and again sat by the bedside of the women in the throes of parturition and listened often with anguish to myself, to their cries for relief from pain, heard their moanings from almost insufferable agony, for hours of such scenes that impressed themselves upon my memory in a manner never to be forgotten. With chloroform at hand, and with my familiarity with its action, I never have to pass through such painful scenes now. . . . I have found it not only a blessing to the patient but to the physician also. Without the means of relieving

human suffering what a dreary, unsatisfactory and repulsive life that of the physician would be.[32]

Dr. Brown's statement of how much easier and more pleasant anesthesia made his own job could not have been a minor consideration. Physicians, as we have already discussed, came into the birthing rooms of women in their own homes surrounded by their familiar friends. The doctors were not always sure of their role and some of them exhibited significant discomfort. When women and doctors could agree on the administration of anesthesia, the relationship between them developed well, giving the medical attendant greater status and increased respect. Doctors must have greatly appreciated anesthesia's benefits because the very process of employing anesthesia enhanced their own role during labor and delivery.

Furthermore, it is certainly possible that women, who so dreadfully feared childbirth and its attendant dangers, became more relaxed and did experience safer—not just less painful—labors with the use of the anesthetic agents. The actual progress of labor must have been physiologically more difficult because of women's fear of death and the extreme tensions they carried into the birthing rooms. These worries undoubtedly exacerbated problems of elevated blood pressure and cardiac function, and they may have increased the likelihood of shock and hemorrhage. Anesthesia would, in eliminating such worries, make labor and delivery safer, at the same time that it might have led to an increase in the possibility of drug-related dangers.

By the beginning of the twentieth century women's expectations about the possibilities of painless delivery had been heightened, and physicians' acceptance of anesthesia was common. But none of the anesthetics then available met all the requirements for comfort and safety. Physicians relied on opium—the drug William Shippen brought to Sally Downing's deliveries back in the eighteenth century—and on the newer chloroform and ether to relieve pain and expedite labor. Drugs and instruments may have made some labors shorter but they probably made others longer. Anesthesia did not necessarily make labor more enjoyable. Most drugs could not be used safely until late in labor, either because they affected muscle function or because they were dangerous for the fetus, so women still experienced pain. The side effects from the widely used chloroform and ether still made them less than ideal agents.

The search for a perfect medical answer to pain, begun when physicians first entered the practice of normal obstetrics in the middle of the eighteenth century and intensified when anesthesia was first introduced in 1847, continued into the twentieth century. Calling for studies to find an ideal anesthetic agent, Dr. Laura H. Branson of Iowa City wrote in 1908: "I know of no suffering that is more dreaded by our sex than that which confronts them as they heroically take their lives in their hands and go down into the very shadows of death itself in order that they may fulfill the plans of the Creator in populating this world of ours! I speak now of the general verdict of women and I declare emphatically that this terror of the physical suffering of childbirth is most intense and were not the weaker sex endowed with indomitable courage, they would succumb at the first onset of pain. Is it necessary that such suffering should be endured?"[33] Into this context of unfulfilled expectation, in the second decade of the twentieth century, came scopolamine.

"At midnight I was awakened by a very sharp pain," wrote Mrs. Cecil Stewart, describing the birth of her child in 1914. "The head nurse . . . gave me an injection of scopolamin-morphin. . . . I woke up the next morning about half-past seven . . . the door opened, and the head nurse brought in my baby. . . . I was so happy."[34] Mrs. Stewart had delivered her baby under the influence of scopolamine, a belladonna alkaloid and amnesiac that, together with morphine, an opiate, produced a state popularly known as "twilight sleep." She did not remember anything of the experience when she woke up after giving birth. This 1914 ideal seemed finally to have answered medical and lay wishes for untraumatic childbirth. As one woman gratefully put it: "The night of my confinement will always be a night dropped out of my life." According to her best expectations, she remembered nothing of her delivery.[35]

In scopolamine deliveries, the woman went to sleep, delivered her baby, and woke up feeling vigorous, "so free from fatigue or soreness that she could leave her bed at once and care for her own baby." The drug altered women's consciousness so that they did not remember painful labors, and women claimed their bodies did not feel exhausted by their efforts. Both the women who demanded scopolamine and the doctors who agreed to use it saw it as far superior to other agents because it did not inhibit muscle function and could be administered throughout the birthing process. It was the newest and finest technique available—"the greatest boon the Twentieth Century could give to women," in the words of Dr. Bertha Van Hoosen, one of its foremost medical advocates.[36]

Women's bodies experienced their labors, even if their minds did not remember them. Observers witnessed women screaming in pain during contractions, thrashing about, and giving all the outward signs of "acute suffering." Residents of Riverside Drive in New York City testified that women in Dr. William H. W. Knipe's twilight sleep hospital sent forth "objectionable" noises in the middle of the night. But few women described such suffering after they emerged from a twilight delivery; the amnesiac properties of scopolamine eliminated their memory of any discomfort.[37]

A successful twilight-sleep delivery, as practiced by Dr. Van Hoosen at the Mary Thompson Hospital in Chicago, required elaborate facilities and careful supervision. Attending physicians and nurses gave the first injection of scopolamine as soon as a woman appeared to be in active labor and continued the injections at carefully determined intervals throughout her labor and delivery. They periodically administered two tests to determine the effectiveness of the drug: the "calling test," which the parturient passed if the doctor could not arouse her even by addressing her in a loud voice, and the "incoordination test," which she passed if her movements were uncoordinated. Once the laboring woman was under the effects of scopolamine, the doctors put her into a specially designed crib-bed to contain her sometimes violent movements (see illustration). Van Hoosen described the need for the bed screens: "As the pains increase in frequency and strength, the patient tosses or throws herself about, but without injury to herself, and may be left without fear that she will roll onto the floor or be

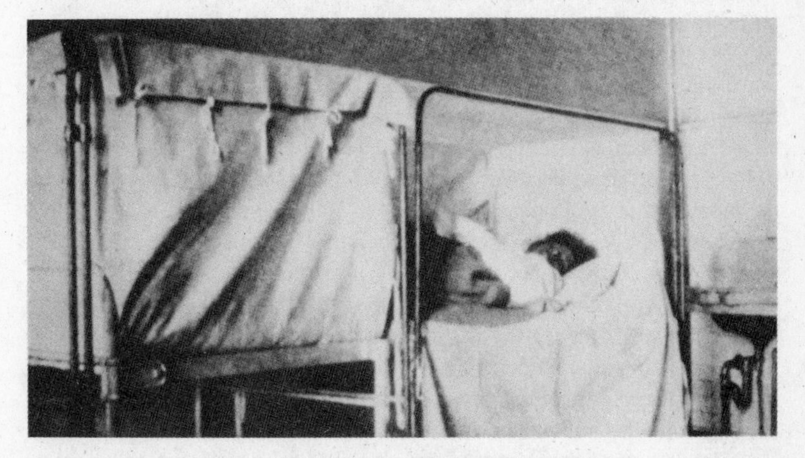

Twilight sleep patient in crib-bed at the Mary Thompson Hospital in Chicago. Source: Bertha Van Hoosen, *Scopolamine-Morphine Anaesthesia* (Chicago: House of Manz, 1915).

found wandering aimlessly in the corridors. In rare cases, where the patient is very excitable and insists on getting out of bed . . . I prefer to fasten a canvas cover over the tops of the screens, thereby shutting out the light, noise and possibility of leaving the bed." Van Hoosen preferred the hospital for a twilight sleep delivery, but she maintained that "when physicians, nurses and the laity understand its action, it will be as possible to give it in a private home as in a hospital."[38]

Twilight sleep became a controversial issue in American obstetrics in June 1914, when *McClure's Magazine* published an article by two laywomen describing this newly popular German method of painless childbirth.[39] In the article, Marguerite Tracy and Constance Leupp, both visitors at the Freiburg women's clinic, criticized high-forceps deliveries (which they called a common American technique) as dangerous and conducive to infection. They contrasted these imperfect births to the safety and comfort of births under twilight sleep, which, they believed, rarely required the use of instruments. The new method was so wonderful, the women asserted, that women having once experienced it would "walk all the way [to Germany] from California" to have their subsequent births under twilight sleep. The physicians at the Freiburg clinic thought the method was best suited for the upper-class "modern woman . . . [who] responds to the stimulus of severe pain . . . with nervous exhaustion and paralysis of the will to carry labor to conclusion." They were less certain about its usefulness or necessity for women who "earn their living by manual labor" and who could tolerate more pain.[40]

Because American doctors were not as quick as German doctors to use twilight sleep, the women who took up the cause in the United States concluded that they were consciously withholding this blessing from American women. Physicians have "held back" on developing painless childbirth, accused Mary Boyd and Marguerite Tracy, two of its most active proponents, because it "takes too much time." They urged women to act in their own behalf. "Women alone," they asserted, "can bring Freiburg methods into American obstetrical practice."[41] Others echoed the call to arms. Journalist Hanna Rion urged her readers to "take up the battle for painless childbirth. . . . Fight not only for yourselves, but fight for your . . . sex."[42] Newspapers and popular magazines joined the chorus, advocating a widespread use of scopolamine in childbirth.[43]

The lay public's efforts to get the medical profession to adopt a technique they believed beneficial to women erupted into a national movement. The National Twilight Sleep Association, formed by upper-

and middle-class clubwomen, was best epitomized by its leaders.[44] They included women such as Mrs. Jesse F. Attwater, editor of *Femina* in Boston; Dr. Eliza Taylor Ransom, active women's rights advocate and physician in Boston; Mrs. Julian Heath of the National Housewife's League; author Rheta Childe Dorr of the Committee on the Industrial Conditions of Women and Children; Mary Ware Dennett of the National Suffrage Association (and later the National Birth Control League); and Dr. Bertha Van Hoosen, outspoken women's leader in Chicago medical circles.[45] Many of these leaders saw the horrors of childbirth as an experience that united all women: "Childbirth has for every woman through all times been potentially her great emergency."[46] Dr. Ransom thought that the use of twilight sleep would "create a more perfect motherhood" and urged others to work "for the betterment of womankind."[47] Many of the twilight-sleep leaders were active feminists, and they saw this controversy as an issue for their sex, not just their class.[48]

The association sponsored rallies in major cities to acquaint women with the issue of painless childbirth and to pressure the medical profession into adopting the new method. In order to broaden its appeal, the association staged meetings "between the marked-down suits and the table linen" of department stores where "the ordinary woman" as well as the activist clubwomen could be found.[49] At these rallies, women who had traveled to Freiburg testified to the wonders of twilight sleep. "I experienced absolutely no pain," claimed Mrs. Francis X. Carmody of Brooklyn, displaying her healthy baby at Gimbels. "An hour after my child was born I ate a hearty breakfast. . . . The third day I went for an automobile ride. . . . The Twilight Sleep is wonderful." Mrs. Carmody ended her speech with the familiar rallying cry: "If you women want it you will have to fight for it, for the mass of doctors are opposed to it."[50]

Department store rallies and extensive press coverage brought the movement to the attention of a broad segment of American women. Movement leaders rejoiced over episodes such as the one in which a "tenement house mother . . . collected a crowd" on a street corner where she joyfully told of her twilight-sleep experience.[51] Many working-class women were attracted to twilight sleep not only because it made childbirth "pleasanter" but because they saw its use as "an important cause of decreased mortality and increased health and vitality among the mothers of children."[52] Some feared, however, that twilight sleep would remain a "superadded luxury of the wealthy mother" because it involved so much physician time and hospital expense.[53] The various groups who advocated twilight sleep—some physicians,

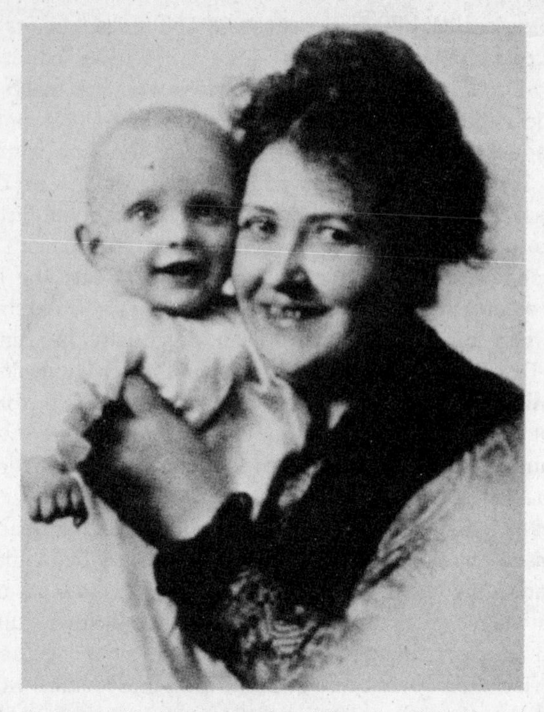

Mrs. Francis X. Carmody, promoting the cause of twilight sleep by exhibiting her healthy son born in September 1914.

Source: Marguerite Tracy and Mary Boyd, *Painless Childbirth* (New York: Stokes, 1915), 143.

middle- and upper-class clubwomen, and working-class women—all united behind the banner of easing the suffering of childbearing women.

Van Hoosen emerged as the most avid advocate of twilight sleep in the Midwest. She had received her M.D. from the University of Michigan Medical School and had worked at the New England Hospital for Women and Children in Boston before setting up practice in Chicago in 1892. Her enthusiasm for the method came from two sources: her strong commitment to the best in obstetrical care and her equally strong commitment to women's rights. Through her use of scopolamine in surgery and obstetrics, she became convinced that twilight sleep offered women a "return of more physiological births" at the same time that it increased the efficiency of physicians, giving them "complete control of everything."[54] She guided many other physicians to the twilight-sleep method.[55] In terms of safety and comfort, she could not imagine a better method of birthing. Moreover, Van Hoosen believed that women had a right to this newest birth panacea.

Slowly American doctors began to deliver twilight-sleep babies. Some traveled to Germany to learn the Freiburg technique and subsequently offered it to both private and charity patients.[56] "If the male had to endure this suffering," said Dr. James Harrar of New York, "I think he would resort very precipitously to something that might relieve the . . . pain."[57] Dr. W. Francis B. Wakefield of California went even further, declaring "I would just as soon consider performing a surgical operation without an anesthetic as conducting a labor without scopolamin amnesia. Skillfully administered the best interest of both the mother and child are advanced by its use."[58] Another physician listed its advantages: painless labor, reduction of subsequent "nerve exhaustion that comes after a prolonged hard labor," better milk secretion, fewer cervical and perineal lacerations, fewer forceps deliveries, less strain on the heart, and a "better race for future generations" since upper-class women would be more likely to have babies if they could have them painlessly.[59] There was also, a physician claimed, an "advantage to the child: To give it a better chance for life at the time of delivery; a better chance to have breast-feeding; a better chance to have a strong, normal mother."[60]

Despite the energy and enthusiasm of the twilight-sleep advocates, medical and lay, significant numbers of American doctors resisted the technique. One reason for this involved the issue of the drug's dangers either to the mother or the child. The *Journal of the American Medical Association* believed that "this method has been thoroughly investigated, tried, and found wanting, because of the danger connected with it."[61] This conclusion, in direct opposition to so much other literature, created confusion in the medical world similar to what it had experienced when anesthesia was first introduced in the middle of the nineteenth century.

With the evidence mixed, many doctors were frustrated in their attempts to find out whether scopolamine was harmful or safe for use in obstetrics. Early experience with the unstable form of the drug led some to refuse to try scopolamine again, although at least one pharmaceutical company had solved the problem of drug stability by 1914. "The bad and indifferent results which were at first obtained by the use of these drugs we now know to have been due entirely to overdosage and the use of impure and unstable preparations," concluded one physician in a report on his successful results with 1,000 twilight-sleep mothers in

1915.[62] Dr. Van Hoosen had successfully performed surgery on 2,000 patients with the help of scopolamine by 1908 and began using the drug routinely in deliveries in 1914.[63] She concluded after 100 consecutive obstetric cases that scopolamine, properly administered, "solves the problems of child-bearing" and is safe for mother and child.[64] But physicians continued to express concern about the possible ill effects of the drug in producing a breathing irregularity in babies whose mothers had been given scopolamine and morphine late in labor.[65]

Doctors trying to understand the evaluation of twilight sleep must have been confused. In one journal they read that the procedure was "too dangerous to be pursued," while another journal assured them that scopolamine, when properly used during labor, "has no danger for either mother or child."[66] Increasingly, by 1915, medical journals published studies that at least cautiously favored twilight sleep. The January 1915 issue of *American Medicine* published nine such articles, although it also ran an editorial warning of the drug's potential dangers and stressing the need for caution.[67] Practicing physicians faced a dilemna when pregnant women demanded painless childbirth with scopolamine.[68]

While physicians debated the desirability of using scopolamine in 1914 and 1915, the Twilight Sleep Association and its allies, surer of their position, demanded that twilight sleep be routinely available to women who wanted it. Hospitals in the major cities responded to these demands and to physicians' growing interest in the method by allowing deliveries of babies the Freiburg way.[69] In order to gain additional clinical experience, and possibly in response to women's requests, some doctors used twilight sleep in hospital charity wards, where small numbers of poor women delivered their babies. But the technique was most successful in the specialty wards where upper- and middle-class patients increasingly gave birth as hospital maternity facilities expanded around the country. By May 1915, *McClure's Magazine*'s national survey reported that the use of twilight sleep, home- and hospital-based, although still battling for acceptance, "gains steadily" around the country.[70]

Because of the need for expertise and extra care in the administration of scopolamine, the twilight-sleep movement easily fed into widespread efforts in the second decade of the twentieth century to upgrade obstetrical practice, eliminate midwives, and move childbirth to the hospital.[71] Both the women who demanded the technique and the doctors who adopted it applauded the new specialty of obstetrics. Mary Boyd desired to put an end to home deliveries when she advocated twilight sleep for charity patients: "Just as the village barber no longer performs operations, the untrained midwife of the neighborhood will pass out of existence under the effective competition of free painless wards."[72] Not only did scopolamine advocates try to displace midwives, but they also regarded general practitioners as unqualified to deliver twilight-sleep babies. "The twentieth century woman will no more think of having an ordinary practitioner attend her in childbed at her own home," said two supporters; "she will go to a [twilight-sleep] hospital as a matter of course."[73] Specialists agreed that "the method is not adapted for the general practitioner, but should be practiced only by those who devote themselves to obstetrics."[74] Eliza Taylor Ransom went so far as to recommend the passage of a federal law forbidding "anyone administering scopolamine without a course of instruction and a special license."[75]

Some obstetricians used this issue to discredit both their general practitioner colleagues and midwives, who still delivered large numbers of America's babies. Others supported twilight sleep because scopolamine births could be managed more completely by the physician. As one succinctly put it, anesthesia gave "absolute control over your patient at all stages of the game. . . . You are 'boss.' "[76] The time formerly spent at the bedside could be used for other pursuits. "I catch up on my reading and writing," testified one practitioner, "I am never harassed by relatives who want me to tell them things."[77]

How do we explain the seeming contradictions in this episode in medical history? Why did women demand to undergo a process which many physicians deemed risky and in which parturients lost self-control? Why did some physicians resist a process that would have given women an easier birthing experience and would have reinforced physicians' control over childbirth in a hospital environment?

Several factors contributed to the disagreement about the use of twilight sleep. One, as already noted, was safety. Many physicians rejected scopolamine because they did not have access to facilities like those at the Mary Thompson Hospital or because they believed the drug too risky under any circumstances. Because of the variability among physicians' use of scopolamine and the contradictory evidence in the professional journals, we know that safety was a guiding motivation of many physicians. However, this itself is not enough to explain physician reluctance since so many doctors administered other drugs during labor despite questionable safety reports. Fifty percent of the 100 general practitioners surveyed in rural districts and small towns in Wisconsin, for example, indicated that they used ergot during labor, although its use was blamed for "a very large per cent of necessary operations for repair of injuries to the floor and pelvic organs of the female patient."[78] Physicians routinely tried many drugs and procedures before their safety had been totally established.

Differing perceptions about pain during childbirth also contributed to the intensity of feeling about twilight sleep in 1914 and 1915. Although many physicians believed that women's "extremely delicate nervous sensibilities" needed relief, others remained reluctant to interfere with the natural process of childbirth. One anti-twilight-sleep physician argued, "when we reflect that we are dealing with a perfectly healthy individual, and an organ engaged in a purely physiological function . . . I fail to see the necessity of instituting such a measure in normal labor and attempt[ing] to bridge the parturient woman over this physiological process in a semi-conscious condition."[79] Women perceived, too, that some physicians used anesthesia only for "suffering when it becomes a serious impediment to the birth process."[80] However, women who felt they had suffered greatly, or who had watched their friends' agony, actively sought relief from their "physiological" births. They thought pain in itself a hindrance to a successful childbirth experience and "demanded" that their physicians provide them with more positive, less painful, experiences in the future.[81]

Most important to understanding the divisions evident between the medical and lay communities, and indeed within the field of medicine itself, was the question of control: who should make the decisions about procedures to be used during confinement? Both sides in the twilight-sleep debate grappled with the issue of whether the women or their medical attendants should determine and control the birthing process.[82] The women who demanded that doctors put them to sleep were partially blind to the safety issue because the issue of control—over pain, bodily function, decision-making—was so important to them. Control became especially important when American doctors refused to allow women "to receive the same benefits from this great discovery that their sisters abroad are getting."[83] Twilight-sleep advocates demanded their traditional right to decide how they would have their children. Tracy and Boyd articulated this issue: "Women took their doctor's word before. They are now beginning to believe . . . that the use of painlessness should be at *their* discretion."[84]

Although women were out of control during twilight sleep deliveries—unconscious and needing crib-beds or constant attention to restrain their wild movements—this loss of physical control was less important to them than their determination to control the decision about what kind of labor and delivery they would have. Hanna Rion, whose influential book and articles garnered support for the method, wrote:

> In the old-fashioned days when women were merely the blindfolded guardians of the power of child-bearing, they had no choice but to trust themselves without question in the hands of the all-wise physician, but that day is past and will return no more. Women have torn away the bandages of false modesty; they are no longer ashamed of their bodies; they want to know all the wondrous workings of nature, and they demand that they be taught how best to safeguard themselves as wives and mothers. When it comes to the supreme function of childbearing every women should certainly have the choice of saying *how* she will have her child.[85]

Twilight-sleep advocates wanted to control their own births by choosing to go to sleep. These women may not consciously have realized that women before the twentieth century traditionally had held decision-making power in the birthing room, but they acted within this long tradition when they voiced their own commitment to retain such power. They were demanding, as women on a more individual level within their own birthing rooms always had demanded, their right to control their own birthing experiences.

This emphasis on a control over decision-making appears clearly in the writings and lectures of the leaders of the twilight-sleep movement.[86] Many leaders were active suffragists whose commitment to twilight sleep was rooted in their belief in women's rights.[87] Although these activists agreed with most physicians that birth should increasingly be the domain of the obstetricians and that women should not suffer unnecessarily, they disagreed vehemently about who should decide what the birthing woman's experience would be. They clearly and adamantly wanted women to have the right to decide their own methods of birthing.[88] Rion believed that women had previously been blind followers and had only opened their eyes over the issue of twilight sleep in 1914, and she used this belief to strengthen her ideas about directions women should take in controlling their own destiny.

The twilight-sleep advocates unconsciously followed in the footsteps of their mothers and grandmothers when they demanded to make their own decisions about how to have their babies. In fact, it is probably because women were very comfortable making decisions about childbirth that the twilight-sleep movement gained the wide support it did in the United States. It seemed natural to most women that birth procedures would be debated among themselves and that resulting decisions should be ones that doctors would be willing to carry out. The transition from negotiating across a birthing bed to public activity was relatively easy for women who had consciously and unconsciously laid the foundations for it in their own birthing rooms.

But doctors perceived things quite differently in 1914. From their point of view, traditional home births had held many problems, the most significant being that physicians could not make medical decisions without the interference of the birthing woman, her friends, and her family. In the new century, physicians sought to change all that. With the help of advancing obstetrical technology, including advances such as scopolamine, which encouraged women to enter the hospital to have their children, doctors hoped to expand their power in the birthing rooms beyond what they had traditionally held. Most important, they wanted the freedom to develop their own professional judgment about the medical indications in each case they attended and to decide the appropriate therapy. They refused to be "dragooned" into "indiscriminate adoption" of a procedure that they themselves did not choose.[89] They lashed out against the "pseudo-scientific rubbish" and the "quackish hocus-pocus" published about twilight sleep in *McClure's* and other lay journals, and they simply refused to be "stampeded by these misguided ladies."[90] These physicians did not believe that nonmedical people should determine therapeutic methods; to them it was a "question of medical ethics." Negotiation was totally out of the question for these doctors who were trying to assert a new kind of control over birthing procedures.[91] Even the doctors who supported twilight sleep in 1914 and 1915 believed that in the final analysis, the method of childbirth was "a question for the attending man and not the patient to decide."[92]

The decision-making emphasis of the twilight-sleep debate, which for the first time brought to the public forum an issue that previously had been settled behind the closed doors of private birthing rooms, reveals the growing strength of the medical profession and of obstetricians in particular in the early twentieth century. The resistance doctors exhibited during the twilight-sleep controversy must be related directly to the period of childbirth history in which it occurred. Physicians stood on the brink of increasing their power over birth processes, but in 1914 they did not yet have the control they desired over procedures and decisions. They knew enough to realize that they did not want to perpetuate the traditional practice of women making these decisions themselves. The vehemence of the medical argument about lay interference thus is attributable to this stage in the development of obstetrics when physicians were beginning to understand the possibility of ultimate control without yet experiencing the reality of it, as much as it is due to the issue of scopolamine itself. While the issues of safety and pain were important to the debate, it was principally this question of power over decision making that separated the twilight-sleep movement's proponents from its opponents.

In the very successes of the twilight-sleep movement lay the seeds for its demise. Pressured by the clubwomen's associations and their own pregnant patients, doctors who had not been trained in the Freiburg method delivered babies with scopolamine. There was an enormous variation in the use of the drug, its timing through labor, the conditions under which the woman labored, and the watchfulness of attendants. As its advocates had feared, problems emerged when scopolamine was not properly monitored in a hospital setting. Following reports of adverse effects on the newborn, the drug fell into ill repute, and some physicians and hospitals that had been among the first to use it in 1914 had by 1915 stopped administering it routinely.[93]

Those physicians who continued to advocate twilight sleep believed that accidents were due to misuse of the Freiburg method and not to the drug itself. Commenting on its discontinuation at Michael Reese Hospital in Chicago, Dr. Bertha Van Hoosen noted that "it is . . . probable that this adverse report demonstrates nothing more than the inexperience of the people using this anesthetic."[94] Dr. Ralph Beach agreed that "there is no doubt that all of the bad results which have been reported due to this method, are due to an improper technic, or the administration of unstable preparations."[95] Simultaneously in 1915, some doctors expanded their obstetric services to offer twilight sleep, while others began cutting back on its use. Either because they judged the drug dangerous or because they did not use it correctly, some hospitals found the method too troublesome to administer on a routine basis to all patients. Most reached a compromise and continued to use scopolamine during labor's first stage, when it was deemed safest, thus preempting their patient's protests without compromising their medical beliefs.

The event that most inhibited growing use of twilight sleep occurred in August 1915 when Mrs. Francis X. Carmody, one of the country's leading proponents of scopolamine, died during childbirth at Long Island College Hospital in New York. Although the doctors and her husband insisted that her death was unrelated to scopolamine, it nonetheless harmed the movement.[96] Mrs. Carmody's neighbor started a new movement to oppose twilight sleep, and women became more alert to the question of safety than they had been before.[97] Doctors and some former twilight-sleep advocates, emphasizing the issues of safety and the difficulty of administration, began exploring other methods of achieving painless childbirth.[98]

The women's movement may have failed to make scopolamine routinely available to all laboring women in 1914 and 1915, but it succeeded in making the concept of painless childbirth even more acceptable than it already was and in adding scopolamine to the obstetric pharmacopoeia. Obstetricians continued through much of the twentieth century to use scopolamine during the first stage of labor in hospital births.[99] The use of anesthesia in childbirth grew in the years after 1915, because women, aware of the possibility of painlessness, continued to want "shorter and less painful parturition" and also because physicians felt they could disregard these desires "only at great risk to [their] own practice."[100] By the 1930s physicians regularly concluded that consideration for the well-being of their patients (and by implication, the physicians' practice) "demands that physicians administer some form of analgesia or anaesthesia during labor in order to render this process less painful." Public and medical opinion agreed that "some form of narcotization" be employed for every labor. "We rejoice," wrote one Ohio doctor, "in this trend toward the universal employment of anaesthesia in this dread hour, because it spares the nervous system and makes for healthier motherhood."[101]

The attempt by a group of women to retain their traditional control over their birthing experiences backfired in 1914 and 1915, and the medical profession gained additional control over childbirth as a result of this episode. Partial acceptance by the profession quieted the lay revolt, and women lost the power they had sought to keep. Ironically, by encouraging women to go to sleep during their deliveries and to deliver their babies in hospitals, the twilight sleep movement helped to distance women from their bodies. Put to sleep with a variety of drugs, most parturient women from the 1920s to the 1960s did not experience one of their bodies' most powerful actions and thus lost touch with their own physical potential.[102] The twilight-sleep movement helped change the definition of birthing from a natural home event, as it was in the nineteenth century, to an illness requiring hospitalization and physician attendance. As a result of the movement, women in the twentieth century who were trying to make decisions about their own childbirth experiences had to fight a tradition of drugged, hospital-controlled birth, itself in part the result of a struggle to increase women's control over their bodies.

Before examining the factors involved when birthing women and their physicians cooperated in moving childbirth to the hospital, discussed in Chapter 7, we need to understand more fully the physician practice of obstetrics in the latter part of the nineteenth century. In addition to their use of anesthesia, which as we have just seen contributed to the desire for hospitalization, other physician interventions paved the way for the emergence of twentieth-century obstetrics practices. Physicians' routines developed to combat perineal lacerations and to restrain the widespread occurrence of puerperal fever contributed in significant ways to the early twentieth-century movement to increase the medicalization of childbirth.

6

Why Women Suffer So

Meddlesome Midwifery and Scrupulous Cleanliness

If pain relief represented the greatest improvement in women's childbirth experiences in the second half of the nineteenth century, continuing postpartum problems and puerperal fever illustrated how much of the experience remained unchanged and dangerous. Women in the nineteenth and early twentieth century continued to die as a result of childbirth, continued to have horrible birth experiences that left them debilitated for the rest of their lives, and continued to fear the event as probably the most dangerous physical trial of their lives. This chapter will examine some of the reasons for women's continuing obstetrical problems through a close examination of three of the most important issues remaining in the second half of the nineteenth and early twentieth centuries: the obstetrical use of ergot, a fungus-derived drug that hastened labor; the medical efforts to prevent and repair perineal lacerations, including the episiotomy; and the continuing incidence of postpartum infection. All of these issues address the role of the physician in causing or increasing women's troubles. The chapter focuses on this question of medical responsibility for women's birth-related problems. The lay and medical responses to these issues help us understand how the climate was set for childbirth to move into the hospital in the twentieth century.

The degree to which women's birthing and postpartum problems were iatrogenic—that is, caused by their medical attendant—is not quantifiable from the records left to us, but we can reach some conclusions by examining the reported practices of birth attendants. The medical record is full of examples of women whose suffering was increased, in the opinion of the medical attendants at the time, by faulty medical interventions. Although many cases of successful interventions were also reported, physicians wrote numerous impressively detailed accounts of the problem deliveries they attended as they sought help from one another in the pages of the medical journals or as they discussed papers at medical society meetings. Letters requesting advice, case reports of complications, articles introducing new techniques, and discussions following paper presentations at medical society meetings reveal some of the parameters of actual obstetric practice among America's physicians. They allow us to analyze physicians' responsibility for continuing the dangers of women's birth experiences.

Dr. Belle Craver of Toledo, Ohio, was particularly sensitive to the possibility of medical culpability. She observed, "The physician's office in the lying-in room is a peculiar and often a very trying one. . . . Too often we are called to see a well woman, but leave her an invalid."[1] Medical practitioners out in America's communities, with limited medical education in practical obstetrics to help them, often stumbled through labors and deliveries, learning as they went. Their texts and journals did not provide sufficient specific guidance in the form of standardized procedures and practices they needed. Many doctors developed expertise in dealing with birth-related complications, but significant variation in skill levels persisted in American medical practice throughout the nineteenth and into the twentieth century.

In many instances physicians, even when using trial-and-error methods, aided women whose deliveries could not be effected without medical help. For example, Dr. Eugene P. Bernardy related a case in his practice in 1885, in which a prolonged labor due to an awkward presentation in a deformed pelvis created particular difficulties. After one night's exhausting labor by the woman during which the physician's efforts did not produce results, Bernardy sought help:

> On my return at 5 P.M., found the condition of things the same. Dr. A. E. Roussell, who came with me, etherized the patient. I again attempted to change the position of the head, but failed. Pagot's long forceps were applied, but on the slightest traction they would slip. Tarnier's forceps seemed to grasp the head in a firmer manner, but they finally gave way. I had now worked continuously for two hours. Seeing there was no other recourse, I perforated the head, and within twenty minutes the child was extracted, which weighed, without the brains, fifteen and one-half pounds.[2]

The physician was able, through much exertion, to rescue the woman from what would have resulted, without aid, in death to both mother and child. Medical aid came to the woman's rescue, although not without putting her at some peril.

When physicians tried to rescue the women from prolonged and difficult labors, they often created new problems, some unavoidably. We have already discussed in Chapter 2 some of the difficult conditions of forceps use and the problems arising from their abuse. Physicians themselves frequently blamed forceps for the postpartum gynecologic problems of their patients, although their not using forceps or intervening in difficult presentations might have caused equally severe problems for birthing women.[3] Physicians' greatest difficulties when called to attend a woman in labor involved judging when and how to intervene. Obstetrics, for all the benefits brought by forceps, anesthesia, and increasing sophistication about the physiological course of labor, remained essentially an empirical art during the late nineteenth century. Physicians' actions at the bedside reflected this lack of system, and the confusions and indecision they frequently exhibited reflected the state of the "science" of obstetrics.

As we have already discussed, physicians often felt compelled to "do something" to aid labor and delivery. One common response to this expectation involved administering drugs to make labor easier or quicker. Physicians trying to effect a timely delivery often resorted to ergot, a drug that caused or intensified uterine contractions. Like forceps, if misused, ergot could cause much postpartum misery. Because the drug caused strong contractions of the uterus, if administered before the cervix was fully dilated, it would force the movement of the fetus against the unyielding tissues and result in severe lacerations of the perineum. It could also be implicated in fetal death from suffocation. However, in a prolonged labor when the uterus seemed to need help in expelling the fetus, ergot appeared to be an attractive alternative to letting the woman suffer. Similarly, ergot was found effective in curtailing postpartum hemorrhages because it forced the uterus to contract. Many doctors believed that ergot could save a woman from a slow postpartum recovery and save a fetus from the dangerous effects of a delayed delivery.

Although most nineteenth-century medical texts taught that ergot should be given only after the second stage of labor, after the baby was born, and some advised its use only after the third stage, when the placenta had already been delivered, many physicians relied on their own instincts and experience and administered ergot early in labor to bring on delivery. Dr. Harriet Garrison of Dixon, Illinois, even while admitting that many physicians used ergot "unscientifically," stated that she preferred the drug to forceps for the second-stage delivery because "it allows the head to rotate and become shaped to suit the pelvic outlet, thus preventing laceration of the perineum." A Philadelphia doctor similarly "used ergot freely [during the first and second stages], particularly where there was inertia, where the pains are irregular, and in hysterical women where we can not get them to regulate the pains."[4]

Most physicians insisted that ergot use before the expulsion of the child was known medically to be dangerous to the child and the mother. These doctors agreed that it should be used only in or after the third stage of labor. But even with this clear message in the medical literature, disagreement existed and practices varied. "The profession is not agreed with reference to this question," wrote Dr. F. M. Johnson of Kansas City in the *Journal of the American Medical Association* in 1887; "some advocate the use of ergot before the close of the third stage, others immediately upon the expulsion of the placenta, and still a third class is not in favor of the entire administration of the drug."[5]

Illustrative of the disagreements within the profession was the reaction to a paper Dr. Ridgway Barker presented at the American Medical Association meeting in 1893. He advocated routine use of ergot immediately following the delivery of the placenta, claiming that it prevented postpartum hemorrhage. His audience roundly disputed his conclusions. Dr. Joseph Eastman of Indianapolis claimed that routine use of the drug would cause "subinvolution" (failure to return to its normal size) of the uterus. This physician believed that because of ergot's dangers "its use should be restricted to the satchel and not used at all," although he admitted that this position might be too extreme. Dr. John Duff of Pittsburgh also argued "against the routine use of ergot." He believed the routine practice of administering ergot after the third stage of labor was "unscientific." Dr. C. S. Bacon of Chicago reported that he had ceased the "routine practice of administering ergot" in his own practice because he found it to be associated with postpartum lactation difficulties.[6] The editors of the *Journal of the American Medical Association*, in which this debate was reported, concluded: "The rule which should govern the use of ergot in labor is hard to define. As with all rules governing the use of drugs, its application depends more upon the judgment of the physician than upon a written law. Ergot must not be used too early lest the child and mother be injured, neither must it be used too late."[7]

Realizing perhaps the differences of opinion within the profession on ergot use, and fearing the routine administration of such a dangerous drug, Dr. Alex Christie wrote to his pregnant sister with advice about how she should conduct her own confinement. "I would shut my mouth to ergot," he recommended, "against any but a first-class physician." He believed that she could safely take ergot after the birth of the baby to control hemorrhage and that "As to the use of opium or morphia you should have no prejudices against that."[8] Women, armed with such information—received either, as in this case, from physicians within their family or friendship networks, or, as was probably more common, from their own or their friends' experiences in birthing rooms—came to their confinements ready to participate actively in therapeutic decision making.

Dr. E. Stuver of Rawlins, Wyoming, had no doubts that ergot led to trouble for parturient women, sometimes even to "speedy death of the patient." He said that although ergot-produced uterine ruptures were relatively rare, the possibility "ever hangs like the sword of Damocles over the head of the physician who uses ergot freely." He continued:

> The danger of laceration of the cervix, perineum and other portions of the parturient tract is greatly increased by the use of ergot. I am firmly convinced that to its free, I might say reckless use, are we indebted for much of that wealth of material that crowds the gynecologic clinics and private hospitals of our large cities and is such a veritable bonanza to specialists in that particular line of work.[9]

The mixed advice on the question of ergot use led one "young physician" to seek help from the *Journal of the American Medical Association.* He related that in medical school he had learned "Never, under any circumstances, give ergot until the uterus is empty." But in 1904, early in his medical practice, he had attended a difficult case of labor in which the woman experienced continuous pain but no advance of labor. He had consulted a more experienced physician, who recommended the administration of ergot, which, indeed, hastened labor and brought about a successful delivery. But, this physician inquired, "Was it or was it not good obstetrics?" The editors provided a not very helpful answer: "Ergot would be a valuable aid in obstetric practice to stimulate uterine contractions if it were not dangerous and uncertain." Despite their reservations, the editors advised that under careful administration in the hands of a skillful physician it could be used "at times with advantage."[10]

Sometimes patients refused to allow physicians to use instruments but allowed drugs, including ergot, which could be used to the same purpose, although with perhaps increased risk. When Dr. Eugene Bernardy arrived at the home of a patient in 1886, he "found she had been in labor since the previous day; she appeared completely worn out, having hardly any strength to bear down; the family refused positively instrumental interference. I gave two doses of fluid extract of ergot, teaspoonful, repeated in half an hour; under its influence the child was born."[11]

Ergot provided physicians with a double-edged sword. In some cases of protracted labor, physicians reported that they used it early in labor without added risk to the mother. If used after the delivery of the placenta, the drug probably caused its least damage, and it might have aided postpartum recovery by hastening the contraction of the uterus and stemming postpartum hemorrhage. In these cases, ergot enhanced the position and effectiveness of the physician in the birthing room. In other instances, however, physicians administered ergot inappropriately before full dilatation, before the birth of the baby, or before placental delivery, and caused harm to the mother that would not have resulted without its use. Ergot in these cases could have produced uterine ruptures, extensive perineal tears, and fetal damage. The evidence that ergot was used during the first and second stage of labor by physicians who did not thoroughly understand how strong uterine contractions could exacerbate the physical dangers of childbirth is extensive. While we cannot quantify how often physicians caused increased damage by their possibly imperfect use of ergot, we can conclude confidently that this did happen.

"Meddlesome midwifery," the inappropriate interference by medical attendants in the form of forceps and drug abuse, can be implicated in some of women's worst postpartum problems. The predominance of didactic obstetric teaching in America's medical schools and the fact that most physicians graduating from such courses of study had at best watched one or two women deliver their babies put physicians at a disadvantage in judging when to intervene in labor. Despite their lack of practical preparation, most doctors forged ahead with obstetric practices. As Dr. Anna Fullerton observed, "we find that almost any physician dares to practise midwifery, although he may stand conscientiously aloof from the management of less critical conditions belonging to other specialties. . . . In the face of these facts, it is not surprising that we should have such statistics of maternal mortality."[12]

Lacerations, childbirth-related tears in the perineal tissues, were often caused by medical attendants' use of drugs and instruments. As Dr. Mary Whery of Fort Wayne, Indiana, noted, "In most cases where lacerations occur it will be admitted that the delivery was too rapid. The fetal head is born suddenly instead of being extricated slowly. This is especially the case when instruments are used. . . . A little extra patience on the part of the accoucheur will save the patient from laceration in most cases."[13]

Lacerations did not necessarily reflect the physicians' lack of skill; they were unavoidable in many cases. But until patients became aware of the necessity of sutures to prevent postpartum gynecological problems, lacerations were a symbol of the attendant's skill. Physicians sometimes were reluctant to admit that their patients had torn the perineum during delivery, because they didn't want to be blamed. As Dr. Olga McNeile of Los Angeles observed, "the physician was often tempted to neglect the repair of such lacerations, as he would acquire the reputation of tearing his women."[14]

Physicians discussed openly in the medical journals the problems of lacerations and their own possible implication in them. Dr. Philip Adolphus of Chicago, for example, presented a paper on perineal lacerations to the Chicago Medical Society in 1884 in which he puzzled over how physicians could prevent this common problem. He believed that rapid labors, during which the head was most likely to tear the perineum, vagina, and cervix, presented the gravest dangers. "More frequently the physician causes the laceration when the labor requires a speedy termination in the interest of mother or child, or of both. For instance, after a difficult forceps labor." Adolphus suggested that extensive lacerations could be prevented if physicians would take more time to rotate the shoulders during extraction, but agreed that in the anxiety of saving the child, this was not always possible. He admitted that "the child . . . is primarily to be saved; the perinaeum secondarily." The editors of the *Journal of the American Medical Association* agreed that physicians should make all efforts to prevent lacerations, but that "it must be distinctly borne in mind, that, under certain conditions, the preservation of the female perinaeum in an intact state, is an impossible task."[15]

A Cincinnati doctor agreed that some fetal presentations made lacerations inevitable, regardless of anything the attendant could do. Despite his desire to free physicians from blame, this doctor admitted in 1884 that many perineal lacerations were caused by physicians: "it cannot be denied that these errors of practice are sometimes perpetrated by well educated physicians."[16] The prominent Philadelphia physician S. D. Gross agreed in the same year that some lacerations were unavoidable, but, he believed, "in the great majority of cases [they are] the effects of gross ignorance, timidity, indecision, or the maladroit use of the forceps and of other instruments." He continued:

> If all accoucheurs were well educated and well versed in the use of the forceps, there might be some justification for the frequency with which they are applied at the present day. There might even be some justification in hitching them on the child's head, when nature is fully equal to her task, to get home in time to a good supper; but to use them on the slightest pretence, as is so often done now-a-days by every sciolist, hardly out of his swaddling-clothes, is, if you will allow me to say it, simply damnable.[17]

Such admissions of physicians' shortcomings appeared over and over again in the medical literature as doctors struggled with their mistakes and tried to improve their obstetric technique. "Meddlesome midwifery is a prime cause [of women's postpartum problems]," wrote Dr. Charles Meigs Wilson of Philadelphia. Physicians, recognizing the problem and their role in causing it, pushed themselves to try to prevent and repair the damage they repeatedly witnessed.[18]

Despite the recognition by many physicians of the imperfections in obstetric practices, the situation only slowly improved. Physicians' actual birthing room practices continued to reflect extreme variations in knowledge about the process of parturition and about planning interventions. A physician who had been in practice for three years in West Virginia wrote to the *Journal of the American Medical Association* in 1903 seeking advice about a delivery he had managed, which had resulted in a craniotomy. "Did the case justify operation?" he asked. The woman had been in labor three or four hours when the physician was called to the case. "After an hour the pains became more frequent and sharp, with no tendency to bearing down. She being a primipara, I suggested that she use all effort to expel contents and not cry aloud." Hours later, labor still not progressing, and the woman experiencing "severe and cutting" pains, the doctor called another physician in consultation:

> Chloroform was at once administered and a high application of the forceps tried, but found to be impossible by either of us, even with external pressure from above. Another physician was called by the husband and he repeated the trial of high application, but failed. I then tried to do a podalic, but could never reach a foot, as did Drs. X and Y, who were also unable to accomplish anything.

With the woman cynotic (looking blue from insufficient oxygenation of the blood) and bleeding slightly (probably from lacerations caused by the repeated forceps attempts), "I decided to do a craniotomy, which was accomplished in a very few minutes." This case, in the opinion of the *Journal* editors, "well illustrates a mistake . . . of premature unnecessary operative interference." The editors asserted that the physicians should not have encouraged bearing down before full dilatation, they should not have applied the forceps before the head had engaged, and they should not have prematurely performed a craniotomy before labor was given a chance to progress on its own.[19]

This early twentieth-century example illustrates the discrepancy between medical teaching and medical practice. The physician, who had been practicing medicine and, presumably, delivering babies for three years, still could not recognize when intervention was indicated. Nor could his two colleagues. Not checking for complete dilatation before encouraging pushing and prematurely inserting forceps were violations of very basic obstetrical principles.

The case also provides an indication of the panic that must have frequently occurred in America's birthing rooms when labor did not meet the expectations of the family and of the birth attendants—the calling in of multiple physicians, the desperate acts the attendants felt called upon to perform, the physical and mental suffering of the patient and her husband. In this case the presence of three doctors must have exacerbated the compulsion to do something to relieve the slowly progressing labor. Combined with their apparent inexperience and the husband's concern, this led to a poorly managed situation and a probably unnecessary fetal death. To the extent that this situation was mirrored during other labors around the country, we begin to understand some of the stresses of the birthing room and some of the effects of "meddlesome midwifery." In the words of Dr. Simon Marx of New York City, "one gift that is possessed by very few obstetricians is the faculty of knowing both the how and the when for operative interference."[20]

Much of the debate about childbirth-related lacerations focused on the question of when and whether to repair the damage. Physicians could not agree on whether or not immediate sewing of the tears was necessary to prevent future gynecological problems. Dr. Rudolph Holmes of Chicago in 1903 vehemently objected to turning simple lacerations into surgical emergencies. "I condemn the promiscuous repair of lacerations of the cervix," he said, insisting instead that only lacerations that caused pathological symptoms, such as prolapsed uterus or sepsis, should receive the obstetrician's surgical attention.[21] Dr. R. B. Bontecou of Troy, New York, took exception to this position and urged upon his colleagues "the importance and necessity of making ocular inspections in all cases—at least, where there is a suspicion of lesion, and repair it at once." "When views so diametrically opposed, upon a question of such practical importance, are presented to the young practitioner," bemoaned Dr. H. V. Sweringen of Fort Wayne, Indiana, "it will be difficult for him to decide which course he had better pursue." Sweringen added his own recommendation to delay suturing until the woman had recovered from the childbirth trauma. "We are still at sea as to what is really necessary to be done in repairing a lacerated perineum," concluded Dr. G. B. Somers of San Francisco in 1905.[22]

Physicians' struggles with the question of perineal lacerations reveal much about the state of obstetric practice and the confusions within medicine on the questions of managing labor and delivery at the turn of the twentieth century. While unskilled and untrained attendants, physicians or midwives, could cause additional problems, it was also the case that even skilled medical attendance did not guarantee that injuries would not result or that they would be adequately repaired. In their efforts to bring about a safe delivery for women they attended, physicians searched for methods that would be effective in all deliveries and repeatedly modified their birthing room procedures. Dr. G. H. Randall of Chicago, for example, over the years of his practice changed his thinking on how women should be positioned for delivery. "Formerly," reported the secretary of the Chicago Medical Society in 1886, "he had delivered most of his cases in the dorsal position, but not being satisfied with the way he was able to manipulate the perineum and head, he had tried the lateral position, and it seemed a great improvement. He could now support the perineum by directing the head with a great deal more ease and effect than ever before, and it seemed to him that the lateral position is preferable to the dorsal."[23] Many physician's efforts to improve their practice developed through such trial-and-error techniques.

As the nineteenth century approached its end and the twentieth century dawned, physicians continued to share with one another their new procedures and their continuing hopes that they could conquer the difficult problems that childbirth presented. They still felt very much that Walter Channing's advice from the beginning of the century described their position in the labor room: they had to "do something."[24] Because it was not always clear even to the best of them what that something was, physicians continued their debates. Their actions in the birthing rooms across the country in this period must be seen within this context: the questions were asked, but the answers were not yet available in any systematic way.[25]

Medical debate over the technique of the episiotomy, an attendant-made cut in the perineum to enlarge the vaginal opening and facilitate delivery, illustrates the dilemma early twentieth-century physicians faced as they tried to develop optimal birth techniques. Physicians first used episiotomies in the eighteenth century, but American physicians became very interested in the procedure only after Dr. Anna Broomall's introduction of it in the 1870s at the Woman's Hospital in Philadelphia.[26] Its general use awaited hospital-based delivery after the 1920s. At the turn of the century, however, many physicians did episiotomies on their patients confined either at home or in the hospital. Dr. Frank Stahl became one of its most eager advocates: "In my hands," he immodestly wrote in 1895, "episiotomy is an instrument, *par excellence,* aiding as no other instrument can in the preservation of life and body, both in the fetal and maternal, and as I grow in obstetrics . . . I am glad to know that there is so effectual and yet simple an instrument as central episiotomy at my command."[27] Dr. J. J. Mulheron of Detroit agreed in 1899 that the "episiotomy is unquestionably one of the most important of obstetric procedures."[28] For these physicians the only question was where to make the cut, not whether to make it.

Other physicians completely opposed the technique. Dr. Mary Whery wrote in 1903, "Episiotomy has often been recommended, but it is only a substitution of the certainty of laceration for an uncertain laceration. The patient, if she were conscious, would object to the incision." Whery preferred the carefully monitored and slow use of forceps rather than the perineal cut.[29] Dr. Emma Neal's practice in rural Iowa in the early twentieth century confirmed patients' resistance to episiotomies. "Most patients," she noted, "will forgive a doctor for almost any degree of laceration if he explains the conditions that caused it and makes an honest attempt at repair, but very few of them fail to be critical of an episiotomy that fails to heal readily. No matter how urgently it was indicated, the family are apt to show some resentment."[30] These examples raise the possibility that women doctors showed more understanding than did men of their patients' reactions to this procedure, although most male and female physicians refused to use the procedure in the prehospital period.

How should we judge the mounting evidence that physicians' actions in the birthing rooms of America were often imprecise, experimental, and sometimes harmful to women? Merely blaming physicians for the state of their art and the quality of their practice does not suffice because our task is to try to understand medical behavior and to put it into its historical context. It is important to separate individual practitioners from the profession at large in our analysis. The last part of the nineteenth and the early part of the twentieth century were the years in which regular medicine was emerging from the weak and divided condition that had earlier characterized it. The profession won exclusive or near-exclusive licensing laws in states around the country and was superseding many sectarian practices (such as homeopathy and hydropathy) and moving toward a more unified medical practice. This emerging professional strength, which may have increased the authority of the doctor within the birthing room, was, however, not directly mirrored by the conditions of private obstetrics practice. Individual physicians still worked at a disadvantage in the birthing room: their education had not prepared them for many medical situations they faced; they had to share their authority with the birthing woman's friends and family; and they most commonly worked alone without other medical consultation. Individual medical practitioners, delivering babies throughout America, then, did not feel themselves to be the beneficiaries of the profession's rise in status.

One woman, in her description of the exertions of her physician during her protracted labor and difficult delivery, revealed the circumstances under which many physicians labored. "The ether cap," wrote Gladys Brooks about her early twentieth-century confinement, "was pressed over my nose and mouth by the faithful Dr. Jackson, who became quite exhausted from the effort of properly dealing with me atop the wide spaces of the immense family bed."[31] Delivering her baby in the same ancestral bed in which her husband had been born was important to this woman; her doctor had to figure out how to maneuver himself and carry out his interventions within the confines that the woman set. Similarly, Dr. Evaline Peo in Boone, Iowa, described a very difficult delivery during which she was forced to administer anesthesia, perform a complicated internal version, and deliver twins "with no help but a neighbor woman."[32]

The drug and instrument interventions that physicians brought with them into home birthing rooms exacerbated the difficulties they faced while attending their patients. Forceps insertions were especially awkward on home birthing beds; anesthetized patients also could present hardships for positioning and support. Dr. Emma Neal of Cedar Rapids, Iowa, explained in 1923:

> We are called to assume responsibility for two lives at a moment's notice, often having no previous knowledge of the patient's condition, no facilities for doing clean work, insufficient light, the patient

> on a low, back-breaking bed, and frequently no assistance, except possibly a neighbor, whose only qualifications as a nurse is that she has had a child or two of her own.[33]

Similarly, Dr. J. H. MacKay of Norfolk, Nebraska, wrote of his frustrations: a doctor's "case may be miles in the country with bad roads or a blizzard prevailing and he may have no knowledge of the presumptive nature of the case until he sees it. . . . He is always called in a crisis and usually at the last moment."[34] Doctors who attended these home deliveries and the women who suffered through them both felt inconvenienced by the less than ideal situation.

Dr. George S. King described how the physical environment of most confinements and his busy schedule affected his practice of obstetrics in the 1890s: "Many a night we slept on a couch or on the floor while the poor horse stood outside covered with a blanket. Often when we had as many as three, and once five, cases in active labor living miles apart, we had to slow this one down with a sedative and hurry that one up with an oxytocic."[35] Because of such conditions of home-based general medical practice, physicians and birthing women struggled for safer and more comfortable deliveries; that they were sometimes impossible to achieve cannot be surprising.

The late nineteenth and early twentieth century represent a transition period in American obstetric history. Physicians and birthing women voiced awareness that childbirth remained dangerous, yet neither seemed to be able significantly to alter the situation. The continuing, and, some believed, expanding problem of puerperal infection, the raging postpartum infection that women so frequently encountered as part of their birth struggles, represented the worst of traditional childbirth that remained to be conquered. Precisely the period when new knowledge about disease transmission by microorganisms was incorporated into the medical corpus, these turn-of-the-century years were also the times when efforts at prevention and control of infection seemed least effective.

Throughout history some women died from consuming septicemia following their confinements. The raw wound of placental separation combined with the trauma of delivery created a ripe environment for the introduction of infected material and its rapid entrance into the blood stream; postpartum women were particularly vulnerable to infection. The incidence of postpartum infection, usually called puerperal fever, is impossible to know from the records. The mortality record, however, indicates that puerperal fever was the single largest cause of death among childbearing women in the early years of the twentieth century.[36] The question arises whether or not the dangers of infection increased when physicians attended normal deliveries. Did physicians, who attended approximately half of American births in the late nineteenth century, by their very presence and by their intervention techniques increase women's chances of death? This is a puzzle, the pieces of which we may begin to reconstruct.

During the nineteenth century physicians became aware that they might play a role in bringing infection into the birthing room. Dr. Oliver Wendell Holmes in the United States and Dr. Ignaz Semmelweis in Austria claimed that physicians carried infection from patient to patient, and in the 1840s both urged the cleansing of the hands to prevent this transportation.[37] Although the actual mechanism of infection remained elusive—until the science of bacteriology began to unlock the doors of understanding microorganisms decades later—some physicians began to follow Holmes' and Semmelweis' regimens of obstetric practice that included hand-washing before touching the laboring woman. Other physicians vehemently opposed any suggestion that they might be carriers of infection and dangerous to their patients. The most famous debate over this issue at mid-century was the one between Holmes and Charles Meigs, who refused to accept any responsibility for his patients' puerperal fevers.[38] The thought of a gentleman's hands being a carrier of such horror was unthinkable to many, especially as there seemed to be no way empirically to "see" the causative agent, the pathologic microorganism.

As the nineteenth century progressed and the medical profession learned about the role of bacteria in causing infection following Louis Pasteur's investigations in the 1860s and the rapid explosion of bacteriological studies in succeeding decades, physicians increasingly accepted the fact that they had to be careful when attending birthing women. Dr. William Lusk, for example, in 1884 told his fellow practitioners of a physician "with a very large obstetric practice, who . . . was forced to the conviction that he had been carrying infection directly from his scarlet fever patients to his parturient women."[39] Dr. Madison Reece of Abingdon, Illinois, similarly advised his colleagues in the same year, "it is my fixed belief, that thousands of women have come to their deaths, from the dirt and other matters under the finger nails of their attendants." Dr. Ida Gridley Case of Collinsville, Connecticut, repeated the warning: "Many lives have been sacrificed because the physician went directly from some contagious disease to attend a woman in labor." By the decade of the 1880s, physicians increasingly accepted responsibility for transmitting infection to their patients in labor. A Pennsylvania physician put it quite simply, "I believe that many a man and woman, going to attend a woman in confinement, carry her death warrant under their fingernails."[40]

Those who accepted that they could be carriers of puerperal fever tried to achieve sterile conditions in the homes of their patients to prevent the horror, and they shared their procedures with each other in the pages of the medical journals. In great detail they wrote about the benefits of hot water, disinfecting their hands and instruments, and vaginal douches.[41]

Autogenesis, or the theory that women could infect themselves, perhaps by the transmission of germs from the rectum into the vagina during delivery, "may be a doctrine full of comfort to the obstetrician," wrote Dr. Theophilus Parvin in 1884, but "it seems more probable, more rational to conclude that puerperal septicaemia is always and everywhere heterogenetic [introduced from without]."[42] His colleague agreed that physicians were more likely to have carried infection to the childbed than women were to have created it themselves:

> I believe that when a man has a case of puerperal septicaemia [in his practice], he has not to look about him for causes that exist in the cellar or other parts of the house. But let him examine his own self, his hands and clothes, and all his surroundings, and see if he cannot trace the carrying of that poison to the woman. . . . There is one precaution against puerperal septicaemia that every man and every woman can take, and that is making sure that his or her hands are perfectly clean before they are introduced into the vagina or uterus of a woman, to make sure that the nails be pared, the arms and hands should be washed with turpentine and subsequently with soap and water or some alkaline solution.[43]

"The disease of which we are speaking, and which kills the woman, is not born in her," Parvin concluded, "It is brought to and deposited in her from a preceding case of puerperal septicaemia. To believe otherwise would be to believe in spontaneous generation."[44] Dr. A. B. Miller of Syracuse agreed that "the infection is carried usually by the physician in attendance. If he has been attending a pus case, a streptococcus infection, our patient will in all probability be infected and is surely going to die."[45]

Some physicians who accepted the general tenets of bacteriology and who believed that infection was transmitted by microorganisms, that is, believed in the "germ theory of disease," nonetheless rejected the idea that childbed fever was always introduced from without. Indeed, the empirical data seemed to suggest that postpartum fever resulted from a variety of causes, only one of which was microorganisms possibly introduced by the birth attendants. Too many cases of women who did not contract puerperal fever, although their circumstances and environment would have predicted it, contradicted the externally introduced germ theory explanation. "I have had patients placed under the most trying ordeal of poverty and filth, minus all the comforts of life," wrote Dr. J. S. Dukate of Pond Creek Mills, Indiana, in 1894, "and yet these would do well, and that in the filth of their uterine secretions, no undergarments for a change, the very kind of soil to foster bacteria; yet these same women were soon up and attending to the duties of the housewife, having had no unfavorable symptoms."[46] The seeming contradiction of women who had clean deliveries contracting infection and other women who had dirty birthing environments emerging from childbed unscathed baffled the medical observers during this late nineteenth-century period, when germ theory was still new.

Revealing discussions about obstetrical infections took place at the Chicago Gynecological Society and the Chicago Medico-Legal Society in 1888; they bear close scrutiny because they touched both on the question of the role of microorganisms in the production of fever and on the value of antiseptic vaginal injections to kill bacteria that might cause postpartum infection. This midwest debate recalls some of the confusion within medical thinking during the early years of bacteriology and illustrates the controversy among obstetricians about how to convert the new beliefs into treatment.[47]

Some of the physicians attending these Chicago medical meetings simply refused to accept the tenets of the new germ theory. Dr. J. H. Etheridge, for example, found the proposed obstetric techniques to counteract the effects of "an alleged microorganism that no one has seen, excepting Pastuer [sic], who *thinks* that he once saw it," astonishing and preposterous. Other physicians more readily accepted germ theory. Dr. C. W. Earle countered Etheridge: "I am exceedingly sorry that Dr. Etheridge has taken us back and given about the same argument that must have been given 45 years ago, when the illustrious Semmelweiss, in the face of ridicule and scorn, advanced his new ideas regarding puerperal fever." Although germ theory had solid defenders at these meetings, many doctors seemed to agree with Dr. C. T. Parkes, who asserted, "we should not be too hasty in putting forth dogmatic assertions in this matter."[48]

Earle urged his fellow physicians to do everything they could to prevent puerperal fever. He believed that "if everybody will go to cases of labor with clean hands, will employ clean nurses, and see that the atmosphere of the room is not tainted, he will bring the mortality down to almost nothing." Few physicians by the latter part of the nineteenth century denied the necessity of cleanliness in the birthing room. But the specifics of how this was to be achieved, and who was to be blamed if the women contracted an infection, remained controversial.

The vaginal chloral douche, an injection of antiseptics into the vagina before and after delivery to destroy any possible growth of pathogenic matter, provoked some of the fiercest debate at the Chicago meetings. Some physicians believed simply that the douching procedure was ineffective: "If after such an antiseptic injection we could take out the vagina and examine it, I think we would find that not more than one-third of its surface had been touched by this fluid." Etheridge challenged the vaginal douche from a more fundamental disbelief: "How long will it be before the Semmelweiss theory will be modified or before something better will take its place? We find all the way through medicine and surgery that theories are taken up and abandoned."[49]

Many physicians, in fact, believed that the interference of douches increased rather than decreased the dangers to women. Dr. G. Frank Lydston, for example, deplored the "septophobia" in the medical world of the 1880s. He claimed that when "the *prophylactic* injections and complicated manipulations were introduced" at the New York State Hospital for Emigrants, where he was resident-surgeon, "the direct and immediate effect [was] of increasing the mortality rate, which became alarmingly high." In general, Lydston found that injections during labor recommended by "some of our antiseptic extremists," were "not only useless, but injurious."[50] Each opportunity for manipulation increased the potential dangers of introducing injury. Another Chicágo doctor noticed in 1884 that "temperature rise and pelvic inflammations follow the use of frequent vaginal injections, and cases which may eventuate in puerperal septicaemia and lead to a fatal issue would often do well and make a perfect recovery if let alone and kept quiet, and free from CURIOUS visitors."[51]

A "Country Practitioner," who read "with awe and not unmixed with incredulity the earnest discussions of his city brethren of the healing art," when the Chicago meetings were reported in the *Journal of the American Medical Association*, wrote a letter reacting to the controversy. He claimed, "I venture the assertion that not one country practitioner in fifty uses any antiseptic precaution beyond cleanliness. . . . I know practitioners who have attended their thousands of cases without a fatal puerperal case, and who have practiced no preliminary antisepsis but strict cleanliness."[52] This country doctor's experiences were confirmed and repeated by numerous physicians who had attended thousands of women over the course of their professional careers without ever using antiseptic technique and without losing women to puerperal fever. William Allen Pusey, writing about his father's Kentucky practice of obstetrics in the 1870s and 1880s, told how his father had maintained an admirable safety record: "his greatest safeguard here was quite unconscious and that was his natural cleanliness. As a result of this his obstetrical practice had few infections."[53]

In this early bacteriological era physicians found it difficult to sift the useful suggestions from the contradictory in the medical literature and to develop their own obstetrical routines to prevent infection. In the words of Dr. Gustav Zinke of Cincinnati, Ohio:

> To-day, when one new measure or remedy succeeds another, when so many are ever ready to announce something new (?) and, being announced, as many, if not more, are ready to improve and add to the new discovery, the perplexity in which the practitioner is placed at times in consequence, is occasionally not only annoying to himself, but it casts a shadow upon the profession at large.[54]

The controversy about douches and other antiseptic techniques continued. Although Pasteur and his associates showed the causal relationship between streptococcus and puerperal fever by 1879, practicing physicians continued through the rest of the century to doubt that it was the only cause of postpartum infections. Too many cases of infection developing even when strict antisepsis was practiced brought into question the single-cause theory and challenged particularly physicians' role in bringing the infection to the women in their practices. But because of the general acceptance of germ theory among America's physicians late in the century, techniques of obstetric cleanliness developed and were increasingly practiced around the childbirth bed.

From the Preston Retreat in Pennsylvania, Dr. Joseph Price reported in 1889 that over a five-year period 540 deliveries had been accomplished without one maternal death. "The great success attending the work of this Maternity is due to the strict enforcement of the law of cleanliness," he said. "Everything and everybody in the house is clean and jealously kept so." Price described the procedures:

> When ready for the delivery room the patient is again given a hot soap bath and an enema and a vaginal injection of 1 to 2000 bichlo-

> ride of mercury solution. She is clothed in a clean nightrobe and drawers and placed upon a new clean delivery bed. Scrupulous cleanliness is observed in all manipulations of the patient, and after delivery a second vaginal injection is given, and a vaginal suppository of iodoform [a local anesthetic and antiseptic] is introduced.[55]

Price urged physicians in private practice to adapt hospital methods to home use, but, he admitted, it was not always possible. He believed that "in private practice the mortality was greater among the rich than the poor," because, he suspected, water-closets might cause some infections among the better classes, who could afford such devices in their homes.[56]

The president of the American Gynecological Society agreed in 1898 that "women in well-conducted lying-in asylums are far safer from puerperal infection than those who are attended in their own houses, even though they be brown-stone fronts." The large majority of septic cases resulted, he believed, "from the fingers or instruments of the physician or the nurse. . . . It is not only the hands and instruments which may introduce infection, but also the clothing of the attendants, which may have been in contact with some infectious case and which have not been thoroughly cleansed and disinfected."[57] Because of the great social differences between women who were confined in hospitals and almshouses and those confined at home in this period, direct comparison of the two groups is impossible. Physicians, however, were eager to use the argument that hospitals could better prevent infection as they began their push to hospitalize birthing women.

At the turn of the twentieth century, Dr. Bertha Van Hoosen of Chicago observed, "So general has been the knowledge of the causes of puerperal fever that a physician almost regards himself a criminal if a case occurs in his practice."[58] Physicians began thinking about birth as if every woman was a potential casualty of infection, as if every birth was pathologic. "Septicaemia or putrid absorption is possible during the puerperium of every woman," wrote one doctor.[59] Taught that each case might be a possible emergency, doctors sought stringent methods of trying to prevent postpartum infection. Dr. Ida Case changed her birthing-room activities accordingly: "It is now my practice to wear while at labor cases a freshly laundered cotton or silk shirt waist, and a long apron of cotton cloth completely encircling my dress skirt. The apron and waist I never wear to two successive cases."[60] Dr. Olive Wilson of Arkansas similarly insisted that the parturient's genitalia be scrubbed with soap and hot water and then the woman be placed on the Kelly pad and not allowed to move from it. Then, she wrote, "The examining hand, with rings removed is thoroughly disinfected before the first examination with dress sleeve and undersleeve pushed well above the elbow and secured, and hand lubricated with soap provided by myself and known to be aseptic. When the head begins to distend the perineum, a towel dipped in hot bichloride solution 1/5000 is kept over the parts." After delivery, Wilson repaired perineal lacerations and placed "a perfectly clean cloth" over the genitals to receive the discharge, insisting that it be frequently changed.[61]

Physicians' directions to each other about how to keep a home-based normal labor from becoming a nightmare of infection were quite elaborate. Dr. Frederick Holme Wiggin, for example, in 1902 explained what he believed physicians needed to do:

> The physician on his arrival should be careful to disinfect his hands before making a vaginal examination and this he can readily do by scrubbing his hands and arms in hot running water, preferably using tincture of green soap and scrubbing them for ten minutes with a fiber brush. The hands should next be immersed in alcohol; the nails being cleansed with a piece of sterilized gauze wet in the alcohol; they should next be immersed in an alcoholic solution of bichlorid of mercury to the strength of 1 to 500, which solution should be rinsed from the hands by sterilized water before the lubricant is applied to them, which lubricant should be contained in a collapsible tube, or the physician after cleansing his hands may put on rubber gloves that have been boiled for at least half an hour and have then been soaked in a one per cent. solution of lysol.[62]

This sort of medical prescription for scrupulous cleanliness, representing the attempt to produce a germ-free environment, exceeded what most physicians could achieve in the homes of laboring women to whom they were hastily called and in which they could hope for only lay attendants. The discrepancy between what physicians could achieve in a hospital setting and in women's homes grew in the period around the turn of the century, in large part as a direct result of the impact of the germ theory. The difficulties that physicians increasingly faced as they tried to implement their new knowledge at the bedsides of parturient patients encouraged specialists to desire hospital-based practice and to discourage general practitioners' attendance at home deliveries. But the fact remained that most of America's babies, still probably 90 to 95 percent at the turn of the twentieth century, were delivered at home, half of them under the supervision of physicians, general practitioners and specialists in obstetrics, and half under the supervision of trained and untrained midwives.

Dr. J. F. Baldwin of Columbus, Ohio, realized that because of the home-based nature of the practice of obstetrics, advice to the medical attendants had to be practical to be useful: "I have seen explicit directions given requiring at least ten minutes for the scrubbing of the hands with soap and hot water, and then three minutes' continuous soaking in a 1 to 1000 bichlorid solution; or a similar scrubbing of the hands with subsequent treatment with permanganate of potash and oxalic acid. Such precautions are not feasible in general practice and will not be carried out." Baldwin suggested, in 1902, that in a normal delivery, sterilizing the instruments by boiling, thorough washing of the hands (on which the nails are clean and trimmed), and cleansing of the vulva would suffice. Fingernails could be the "main source of danger":

> Many physicians, especially in country practice, are obliged, to a considerable extent at least, to care for their own horses and to do more or less work about the garden. Such men are very apt to have horny hands which in bad weather are quite liable to become more or less chapped and fissured. It is quite impossible to render such hands absolutely sterile. In such cases rubber gloves cannot be too highly recommended.[63]

At the turn of the twentieth century, rubber gloves, a rubber Kelly pad, and shaving the perineum of the birthing woman became standard in the medical advice to physicians. Despite the increased understanding of germ propagation, however, variations in physicians' birthing practices continued. Even as late as 1912, after asepsis—that is, creating a germ-free environment as opposed to antisepsis, the attempt to destroy present germs—provided the model for physician-attended births, an article in the *Journal of the American Medical Association* recommended the use of petrolatum as a perineal rub, even though it was a known bacterial medium. Furthermore, the article did not recommend the use of sterilized gloves. A number of physicians writing letters to the editor protested this (unnamed) author's "antequated" obstetric technique and claimed his methods would increase infection, although a few doctors came to his defense and indicated that they followed similar techniques in their own practices.[64] Obstetric practice throughout the country was in no way standardized. Actual use of the methods needed to create a sterile birthing environment varied from physician to physician and depended in large part on patient cooperation.

Physicians who delivered in patients' homes learned to compromise in the face of family resistance to the new methods. Dr. Emma Neal, practicing in rural Iowa, resigned herself to the imperfections of the conditions in which she had to work. "Most of the patient's surroundings cannot be kept sterile, as she will be certain to disarrange the coverings during pains, but the operator's gloves may be dipped frequently in lysol and must be kept clean. If he has insufficient help, he may be compelled to use one hand in touching non-sterile articles, but the examining hand can, and must be kept sterile. . . . A Kelly pad or rubber sheeting cannot be made completely sterile, and may be the means of carrying infection from one patient to another. The fact that some women are confined in filthy surroundings, with no care afterward, and never have a temperature above 99, and that other women confined in the midst of ideal surroundings and with every facility for skilled care will go through a very stormy puerperium is no argument against doing our very best in every case to protect the interest of the patient."[65]

Dr. Eliza Root, the obstetrics editor of the *Woman's Medical Journal*, observed that, contrary to its expected benefits, attempts at achieving sterile conditions might in fact mask the still-present dangers to birthing women. Physicians may claim that they used aseptic methods, but, Root believed, the naming of their procedures "may mean much or little as to the aseptic methods employed. A careless and faulty technique might ease its conscience by [the use of the phrase] without committing an absolute falsehood."[66] In addition, physicians might be reluctant to admit sepsis cases in their practices for fear of being stigmatized. Dr. Edward Reynolds of Boston tried to prepare a statistical survey of puerperal sepsis in his home state, but he could not do so. "The practitioner is too apt to be unwilling to diagnose sepsis in his own cases," noted Reynolds; "he is too prone to shut his eyes to the possibility of infection, to adopt every other explanation of the condition of his patient, and admit the existence of sepsis only after it has reached the incurable stage."[67]

The editors of the *Journal of the American Medical Association* believed that the rush to antisepsis and asepsis at the turn of the century led itself frequently to greater infection than had existed before the physicians were so aware of the dangers of the germs:

> The physician feels that if he is aseptic in his work . . . he can do practically what he will. The old rule of 'meddlesome midwifery is bad' is cast aside. With improved forceps of several patterns, with

> chloroform given with practically no danger, even the careful physician feels justified in early instrumental interference, resorts to version on slight provocation, is indifferent to lacerations because he can sew them up immediately, is digitally diligent in determining the progress of labor; in fact, he hesitates at none of these because he has practically no fear of sepsis. And why? Because by his side is a bowl of bichlorid solution or of carbolic acid or of some other favorite antiseptic into which he dips his fingers, his silk, his forceps, perhaps, flattering himself that in this way he is rendering himself clean and protecting his patient from harm. . . . There is a slip somewhere in the technique of his asepsis and the deed is done. . . . These tragedies are occurring every day . . . a careless obstetrician, overconfident because of his fancied protection by his so-called asepsis, may be a breeder of the most serious mischief.[68]

Physicians became bolder in their interventions because of the protection they thought they received from their attempts at scrupulous cleanliness, and this, in addition to any mistakes in their sterile technique, led, in the opinion of the editors, directly to increased problems for birthing women.

Ironically, physicians created some additional problems for women at the very time when they increased their own understanding of disease transmission and in the very process of trying to avoid that transmission. Observers had to agree at the beginning of the twentieth century that "puerperal infection in private practice is still much larger than it should be and not on the decline," and that much of it was due to physicians' overeager interventions and carelessness. Although some physicians found the accusation of physician blame "altogether too sweeping in its nature," most had to acknowledge the role of the profession in keeping the rate of postpartum infection high.[69] Physicians discussing the subject before the Wisconsin State Medical Society in 1902, for example, concluded that "nine-tenths of the vaginal examinations were absolutely unnecessary," and that the medical profession could be blamed for "frequently infecting patients by means of digital examinations."[70]

Dr. M. Howard Fussell of Philadelphia lamented the conditions under which physicians had to attend their private patients but nonetheless urged physicians to take responsibility for cleanliness. "I have often wondered whether the use of antiseptic solutions is an unmixed good, so frequently have I seen gentlemen simply rinse their hands with soap and water, immerse them in antiseptic solution, and be fully convinced that their hands were aseptic, that I have often wished they knew nothing whatever of bichlorid of mercury and its like," he wrote. Fussell understood the pressures under which general practitioners labored:

> The man in general practice is constantly called in the middle of a busy day to attend a case of labor; he is hurried; he does not wish to remain if it is necessary; indeed, he can not do so, but he should never allow his hurry and his desire to get through to interfere with the first law of cleanliness.

Fussell urged scrubbing hands thoroughly five or ten minutes, dressing in clean clothes, and using the Kelly pad. He worried that physicians often could not or did not observe the strict routine. "I have seen a man carefully boil his forceps, just as carefully scrub his hands, take the forceps from the receptacle, deliberately pick a towel up from the floor and wipe off the forceps," he related. "Certainly all the precautions of boiling and of scrubbing the hands had been made useless by this act."[71]

Birth attendants (physicians and midwives) were only some of the possible agents of infection in the birthing rooms. Dr. Frances Lee puzzled over a postpartum infection in one of her patients in 1898 because she thought she "had observed all the precautions necessary to an antiseptic and aseptic conduct of the case." Then she realized that the husband had been "surly and glum," and suspected he might be the key to understanding his wife's situation: "Putting the question directly, I found the patient had been submitted to sexual intercourse on the night of the third day, and morning and night of the fourth day, three times in thirty-six hours. . . . The patient stated that she had been submitted to intercourse on the third and fourth days after each confinement." The doctor questioned, "Is the physician always guilty of conveying the infection to the lying-in patient? If this patient had died who would have been held responsible? The physician, of course."[72] Dr. S. H. Blakely of Severance, Kansas, similarly reported a case of postpartum infection that he thought was caused by "a horse with a suppurating sore. The husband of the woman was treating the horse and the transmission was probably by him via the family wash pan, or perhaps still more directly. I consider the husband to be frequently the most dangerous source of trouble not excepting the old granny nurse, who, though ignorant, does generally clean up a little on such occasions."[73]

The prevalence of gonorrhea in the general population affected the incidence of postpartum infection and added to the dangers women faced in pregnancy and childbirth. Not only did the disease make it difficult for an affected woman to carry to term, it also led to increased infections. Physicians reported women whose postpartum danger increased because of recent gonorrheal infections. "Who of us having daughters," asked Dr. Albert Burr of Chicago, "do not look with apprehension as to their future health and safety in the relation of wives and mothers?" Burr did not try to estimate the extent of gonorrhea in the population, but he said it was "of very frequent occurrence." He cited estimates of up to 80 percent of males having been infected at some time of their lives. Thus, "a large number of prospective mothers in or out of wedlock, innocent victims or *particeps criminis*, become the unfortunate hostesses of pathogenic germs that place them in dire perils at childbirth."[74] Dr. Anna Blount, an obstetrician in Oak Park, Illinois, reported the case history of one of her patients whose delivery was complicated by the fact that her sexual partner had given her gonorrhea. In managing this case, Blount became aware of a medical "conspiracy of silence" about the existence of gonorrhea in the population, although, she insisted, "you do not need statistics to convince you that this malady is common."[75]

Today physicians and historians have joined the debate about the extent to which venereally transmitted infection may have contributed to women's postpartum infections during the nineteenth and early twentieth centuries. Dorothy Lansing, Robert Penman, and Dorland Davis have suggested that physicians may have been unfairly blamed for women's severe sepsis problems, and that the cause might well have been the Group B Beta Hemolytic Streptococcus, which is transmitted venereally.[76] Their evidence does not negate the evidence that physicians brought some new infection to the birthing women they attended, but it adds a new dimension to our thinking about the extent of medical culpability in the propagation of postpartum fevers. Physicians inevitably brought some new infection into America's birthing rooms with their new procedures and imperfect technique, but they were not the sole cause of the high rates of postpartum infection suffered by women.

Called to cases of postpartum women suffering from high fever and raging infection, physicians developed strategies to try to insure that the infection did not lead to death. Dr. Madison Reece, for example, of Abingdon, Illinois, was called in 1881 to a woman's bedside:

> I found her in a small bed-room, only large enough for the bed upon which she was lying, with but one window in the room. She had been confined a week previously. Her pulse was 160, her tempera-

> ture 106, the tongue dry, abdomen distended to the size of a woman at full term, the secretion of milk suppressed. She was delirious, and an odor filled the room like that of a body far gone in putrefaction.

Informing the husband that "there was no probability whatever for the recovery of his wife," Reece set about injecting antiseptics into her uterus. "The discharge from the uterus was of such a peculiarly strong odor, that it was impossible to free the hands from it. It was like that one acquires in the dissection of bodies." Unexpectedly and immediately following the cleansing process "the delerium passed off, the temperature fell, the pulse came down—in short, the effect was simply magical," Reece reported. The woman recovered, and Reece became an eager advocate of antiseptic douches following delivery.[77]

Surgery emerged as another possible cure for particularly difficult cases of infection. In 1895, Dr. Charles Noble of the Kensington Hospital for Women in Philadelphia advocated "the performance of hysterectomy for infection of the uterus, when in spite of thorough curettement, followed by copious irrigation of the utero-vaginal canal, and the use of an iodoform suppository and gauze within the uterus, the septic symptoms increase in severity." He believed less radical measures should be attempted for 24 to 48 hours, but that if women did not respond, hysterectomy might prove the only possible way to save their lives.[78] Dr. Reuben Peterson of Grand Rapids, Michigan, agreed that prompt hysterectomy, performed before the infection invaded other organs, could save women's lives.[79] Dr. R. R. Kime of Atlanta, Georgia, however, thought hysterectomy too radical and risky a procedure for most puerperal infection cases, instead he advocated a thorough antiseptic regimen before and after labor.[80] Similarly, Dr. C. S. Bacon of Chicago, found the surgical cure for puerperal infection "exceedingly limited."[81]

Less radical than surgical hysterectomy, and more commonly employed at the turn of the twentieth century, was cleansing and scraping the uterus with the curette. But this procedure also was not without risk to the patient, because of the possibility of perforating the uterus with the sharp instrument, and physicians frequently argued against the curette.[82] "I am aware that many advocate the use of the curette in septic conditions of the uterus following abortions or after labor," wrote Dr. D. S. Fairchild, of Clinton, Iowa. But, he continued, "I have of late years been led to believe that this is not an altogether safe practice to follow." Fairchild believed that if placental tissue was retained in the uterus following delivery, physicians could safely remove it with a curette using antiseptic precautions. But after infection developed, the curette could inflict increased trauma and facilitate faster absorption of the infection. "This paper is presented," he said, "as a protest against what I believe to be an indiscriminate use of the curette in acute infection of the uterus."[83]

Dr. J. T. Priestly, a general practitioner from Iowa, described his practice following a septic delivery: "I . . . take a Munde curette, which is very large, almost the size of the curve of my finger, and use it to curette the uterine cavity. It has no sharp cutting edge, and with it the uterus can be easily scraped. At the same time I flush it with sterilized hot water. . . . I think I have benefited a great many of my patients by this procedure."[84] Dr. Morcedai Price of Philadelphia believed the curette and its accompanying intrauterine irrigation to be very dangerous to women: "The mortality and the danger following such procedures," he said, "is probably the result of at least 50 per cent. of the deaths from puerperal fever."[85] To the extent that physicians employed indiscriminate use of the sharp curette, postpartum infection may have been enhanced rather than stemmed.

Physicians' efforts in the birthing rooms, especially those aimed at creating a sterile environment for birth, frequently met with resistance from their patients or their patients' friends. As Dr. Norman Roberts of Fort Stanton, New Mexico, wrote, "It is easy to scrub one's own hands, while it requires more than ordinary tact and courage to succeed in inducing a frightened woman to submit to a disagreeable procedure which all her female friends assure her is unnecessary."[86] Yet some doctors were able to create the atmosphere they desired. "I find the people, however ignorant they may be," wrote Dr. Ida Case in 1895, "ready and willing to assist me in carrying out any plans which will prevent child-bed fever; so I meet with no opposition on the part of the patients I attend. This is the more remarkable because I am the only physician in this place who uses this method."[87] Similarly, a Wisconsin physician urged his colleagues not to hesitate in enforcing their own ideas of cleanliness in the birthing rooms they attended. Proper medical authority, he believed, could insure that a birth be carried out under ideal aseptic conditions.[88]

Other physicians did not find it so easy to gain cooperation around their efforts to be scrupulously clean. "The dirty hand of an officious though kind neighbor may at the critical moment upset our closely observed technique, or render an indifferent technique fatally faulty," observed one doctor.[89] This physician worried not about resistance on the part of the woman's friends, but their lack of understanding of the requirements of the sterile technique.

"We who are in private practise," wrote Dr. Emma Neal of Iowa, "must work under the more or less close scrutiny of the patient's relatives, who all too often have been brought up in the belief that nature should be allowed to take her course unaided, and that interference of any sort is flying in the face of Providence. . . . Probably none of us will live long enough to see all of our patients willing to follow all the advice we give them, but there is considerable satisfaction in knowing that we have done our best."[90] Dr. Benjamin Washburn optimistically recorded that his obstetrical work in 1910 brought about "marked improvement" in his North Carolina community: "The women were quick to recognize the benefits of cleanliness and to note the decrease in childbed fever as well as the more rapid convalescence in cases where the superstitious practices of midwives were not employed."[91]

Many physicians concluded from their experiences that doctors had to become educators and take the time to teach women the importance of cleanliness in the birthing room. "The time was when the doctor's dirty finger was believed to be almost the sole source of infection," wrote Dr. Olive Wilson. "I believe it is not true to-day. The majority of women are ignorant of true cleanliness at such a time. It is a duty we owe the parturient patient to instruct her in the surgical cleansing of her body and preparing her to resist this preventable catastrophe, puerperal septicaemia."[92]

The escalation of the level of difficulty in managing normal labor and delivery at the turn of the twentieth century due directly to knowledge of germ transmission caused physicians and, increasingly, their patients to believe that "all obstetric cases should be treated like surgical cases, and the same precautions taken as in a surgical operation."[93] The requirements of asepsis were severe, and physicians bemoaned their inability to meet them all. Doctors might have encouraged one another to enforce their own ideas in the birth rooms, but when that meant removing all carpets and draperies, washing furniture in lysol, providing new mattresses and bedding, spraying daily prior to accouchement, cleansing of all attendants, shaving the pubic hair surrounding the genitalia, sterilizing clothing, instruments, and other accoutrements of the birth room, enforcement remained virtually impossible. The hospital, a controlled environment in which sterile conditions appeared more easily attainable, increasingly beckoned.

At the beginning of the twentieth century, when physicians became conscious of the added burdens of their obstetric work, they began to notice that they did not get adequate compensation for these additional labors. Dr. J. F. Baldwin in 1902 called obstetrical fees "ridiculously inadequate." He claimed that Ohio doctors received only about $10 per case. "An obstetric engagement, carrying with it the responsibility which it does," he concluded, "should certainly furnish as much compensation as a mere broken leg." He realized that poor patients could not afford larger physician fees, but he hoped that the "fees of the rich should make up for the lack among the poor."[94] Dr. C. S. Bacon of Chicago concurred about the inadequacy of obstetric fees. He thought that "hasty obstetric work" was attributable to the "insufficient compensation which is almost universally given physicians for the management of cases of labor." He continued:

> Why should one agree to take charge of a case for a certain fee not knowing whether the labor will last two hours or two days? The result of this practice is to induce the physician to hasten the labor with [adverse] effects. How can a physician be expected to watch a case carefully and patiently when he knows that his fee for twenty hours of work which have kept him from his sleep and his office and other practice will be $10, this also including his compensation for previous and subsequent visits? It is no doubt true that much of the obstetric work pays less than 50 cents an hour, less than the wages of a carpenter or plumber.

Bacon, and much of the profession with him, asserted that the quality of physicians' obstetric work might improve if the quantity of compensation for it increased.[95]

The economics of obstetric practices underline the precarious state of the art at the turn of the twentieth century. Physicians were not yet meeting the needs of the birthing women who had invited them to attend their deliveries, and an enormous variation in medical abilities and practices persisted. Some women, when they suffered at the hands of inexperienced, inept, or harassed physicians, understood first hand the limitations of medical midwifery. Other women believed from their positive experiences that medicine at its best could offer them a safe and expeditious labor and delivery. But the practice of obstetrics was not standardized, and it could not always deliver the promises it made. Childbirth remained hazardous and difficult in the very era when medicine at large was beginning to show its mettle. The pressures exerted by women and by physicians to improve these imperfect birthing conditions ultimately encouraged the move into the hospitals, where both groups believed birth could be more safely managed. This twentieth-century transition will be explored in the next chapter.

7

"Alone Among Strangers"

Birth Moves to the Hospital

Modern hospital births, streamlined and under the observation and control of specialist nurses and doctors, became increasingly attractive to middle-class American women in the second and third decades of the twentieth century. Some hospitals were so enticing, in fact, that author Betty MacDonald, giving birth in the 1920s, recalled, "The prospect of two weeks in that heavenly place tempted me to stay pregnant all the rest of my life."[1] The hospital offered what many considered to be the safest application of the newest technological and scientific methods of birth. Furthermore, the environment, the food, the total care from the nurses all made the hospital stay seem like a vacation from domestic chores and greatly to be desired. Because of the dual attraction of new medicine and comfort, of safety and convenience, upper- and middle-class women increasingly sought an institutional location for their confinements. By 1940, 55 percent of America's births took place within hospitals; by 1950, hospital births had increased to 88 percent of the total; and by 1960, outside of some isolated rural areas, it was almost unheard of for American women to deliver their babies at home.[2]

This chapter will examine the transition that first upper- and middle-class and later almost all American women made from home to hospital deliveries and will analyze the role that birthing women played in the transition. Second, the chapter will look at what women found once they got to the hospital and assess the extent to which their expectations for safer and more comfortable births were met.

Before the twentieth century almost all American women had their

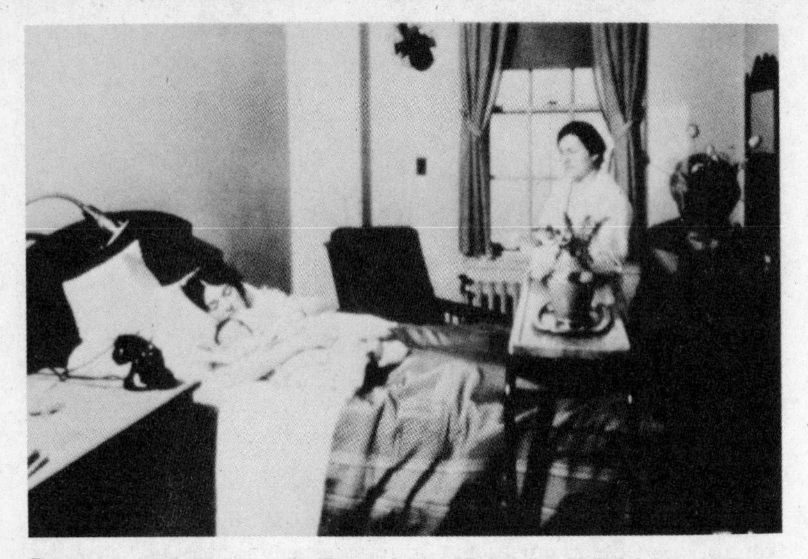

Private maternity room at the Pennsylvania Hospital in Philadelphia, 1930. Source: Pennsylvania Hospital Archives.

babies at home.[3] A few poor urban women went to charity hospitals or medical school dispensaries in the late eighteenth and nineteenth century (probably not more than five percent of the total), but this was rarely because of choice. Women considered their own homes, surrounded by familiar women friends and relatives, to be the most desirable birth setting, and both midwives and doctors entered this domestic woman-centered environment to attend labor and delivery. The system worked well because it was cost-effective and in most cases it resulted in live deliveries. Furthermore, it allowed women who had some financial options to combine traditional practices with medicine's ever-evolving innovations. Women could keep their comforting bedroom location and their women helpers and at the same time take advantage of medical technology and expertise. They could, in short, get what seemed to be the best of both worlds of women's tradition and men's medicine. Anita McCormick Blaine, for example, whose economic and social position in Chicago allowed her to choose optimum care when she first became pregnant in 1890, determined to have her baby in her childhood home and to be surrounded by her friends and relatives. While two women supported her, and her husband waited outside, a doctor administered chloroform to make her more comfortable while he delivered her child. She wanted and got the traditional home birth experience accompanied by the most that medicine had to offer.[4]

In the twentieth century, however, middle- and upper-class women like Anita Blaine and the growing number of physicians specializing in obstetrics increasingly found fault with these home-based childbirth practices. The application of new notions of germ transmission particularly made home deliveries difficult to manage. From both birthing women and their physicians came pressure to change procedures and to modernize birth by moving it to the hospital.

In part women's desires to go to the hospital in the first third of the twentieth century reflected merely one more instance of a movement that had begun in the eighteenth century, when male physicians first began attending normal births in this country. Since that time, women who could afford them sought out the newest technological and medical advances in obstetrics. Middle-class women invited male physicians into their home birthing rooms to use forceps, ether, and chloroform and to perform surgical operations because they believed this would help them become living mothers of living children.[5] Motivated in large part by fears of death and long-lasting debility that seemed the all too common results of childbirth, women sought the promise of improvements, of hope, of "science." The expectation that death could just as likely result from childbirth as could life led women on a long search for better and safer births. In the eighteenth and nineteenth centuries the search for improved birthing conditions led women to seek medical help in their homes. In the twentieth century, it led American women into hospitals.

A close examination of the experiences of the early generations of hospital-going women, however, reveals a significant difference between nineteenth-century, medically managed home births and twentieth-century hospital-based obstetrics. Through all the innovations of the nineteenth century, doctors were invited guests in women's homes, and birthing women or their representatives retained the ability to make critical decisions about the conduct of labor and delivery. In the early twentieth century, however, women were ready, willing, and even eager to give up the control they had in their own homes and to put themselves more completely in the hands of obstetricians and medical institutions, putting their faith and their bodies more entirely into the hands of science.

Why?

The traditional answers to this question have centered on medical progress and doctors' convenience. Hospital use increased, it is argued, because at last science, following the bacteriological and surgical revolutions, had something to offer: people flocked to take advantage of the expertise of the new medical scientists.[6] I believe that an important part of the explanation is rightly placed in the realm of scientific advances. However, in obstetrics it was more the image of science's potential, the lure of what science could offer, than any proven accomplishments that attracted women to the hospital. When most middle-class women like Betty MacDonald decided to go to the hospital to deliver their babies in the 1920s and 1930s, there were no statistics proving to them that science applied in the hospital had in fact made birth safer. Maternal mortality remained high during this period. To understand why women wanted to go to the hospital to have their babies in the 1920s and 1930s, we must take into account two factors other than proven safety, both of which are difficult to trace but essential parts of the transition. First is the increasing mystification of medical knowledge in the post-bacteriological era; second is the declining ability of women's traditional networks to meet the demands of childbirth.

Turn-of-the-century laboratory-based medicine showed that health could be enhanced by the application of scientific principles. Surgery was the most promising example of the new medicine, but the control of certain infectious diseases and the declining rate of infant deaths indicated a broad scope of possibilities. The lure of what could happen in obstetrics if the scientific principles could be applied within medical institutions seemed to hold out the potential of making safe—at last—women's most dangerous moments. The price of the new science was a growing separation between expert and layperson, between obstetrical specialists and birthing women. Medical scientists understood bacteriology and surgical procedures, but birthing women did not have access to the intricacies of the new science. The knowledge gap produced when medicine became increasingly technical put the uninformed in awe of medical science. Patients seeking the newest that science had to offer were intimidated in the face of the language and aura surrounding "Science," in their minds spelled with a capital S, and they came to accept the benefits of medicine without knowing how they worked.[7] "I have placed myself in the hands of . . . a specialist in obstetrics," wrote Lella Secor to her mother in 1918. "I have every confidence in him, and it is a great relief."[8] The distancing of scientific knowledge and technical expertise from the general population enhanced its appeal for millions of Americans.

Instead of trying to keep medical science within women's control, as women had wanted in the nineteenth and very early twentieth century, by the 1920s and 1930s women urged one another to follow specialists' directions without necessarily understanding them. "See an obstetrician early," *Hygeia* urged its readers, "He will take care of the rest."[9] Dr. Josephine Kenyon told *Good Housekeeping* readers, "choose a doctor you have faith in. You can trust him to guide you through."[10] Despite continuing high maternal mortality rates, women's journals repeatedly argued that the new hospital-based childbirth meant real progress. "Slowly but surely," *Good Housekeeping* proclaimed, "childbirth is being lifted out of the realm of darkness into the spotlight of new science."[11]

Seeking the newest and best way to have babies and convinced that traditional ways of giving birth had been superseded, women wanted to believe that progress had finally come for them. The popular literature on childbirth in the 1920s and 1930s reveals the hope of women that the almost universal experience of womankind could be made less dreadful through science. Articles in women's journals were filled with heart-rending personal examples of women whose lives would have been saved if they had been in the hospital for their confinements. For example, Ann Hamilton, an American of "pioneer stock" who "loved America, its traditions, its ideals, and its promises for the future in which her children would have their part," had a protracted labor at home in 1920 attended by a general practitioner who "did his best, but . . . had nothing with which to work" and by a neighbor who "was not a trained nurse and did not know what to do." Her 60-hour labor ordeal resulted in her death and in the death of her baby.[12] Through such emotion-laden examples, the possibilities of scientific obstetrics captured birthing women, who, like the rest of the population, were determined to join the march of medical progress.

If promises and hope pulled women toward medical institutions in the early twentieth century, an equally potent force pushed them away from their traditional confinements. The hospital beckoned the growing number of women who found their home births logistically difficult to manage. Hallie Nelson's experiences in drought-ridden rural Nebraska emphasized some of the reasons women had begun to dread the ordeal of childbirth at home. Recalling when she was pregnant with her fifth child in 1936, Nelson wrote: "We had been at wit's ends to find a woman to take care of me and the baby and to help take care of the children." While she had been relatively successful in finding neighboring friends and relatives to attend her during her first four births, this time Hallie lamented: "The Clines had left the hills. . . . My sister Beulah was not available. . . . The other neighbors had children of their own to care for." Similarly, Ida Wolsey wrote after her fourth confinement that her husband Tom had "hired a woman to come from Payson to help me. She stayed a few days—it was about Christmas time—and then went home to spend Christmas. Tom came home from his work on the railroad to spend Christmas. She did not come back because she was ill. Tom had to leave and we were on the spot."[13]

The traditional woman-centered event in the home, called by historians "social childbirth," had been predicated on women being available when parturients needed them. With the help of her friends and relatives, a birthing woman could manage both the birth itself and her household. Domestic life swirled around the birthing bed while the confined woman received the ministrations of her friends. She was part of the household and at the same time the recipient of special favors. Her friends and relatives took care of her during and after labor and delivery, watched her children, fed her husband, and did her domestic chores. In turn, she would be expected to reciprocate when her friends' time came.

The mobility and urbanization of the nineteenth century had strained these traditional practices. Women had fewer friends around them during and after labor and delivery than their eighteenth-century foremothers, but adjustments to the system did not change its basic structure. Nineteenth-century women were able to maintain the crucial elements of female-centered birth, as countless diaries and autobiographies reveal. Sister Eva, Cousin Sarah, or Mrs. Campbell from down the road came for the confinement and stayed to do the domestic work that the parturient usually did.[14]

But the forces that made traditional practices difficult in the nineteenth century finally destroyed the women's social networks in the twentieth century. Increased physical and psychological isolation left women in situations in which they simply could not find the help they needed. Helen Whiting of Winchester, Virginia, believed that "If there are other children, the mother cannot have the peace and rest she needs [at home]."[15] Getting out of the home for confinements seemed the only way of coping with the stress that developed when a woman was ready to deliver her baby.

The growth of hospitals around the country during these early twentieth-century years when women began to feel the need to leave their homes for their confinements gave added force to their argument. The transformation of hospitals from their nineteenth-century public-

and private-charity focus to their twentieth-century private-paying-patient emphasis provided an alternative for birthing women, just at the moment in their history when women most needed it. Hospitals, and the specialist doctors they recruited, encouraged birthing women to consider the institutional alternative by praising the institutional potential of managing sterile and infection-free deliveries.

The hospital, lauded as the newest and best place for delivery, looked doubly attractive to women who could not create a supportive home atmosphere. As one woman put it: "Sure! It would be nice to have babies born at home! But who is going to bathe the baby . . . bring the mother's tray . . . change her sheets? Who?" The home did not hold for the twentieth-century women the same comforts and sustenance that Anita McCormick Blaine had found so reassuring in 1890. The "hospital is equipped with every modern device for the safe delivery of babies," wrote one mother, "nursing and medical attention is available at any hour of the day or night. How much simpler—and more restful—to be in a hospital where babies are an accepted business."[16] Another woman found, "My stay in that hospital was like a lovely vacation." "I can't tell you the relief I feel as I walk out my door headed for the hospital to have a baby," wrote another. "I have nothing to worry about . . . and have only to concentrate on giving birth. All this peace of mind, plus expert medical attention, makes me wonder why anybody would consider it a 'privilege' to have her baby at home."[17]

So growing numbers of women went to the hospital to give birth.[18] They were welcomed and encouraged by physicians specializing in obstetrics who also found the hospital environment attractive. Filled with equipment and supporting staff, hospitals made delivering babies easier and less time-consuming. But more important than their convenience, doctors argued, hospitals made birth safer.[19] Physicians found it difficult to achieve infection-free deliveries at home births, in part because the home did not easily allow for sterilization and proper positioning of the parturient. "Little, very little, can be offered in favor of attending women (rich or poor) in the act of birth at their homes," claimed Dr. Gustav Zinke of Cincinnati, Ohio:

> The argument that women love their homes and abhor the idea of going to a hospital for the purpose of confinement is only a sentiment begotten of custom and deserves no special refutation. Let women once appreciate that the hospital is the safest place for them to pass through the ordeal of labor, they will seek it of their own accord.

Zinke's conclusions received general approval at the 1901 meeting of the American Medical Association. Dr. Philander Harris of Paterson, New Jersey, for example, agreed that "When I and others of my age studied medicine, hospitals were regarded as death-traps," but at the turn of the new century he believed "a well-ordered hospital is the very safest place for a woman during her confinement."[20] Beginning in the early part of the century and increasing throughout the 1920s and 1930s, popular journals as well as medical journals urged women to go to the hospital to receive the best possible obstetrical care and to insure the safety of both mother and child.

Physicians trained in the new century found a great contrast between their hospital training and obstetrics practice in women's homes where they could not maintain sterile conditions or have trained help. Dr. Charles Fox Gardiner described one home birth he attended near the turn of the century in Colorado, contrasting it to his previous hospital experience:

> As I sat there in that cabin, all alone with my patient, I could not resist a smile at the contrast between my present position and the maternity room of the big hospital where I treated such cases in New York, and, as I watched, by the light of the stove, the little drifts of snow came sifting in through every crack, heard the roar of the wind, and felt the deadly cold increase hour by hour, I pictured that white and spotless delivery room, so warm, so sheltered from any noise or draught; those white robed nurses, so alert and skilled in their duties; that trained anesthetist, so sure and safe; that chief in charge ready to help a novice over the hard places; all so complete, so restful, that one was merely part of a well-oiled machine, while here I was completely cut off from any help, no matter what happened.[21]

For the attending physician, deliveries in the hospital held the prospect of security and safety. Dr. "Bessie" worried about the ill-equipped homes of her Iowa patients and realized how much rested on her shoulders: "what ever the situation demanded, I had to improvise and find some solution. I had no anesthetist, nurse, or intern standing by. Whatever garment, sponge, towel, instrument, or vessel I needed, I had to take care of myself." Dr. Henry P. Newman of Chicago concluded simply, "the appointments of the modern hospital should be preferred to the makeshifts of home treatments." Similarly, Dr. Mabel Gardiner, writing in 1924, found the hospital far superior to the home:

> In the course of the delivery of a condition that would in the home constitute anything from an inconvenience to an emergency, with serious consequences, such as posterior position, failure of the head to descend, postpartum hemorrhage or second degree laceration, may in the hospital be cared for as a mere incident of the delivery, because the proper assistance, instruments, and lights are at hand. . . . the home can never equal the hospital. The "lying-in-chamber" is pictured down through historical scenes as the bed chamber in the home, but as the barber applying leeches has given way to the surgeon, so the bed chamber must give way to the hospital delivery room, and our united efforts should be to encourage women to know that hospital care is the best care, and to be obtained, if possible, even at a sacrifice, and home care is second best, even though more sociable in its family relations.[22]

The move to the hospital was hastened by specialists' attempts to wrest birth away from general practitioners by systematizing birth procedures within the hospital setting. One very influential move in this direction was made in 1920 by Joseph B. DeLee of Chicago in the first volume of the new journal for specialists, the *American Journal of Obstetrics and Gynecology*. DeLee argued that birth was a "pathologic process" and that "only a small minority of women escape damage during labor." He continued: "So frequent are these bad effects, that I have often wondered whether Nature did not deliberately intend women should be used up in the process of reproduction, in a manner analogous to that of salmon, which dies after spawning?" DeLee believed that birth, because of its dangers, needed careful monitoring in skilled hands. He recommended reducing birth to predictable patterns by using outlet forceps and episiotomy routinely and prophylactically in normal deliveries. DeLee sedated the parturient with scopolamine, allowed the cervix to dilate, gave ether during the second stage, performed an episiotomy, and lifted the fetus with forceps. He then extracted the placenta, gave ergot to help the uterus contract, and stitched the perineal cut. DeLee believed this new obstetrical practice could save the lives of many women and make their postpartum experience less traumatic. He recommended that only obstetric specialists perform the operation of prophylactic forceps. "I have always felt," he confessed, "that we must not bring the ideals of obstetrics down to the level of the general practitioner—we must bring the general practice of obstetrics up to the level of that of the specialist."[23]

DeLee's prophylactic operation represented the new move in the 1920s and 1930s to make obstetrics scientific, systematic, and predictable by putting it under the control of the specialist, a move that occurred simultaneously in other medical specialties. The reaction to DeLee's paper indicated, however, that not all obstetric specialists wanted to use prophylactic forceps. J. Whitridge Williams strongly objected that DeLee proposed too much interference. He called the Chicago obstetrician "perniciously active," asserting that "it seems to me that he interferes 19 times too often out of 20."[24] Despite some significant objections among DeLee's colleagues to his particular regimen, the idea of systematic interventions in normal labors in hospitals did take hold in the obstetric community. Hospital-based obstetricians developed routines for managing childbirth that incorporated systematic use of pain-relieving drugs, labor inducers, and technological intervention.

Mothers-to-be learned they could plan when they would have a baby, and doctors could predict the course of labor because they controlled it. "The old way [of having a baby] was no fun," wrote one father about the 1916 birth of his first daughter. Twenty-two years later, in 1938, his second wife gave birth to another daughter, who "was born the new way—the easy, painless, streamlined way." His wife, in consultation with her doctor, decided which day to deliver, and after a matinee and dinner went into the hospital. Pituitrin induced her labor, Nembutal and scopolamine deadened her perceptions of it, and the doctor delivered her baby. "Why, I wouldn't mind having another baby next week," she said, "if that's all there is to it."[25] Increasing numbers of middle-class women turned to the hospital and the specialist for their childbirths, believing, as one of them put it, "the vexation of hospital routine shrinks to infinitesimal importance beside the safety of the delivery room."[26]

In ideal hospital deliveries women left their families and friends at the door of the labor room and faced their birthings alone, as one account of birth in the 1930s indicated:

> Arriving [at the hospital], she is immediately given the benefit of one of the modern analgesics or pain-killers. Soon she is in a dreamy, half-conscious state at the height of a pain, sound asleep between spasms. . . . She knows nothing about being taken to a spotlessly clean delivery room, placed on a sterile table, draped with sterile sheets; neither does she see her attendants, the doctor and nurses, garbed for her protection in sterile white gowns and gloves; nor the shiny boiled instruments and antiseptic solutions. She does not hear

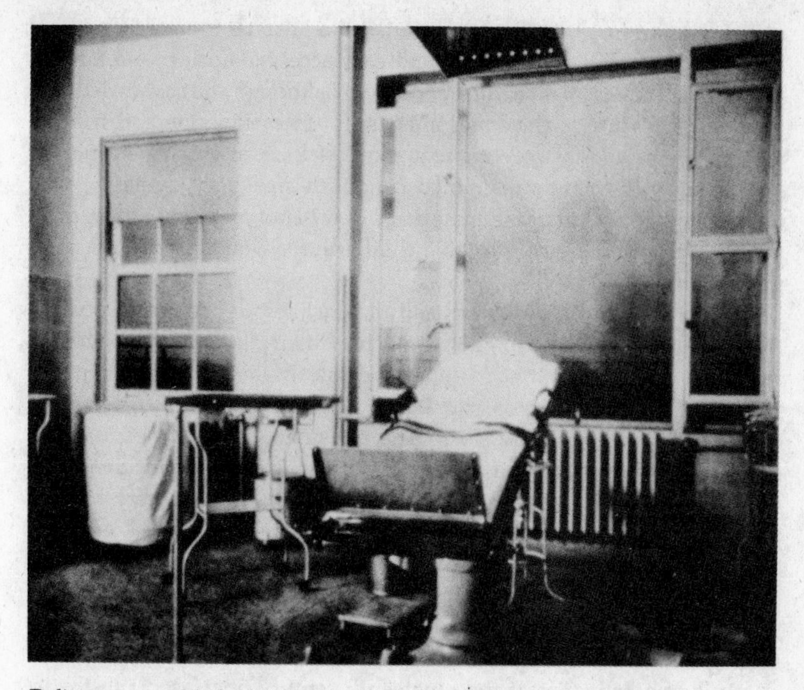

Delivery room, Methodist Hospital, Madison, Wisconsin, ca. 1929.
Source: Methodist Hospital, Madison, Wisconsin.

> the cry of her baby when first he feels the chill of this cold world, or see the care with which the doctor repairs such lacerations as may have occurred. She is, as most of us want to be when severe pain has us in its grasp—asleep. Finally she awakes in smiles, a mother with no recollection of having become one.[27]

This woman was separated from the people she loved; she was in an unfamiliar environment controlled by others; and she was unconscious during parts of her labor and delivery. She was also without the fears and anxieties that had haunted generations of her foremothers. Women did not view the stay in the hospital as a time when they lost important parts of the traditional birth experience, but rather as a time when they gained protection for life and health, aspects of birth that had been elusive and uncertain in the past. They gave up some kinds of control for others because on balance the new benefits seemed more important. Erva Slayton refused her mother's and sister's offers to be confined at their homes, assuring them in 1919, "I really selected the hospital from choice." She believed the sterile environment and easy access to doctors and nurses offered her the optimal birthing conditions, although she acknowledged "the worst feature is the lonesomeness."[28] In seeking life and health, women were willing to relinquish some of their traditional supports.

But was the new streamlined childbirth safe? Did increasing the use of the hospital increase maternal safety? Had medicine at last provided safer and more comfortable childbirth for women, as it had promised since the 1760s?

Observers in the 1930s realized that, while the practice of obstetrics now could relieve women of much of their discomfort, childbirth remained as unsafe as it had been in the past. Maternal mortality in the 1930s remained "unnecessarily high," according to a group of concerned physicians in New York. The physicians claimed hospital deliveries contributed to the high mortality with a "high incidence of operative interference during labor . . . undertaken when there was no indication or a plain contra-indication." Birth in the hospital encouraged interference because the equipment and staff were readily accessible. Rather than making childbirth safer, physicians in the 1920s and 1930s, according to their own evaluation, were responsible for maintaining unnecessarily high rates of maternal mortality.[29]

In home deliveries of the nineteenth century, increased anesthetic use had not caused an increase in forceps deliveries, but in hospital deliveries of the early twentieth century, a direct relationship existed between anesthesia and forceps. The New York doctors noted that "The frequent use of instrumentation is based upon the easy accessibility of anaesthesia. . . . the increase in the use of anaesthesia is a factor in keeping the maternal mortality rate stationary." According to the New York study, use of anesthetic agents led directly to increased instrumentation because drugged women were less effective at pushing the baby out. Approximately 25 percent of hospital deliveries were operative. "The increase in the use of instrumentation brings with it an increased hazard," the doctors found. "Clearly a reduction of the mortality rate can be achieved through a reduction in operative interference."[30]

If the hospitals were safer for childbirth, maternal mortality rates should have begun to decrease as more women entered the hospitals; in fact, the death rates stayed the same or even increased in the years when women began going to the hospital to give birth.[31] Urban rates of puerperal infection increased particularly during the decade of the 1920s, indicating that hospitals may have increased maternity-related infection risks for women. (See graphs.) The direct relationship is im-

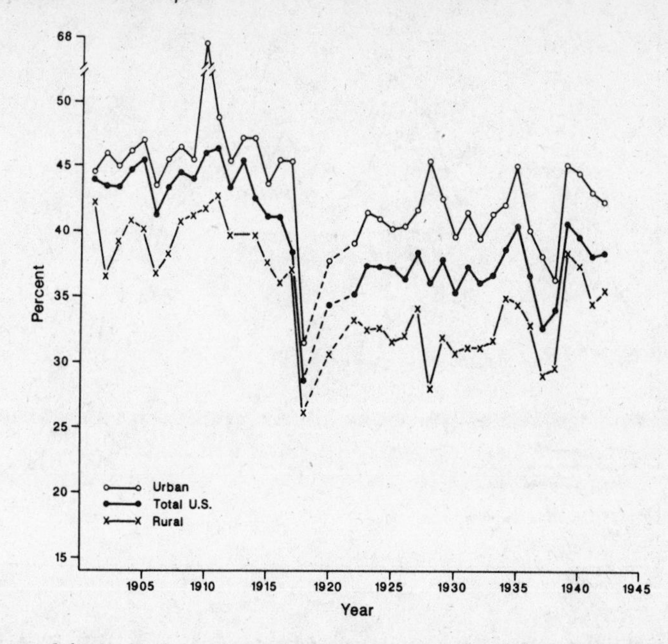

Puerperal fever deaths as percent of total maternal mortality. Notice that rates did not decline during the 1920s, although increasing numbers of women were going to the hospital to deliver.

Source: My thanks to Charlotte Borst for constructing this graph.

possible to reconstruct with available data, but the rise in postpartum infection during the very decade when thousands of women were for the first time choosing the hospital for their place of confinement is suggestive.

Not eager to admit it even among themselves, doctors and public health officials in the 1920s tentatively groped for answers as to why modern medicine—showing its mettle so strongly in areas outside of obstetrics—could not control, within its own halls and by its own experts, the ravages of puerperal death. Dr. Joseph B. DeLee of the Chicago Lying-In Hospital, who earlier had encouraged operative interference in most births, was one of the most outspoken when he faced his own and his profession's shortcomings.[32] Humbled by the apparent truth that infection spread in the hospital despite careful aseptic and antiseptic techniques, DeLee accused himself and his colleagues of bringing about the deaths of thousands of women each year.

Drawing on his thirty-four years of experience in eight Chicago

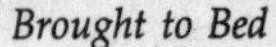

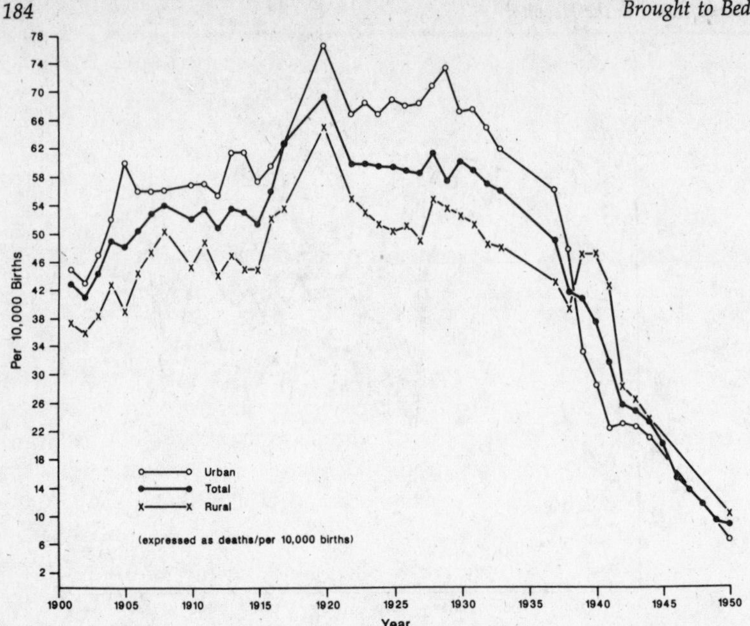

Maternal death rates from all childbirth-related causes, U.S., 1901–50. Notice the divergence between urban and rural in the 1920s. As more urban women delivered in the hospital, their risks did not decline.

Source: My thanks to Charlotte Borst for constructing this graph.

hospitals, DeLee in 1926 blamed the "great evils [which] swell the mortality and morbidity of the mothers and babies in the United States" on both physicians' practices and hospitals' physical structure. He observed that the "service rendered the patient in the obstetric ward is nearly always poorer than that in the rest of the hospital"; that, whereas general surgery had been standardized and regulated, "in the obstetric room each man does as he pleases"; and that "the aseptic technique is not insisted upon as it is in the surgery." He drove his argument home with his most important finding: "The peril lies in the infective influences which emanate from the wards devoted to medicine, surgery, gynecology, pediatrics, the laboratories and the autopsy room." DeLee, sounding much like Ignaz Semmelweis almost 100 years earlier, believed that nurses and doctors most frequently carried the infection from one place in the hospital to another, and that insufficiently disinfected linen also was responsible for distributing infection all over the hospital. Convinced by "numberless proofs that it is impossible to keep infections in bounds in our hospitals today, and that it will continue to be so long as human nature is what we know it to be," DeLee concluded, "the maternity ward in the general hospital of today is a dangerous place for a woman to have a baby."[33]

Seven years later, in 1933, DeLee, even more depressed by the situation in hospital obstetrics, noted, "the increasing preference of the hospital as a place of delivery, one of the most marked changes that has taken place during the last few years and is growing, seems not only not to have bettered the results but seems actually to have made them worse. . . . This development is increasing maternal mortality and morbidity." This specialist in obstetrics, drawn to the potential of scientific medicine but able to acknowledge its grave shortcomings, agreed with the conclusion that "home delivery, even under the poorest conditions, is safer than hospital delivery." But DeLee did not want to abandon hospitals as the location for medically directed childbirth. He called rather for major alterations in the physical structure of hospitals to separate obstetrics wards completely from all other parts of the hospital by an air corridor and by cutting all human and material communication. A separate building, separate staff, and separate laundry seemed the only way to insure that cross infection would be stopped. To his critics who said his plan was too costly, DeLee answered, "I will say only this: Nothing compares in value with human life."[34]

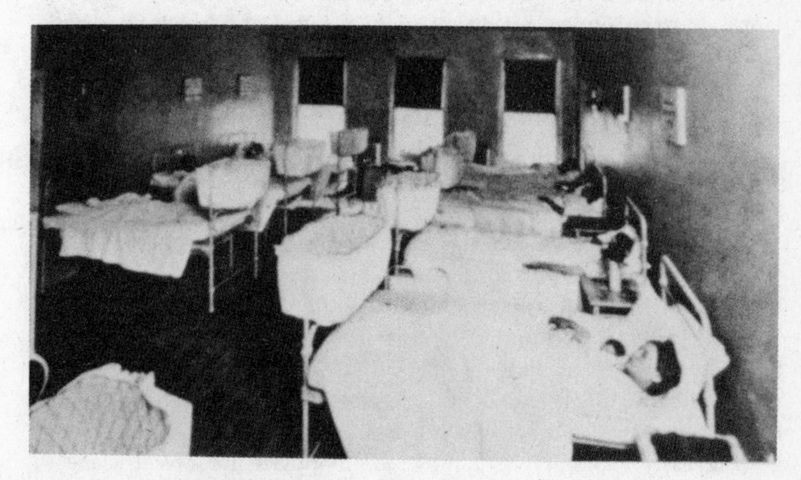

A charity ward at Jewish Maternity Hospital, New York, 1912.
Source: United Hospital Fund.

DeLee listed numerous outbreaks of hospital puerperal fever epidemics, and the medical journal reports bore him out. Around the country, general and maternity hospitals reported raging hospital infections among childbearing women that doctors could not prevent. DeLee believed that the reported epidemics represented only the tip of the iceberg, because most "hospital authorities use every effort at concealment."[35]

An uproar greeted DeLee's call for radical changes in hospital architecture in order to isolate birthing women from medical and surgical patients as the only way to make hospitals safe for confinements. Doctors led by the notable J. Whitridge Williams of Johns Hopkins vehemently opposed DeLee's costly innovations, countering that aseptic deliveries could be carried on within hospital wards. Williams based his views on his own equally impressive years of experience at the Johns Hopkins Hospital. Insisting that it was possible to stop cross infection by maintaining strict aseptic techniques in obstetric wards, Williams said that DeLee's insistence on sterilizing even the history charts of patients "represents a degree of caution that approaches 'infectio-phobia.' " But Williams did not want a fight: he thought that if the two of them could talk face to face they would discover that "our differences are less radical than they appear at first glance and are really more apparent than real."[36]

Other doctors entering the debate, however, took the disagreement between the two obstetric giants as real and significant, and virtually all of them who put their feelings in print sided with Williams. As one Connecticut doctor pointed out, DeLee's solutions harkened back to "the days of the miasmatic theory of the transmission of infections, and had thrown into discard all of the knowledge of aseptic technique that had been gained since that age in the history of medicine." Besides, this doctor concluded, DeLee's proposals were not "practical, workable and within the limits of the things possible for the average hospital or community."[37]

Despite the general disagreement with DeLee's solution to the problem, virtually no doctor disputed his claims that general hospitals when used for maternity cases (representing about 85 percent of all hospital births) could and did threaten women's lives. Dr. Florence Sherbon of Iowa concluded in 1917 that normal uncomplicated cases should stay at home and that "a certain menace [existed] in the intimate grouping of mothers [in hospitals] at the time of confinement." By the early 1930s it was almost commonplace for obstetricians to blame themselves for a large percentage of the preventable deaths of parturient women. The New York Academy of Medicine, the Philadelphia County Medical Society, the White House Conference on Child Health and Protection, and countless individual physicians went on record in the early 1930s proclaiming physicians themselves responsible for over half of America's preventable maternal deaths and claiming that the hospitals exacerbated these dangers.[38]

The medical profession confessed publicly and repeatedly the shortcomings of its obstetric practices. Dr. Rudolph Wieser Holmes declared at a crowded American Medical Association meeting in 1936: "I have seen hundreds of women die on the delivery table because of the wrongful use of drugs." Holmes blamed his own role in accelerating scopolamine use for many of these deaths. The public health commissioner for the state of New York calculated that maternal deaths were actually increasing during the first thirty years of the twentieth century and concluded that "they represent the results of meddlesome and unskillful obstetrical practice."[39] Philadelphia doctors agreed that the midwife was "an almost negligible factor in mortality," but that 56 percent of preventable maternal deaths could be blamed on physicians' errors of judgment and technique.[40] A national study concluded similarly that "artificial delivery is becoming increasingly frequent, especially in hospital practice," and that "interference with normal labor is accompanied by some added risk to both mother and child." Although the indictment was not universally accepted by physicians in the early 1930s, statistics indicated that going to a hospital to give birth under the influence of twentieth-century drugs and instruments did not necessarily give a mother an advantage and may have put her in greater jeopardy than her neighbor who stayed home.[41]

Although obstetrics by the mid-1930s had not achieved a record of safety commensurate with its potential abilities, the practices of specific physicians and clinics showed it could be done. The Chicago Maternity Center, serving the inner city with a predominantly home-based service, continued its unsurpassed record of safely delivering poor mothers through strict regimens that discouraged infection. The Center's program of active prenatal care identified and closely monitored high-risk cases. Their records revealed that maternal mortality could be significantly reduced through such care.[42]

Aided by the New York Academy of Medicine's 1933 revelations about preventable maternal and infant deaths, physicians moved toward regulation and standardization of hospital obstetrics in their attempts to decrease the overuse and misuse of drugs and operative procedures. Their success in establishing minimum standards for delivery procedures is evident in the fact that hospital births increased from

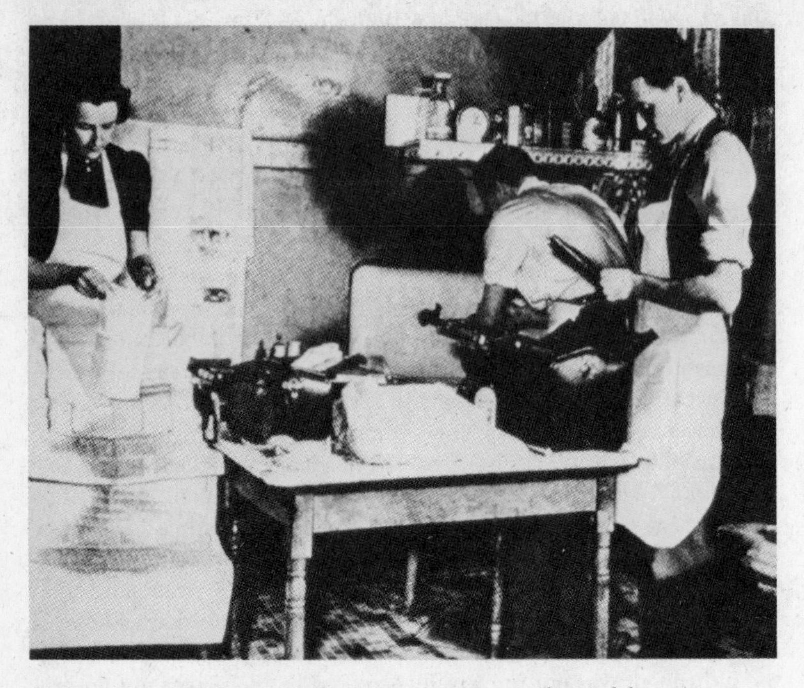

Chicago Maternity Center staff prepares to assist at a home delivery.
Source: *Hygeia* 16 (1938).

35 percent of all births in 1933 to 72 percent ten years later and "for the first time [the hospital] was not associated with higher rates of puerperal death."[43]

The medical debate acknowledging the profession's shortcomings during the 1920s and 1930s reached the popular press and women's magazines in much milder form. DeLee himself, in the same year he proclaimed hospitals dangerous places to give birth, wrote a series for the *Delineator* in which he encouraged increased medicalization, including hospitalization, of childbirth. "The main object of this [article]," DeLee wrote, "is to show the need for proper supervision of the expectant mother and how safe the function of childbirth can be made if the individual patient will cooperate with her doctor." He urged women to exercise care in selecting their doctor and their hospital, but only tucked away in the middle of one of his articles did he mention the physicians' investigations showing that "many hospitals were not good places for women to have babies."[44] In a private communication, De-

Lee admitted his duplicitous argument. "I am perfectly willing to repeat that general hospitals are cesspools of infection," he wrote to journalist Paul de Kruif in 1935, "but only in a medical journal." He did not want to "frighten the women too much" by revealing the full story in the lay press.[45]

DeLee's associates, Drs. Beatrice Tucker and Harry Benaron, wrote of the wonderful results of the home delivery service run by the Chicago Maternity Center in the 1930s. But they, too, concluded: "We do not wish to leave the impression that a reversion to home obstetrics is desirable. The well-equipped maternity hospital is undoubtedly the ideal place for a woman to have her baby." Paul de Kruif's series on childbirth in the *Ladies' Home Journal*, clearly influenced by DeLee himself, similarly put the promise of the new science and the specialist-run hospital at the pinnacle of what safety science could offer women.[46] Most articles in the popular press still referred to the potential of obstetrics rather than to its actual record; but the distinction was not clearly expressed to readers.

Thus women continued to be encouraged to trust specialists and to choose the right hospital, but their image of what to expect in the hospital differed significantly from what the physicians knew about the dangers of many hospital births. Women expected to be whisked from the hospital door into shining, clean delivery rooms where modern scientists worked their mysterious ways to produce a safe, short, and painless birth. They expected to emerge from this dream healthy and vigorous, the main work of the ordeal having been taken over by expert technicians.[47] But doctors knew that agents of infection, hidden in the seemingly clean atmosphere, could be transferred into the raw wounds of the women and that epidemics of puerperal fever still plagued the maternity wards. Hospitals, as Williams and DeLee could agree, could be and often were the sponsors of death.

Yet another menace greeted women who gave up their home deliveries and went to the hospital to give birth: the psychological costs of leaving their own domestic world and entering a world controlled by others. Thinking they were increasing their chances and their babies' chances of survival and unable to overcome the difficulties of preparing for birth at home, women found hospitals attractive answers to both concerns. Yet when they got to the hospital, when they said goodbye to their husbands and family and went up to the labor rooms, women found themselves abandoned to the impersonal routines of impersonal institutions. Instead of being comforted by the efficiency of the hospital, many laboring women agreed with the Bozeman, Montana, woman who felt, "The cruelest part of [hospital] childbirth is being alone among strangers." She found nothing familiar to comfort her through the difficult hours, only the routine of hospital life she and others described as an assembly line. Margaret Budenz, in labor with her third child in 1943, was told by her doctor that "books were not allowed in the labor room." A woman from Elkhart, Indiana, wrote to the *Ladies' Home Journal*, which exposed the impersonal conditions, "So many women, especially first mothers, who are frightened to start out with, receive such brutal inconsiderate treatment that the whole thing is a horrible nightmare. They give you drugs, whether you want them or not, strap you down like an animal." A woman from Columbus, Ohio, concurred that a new mother was "foiled in every attempt to follow her own wishes."[48]

These women realized, perhaps too late, that the physical removal of childbirth from the woman's home to the physicians' institution shifted the balance of power. Birth was no longer part of the woman's domain, as it had been during all the years it remained in the home. It had become instead a medical affair run by medical professionals. Women were no longer the main actors; instead, physicians acted upon women's bodies. Women who were attended by physicians in their own homes could still determine what would happen, could refuse to be shaved or could demand ether. They still controlled much of the birthing process. But women who entered the birthing rooms of medicine were captured by the routine and by the expertise surrounding them. They could not decide the specific events of their own confinements. A woman wrote from Ohio:

> Many normal deliveries are turned into nightmares for the mothers by "routine" obstetrical practices. I have had two such experiences. My third baby will be born at home, despite the sterile advantages of a hospital confinement, for I feel the accompanying emotional disadvantages are just not worth it.[49]

Women who went to the hospital missed the companionship that had been theirs at home and early felt alienated from the hospital environment. Perhaps they could not have predicted ahead of time that the domestic comforts could not be replicated in the hospital, but they certainly missed them when they were gone. Upon entering the hospital women found that hospital routine put them on an assembly line and took away their individuality.

All of a sudden the familiar supports disappeared, and in their place, little comfort; only the bustle of starched skirts, the thermometer poked in the mouth, and the whispers of strange people speaking among themselves. One woman remembered her 1935 confinement as a "nightmare of impersonality," during which she felt "helpless" and "like a pawn in a strange game." Others remembered being "all alone" "abandoned," and "lonely . . . knowing no one." Hospitals seemed unable to provide a supportive atmosphere for women in labor; perhaps more significant, hospital staffs did not notice that such an environment was needed or desired by their maternity patients. Women felt too intimidated by institutionalized medicine to make their feelings known; doctors and nurses did not show a personal empathy for women's ordeals; and routines and schedules did not encourage providing the comforts of home. One woman found her hospital experience so traumatic that, she wrote, "Months later I would scream out loud and wake up remembering that lonely labor room and just feeling no one cared what happened to me, no one kind reassuring word was spoken by nurse or doctor. I was treated as if I was an inanimate object."[50] Birth in the hospital for many American women was no blessing at all. It was still dangerous, perhaps more dangerous than being at home, and it was psychologically alienating.

Listen, for example, to Lenore Pelham Friedrich, disillusioned by her three "scientific" and expensive hospital deliveries in the 1930s:

> I had submitted to the routine proceedings. Each time it had been an unpleasant, upsetting and baffling experience. . . . I experienced the sensation which has always seemed to me worse than any pain—of struggling for consciousness, going down into blackness, coming up only to know that something big and dreadful is happening, to feel fear, to hear oneself moaning, to sense strange people, with offensive professional voices. . . . it became obvious to me that . . . an important thing had happened to me and I knew nothing about it. . . . The days in the hospital after the birth had been a further ordeal. The routine, the early morning waking, the constant running in and out of strange young women on errands such as counting blankets, are painful memories to nearly every sensitive maternity patient.[51]

Or listen to Ann Rivington, who delivered her baby in a city hospital in 1933:

> I went there with no false expectations of luxury or coddling, with no fond hopes of ease or comfort even. But a certain adequate minimum of care I did consider my right. . . . [I was] left lying in the emergency room. . . . The nurses were cynical and cruel to everyone on

> the ward. . . . We were all obsessed with a mad desire to get away. . . . My next baby's going to be born at home.[52]

These two women, representing different socioeconomic classes and birth experiences, one able to pay for the best care and the other on the public purse, found their hospital births inhumane. While American women did not in huge numbers make concerted efforts to change the hospital routines until the 1950s, this earlier generation of hospital-delivered women found that an important element of birth, which had been present in home deliveries, was noticeably absent in medical institutions.

Of course, some women, like Betty MacDonald, coddled in her small mountainside retreat hospital, had positive experiences in hospitals and kept alive the dream of what birth under ideal conditions could be. These women dismissed women's desires to go back home to give birth as "nostalgic gestures." They welcomed all the efficient people—representing science's best influence—bustling around their hospital beds. This group of birthing women may have been limited to luxury hospitals and be representative of only the most elite birth experiences. Many other women tolerated the unpleasant routines and impersonal treatment in order to receive what they believed to be the best in scientific care. They could not wait to get home and forget their hospital ordeals.[53] But the outpouring of unhappiness that erupted during the 1950s as thousands of American women demanded improved and more humane treatment from doctors and nurses in the hospitals indicated that the impersonal routines must have been more common than the satisfying experiences. Physician-directed hospital obstetrics had not met the expectations of American women for protecting a woman's dignity and integrity at the same time as it insured her safety. Women wanted the psychologically comforting practices of their traditional birthing rooms to be incorporated into the modern practices of the birthing rooms of medical science.[54]

Actress Julie Harris, who delivered her baby in a New York hospital in the 1950s, captured both the positive and negative aspects of hospital birth as she related her story to Betty Friedan. As a result of her position, she was able to persuade the hospital to go against its usual policy and allow her husband into the labor room. Because of this Julie Harris had an elated labor. She felt in control of her contractions and able to laugh off the nurse's efforts to get rid of her husband. She was aided greatly by his coaching and support. But when it was time to go to the delivery room, her husband was removed:

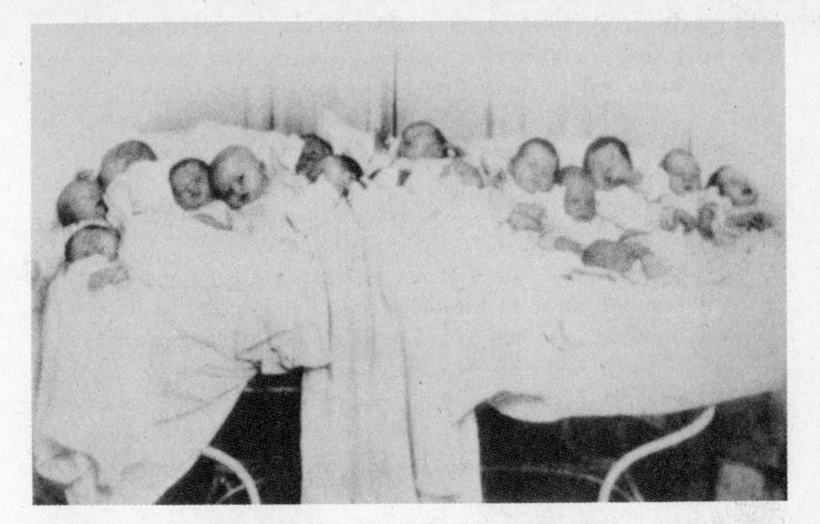

Babies on the cart at the Manhattan Maternity and Dispensary, 1912. One common maternal fear was the danger of going home with someone else's baby.

Source: United Hospital Fund.

> I begged, but they wouldn't let him go with me. . . . They were wheeling me into bright white light, lifting me onto another table, strapping my legs down in long white leggings, clamping my feet and hands in stirrups. For the first time in my whole labor I felt helpless and afraid. And then the doctor tried to clamp an ether mask on my face. I was terrified, then angry. They were going to make me miss the climax. . . . I fought so that when they took the mask off I was still conscious.[55]

This birth account, by an actress who got so entirely caught up in the process of becoming a mother that she described motherhood as "the most courageous, difficult profession," reveals the essence of the twentieth-century hospital experience for women. Medical institutions had the potential of taking away the control over birth that women had always had, and women missed this control precisely because it was an important component of their traditional expectations. Although traditional births had been dangerous, they had not robbed women of one of their most important social functions. Julie Harris had decided she wanted to deliver with her husband's assistance and with no drugs. As long as she could prevail, she felt in control and able to deal with hospital routine; but when they took away her support and tried to force drugs on her, she felt trapped, out of control, and terrified. More articulate than most, she put into print the positive aspects of the process of becoming a mother alongside a moving account of her inability, and the inability of any individual woman, to challenge the medical system in its institutionalized mid-twentieth-century form.

The particulars of Julie Harris's experience—that she wanted her husband and did not want anesthesia—are unimportant for this analysis. Each individual woman would have had her own expectations and desires. In home deliveries, women could have insured that many of their expectations became realities, but in the institutionalized setting, the probability of transforming expectation into reality disappeared. Women giving birth within their own homes could decide the circumstances of the births; women giving birth in the hospital could only hope to be able to do this. When hospital routines usurped a woman's ability to determine who could accompany her through labor and delivery, or to decide what procedures she would endure, they took away an essential ingredient of a woman's identification as a woman and as a mother-to-be. They erased a woman's powers over the processes of childbirth, which to her marked the beginning of her maternal responsibilities, and thus threatened her competence for her new job of motherhood. They obliterated millennia of women's own birthing traditions.

In the 1920s and 1930s when women in alliance with obstetrical specialists decided to move childbirth to the hospital, they made the decision because they believed in medical science. But birthing women and their doctors in the first third of the twentieth century compromised both the physical and the psychological aspects of the birth experience even while they thought they were extending the frontiers of science. Maternal mortality remained high in the hospital, and women suffered severe psychological dislocations.

By the 1940s and 1950s, maternal mortality had fallen in the wake of increasing hospital regulation of obstetrics practices, antibiotics to treat infection, transfusions to replace blood lost by massive hemorrhaging, and prenatal care to identify many potential high-risk cases. Medicine had combated successfully infection and hemorrhages, two major sources of maternal deaths, and by the middle of the twentieth century, childbirth at last became a demonstrably safer event than it had ever before been. With this major increase in physical safety, women could concentrate more on improving the psychological dimension of the experience. The natural-childbirth movement, and the various alternative modes of delivery available at the end of the twentieth century, although not the subject of this book, should be viewed in this context. They represent women's efforts to retrieve some decision-making control over their confinements, an element that had been traditional but was missing from early twentieth-century hospital experiences.

For most of history, birthing women, accompanied by their women friends and relations, had controlled the birth environment and had felt comfortable in it because it was part of their own domestic world. The medical institutionalization of birth in the twentieth century took away the parts of the birth experience that had been traditionally under women's control and left women vulnerable and alone. The move to the hospital thus emerges, in my analysis, as the single most important transition in childbirth history. More than the entrance of male physicians and their medical interventions, the location of childbirth uncompromisingly and directly altered women's birth experiences, replacing the traditional female-centered domestic childbirth with a physician-directed medical and surgical event. Women realized that in the earlier period, with either midwife or physician attendants, they had been "brought to bed" by their friends while by the middle of the twentieth century they were "alone among strangers" in an alien hospital environment.

8

Decision-Making and the Process of Change

Two images of birthing women in America—one "brought to bed" in her own home by the women she had called together and the other drugged and "alone among strangers" in an impersonal hospital—frame the American obstetric experience. The eighteenth-century woman felt vulnerable to death and debility despite the strength she derived from her friends; the twentieth-century woman felt vulnerable to the institutional routine despite the strength she derived from believing birth was safer for her than it had been for her foremothers. Neither woman had what she needed at the time of her confinement: the confidence in a healthy outcome with the freedom to make choices about how to conduct the important event.

This book has examined how women moved from being brought to bed by their friends to being alone among strangers in the hospital. It has argued that birthing women themselves played a crucial role in bringing about these transformations and that many of the changes directly reflected women's needs at various points in history. This chapter analyzes the processes by which women and their medical birth attendants altered women's birth experiences and concludes that, because of the long traditions of female-dominated confinements, the particular history of childbirth is unique in the annals of women's relationships with the medical profession.

From Mary Holyoke, who epitomized the eighteenth-century home-based experience, to Julie Harris, who struggled with a mid-twentieth-century hospital confinement, women have been able to make many choices about their deliveries, but they have found other options out of reach. Succeeding generations of women have emphasized different aspects of childbirth that concerned them, and their interests reflected the particular circumstances of their own lives and times. Reviewing chronologically the experiences of individual women whose lives this book has documented, we can identify patterns in the scope of women's choices and understand how the interactions between birthing women and their medical attendants produced changes in childbirth history. We also can see how women's age-old knowledge about childbirth strengthened their position in relationship to their medical attendants.

When Mary Holyoke delivered her twelve children between the years 1760 and 1781, she followed routines traditional to colonial women. During this period of obstetric history, childbirth was almost exclusively under women's jurisdiction. Midwives and women friends and relations, using minimal techniques of aid and intervention, attended childbearing women in their own homes. Traditional births encompassed some female-centered comforts within the context of ever-present dangers. For each of her confinements, Mary Holyoke was attended by a group of her friends and relatives; she in turn regularly attended the deliveries of others. She recorded in 1770, for example, "Mrs. Brown Brought to Bed 1/2 after 7 A.M. I was there." Or about her own delivery in 1769: "Taken very poorly. Mrs. Jones, Mascarene & Epps here. I was brought to bed 1/2 after 11 P.M." As with her contemporaries, Mary Holyoke seems to have had very little choice with regard to the frequency of her pregnancies. Once married, she was subject to repeated confinements. There is no mention in her diary of attempted birth control or abstinence; and the number of pregnancies indicate that if she did try to limit her conceptions she was unsuccessful. The historical context of her life, then, was paramount to our understanding the limitations and freedoms available to her. No hospitals provided maternity care; few if any physicians provided maternity services. The choices Mary Holyoke could make as she prepared for her confinements were in seeking familiar faces across the birthing bed and in obtaining knowledgeable attendants. These choices she made; when they were taken out of her hands by an unexpected or precipitous labor, as in 1771 when she found herself "quite alone" during her delivery, she felt vulnerable and afraid.[1] Her security rested on her choice of attendants and the arranging of her household; Holyoke had little power to determine other aspects of her confinements.

In the early and mid-nineteenth century, women who had the financial ability took some additional authority over their confinements by inviting physicians to attend them. The physicians who attended birthing women, "male midwives" as they were called, brought some new drugs into the birthing rooms, and most important in this period, they brought forceps. These instruments created powerful images in the minds of the women on whom they potentially would be used and in the minds of the physicians themselves. Forceps could be the saviors of women and babies, and their presence symbolically and practically changed the face of the childbirth experience. Now birth could be managed and directed, saved perhaps, by the action of people, specifically by the action of men. The traditional female event, which had resorted to men only when emergency warranted it, now routinely included men. While birth remained traditional in this period in the sense that it still occurred in women's homes and still took place in the presence and under the authority of the women of the community, it became a different kind of event, one that could be shaped and influenced by women and by the attendants women called to help them.

The pregnant Emily Hale, daughter-in-law of Sarah Hale and wife of Edward Everett Hale, took advantage of medical attendance during her two confinements in the 1850s, and Sarah recorded in detail some of her daughter-in-law's concerns. Emily wanted her mother-in-law and midwife or friend to help; she made arrangements also for a physician and nurse to be in her home. She thought about her neighbors as possible helpers if labor came on rapidly. She considered, too, whether moving to her country home, which would make it easier for Sarah to join her, might be preferable to giving birth in her Boston home. Sarah wrote Edward warning against moving Emily out of town, because the doctor would have longer to travel and the physical layout of the alternative house was not as favorable: "at home all her things are convenient and at hand."[2]

Emily Hale's choices, which were numerous, illustrated the choices of the privileged at the middle of the nineteenth century. She could afford the services of a physician, thus utilizing what medicine could offer; at the same time she could arrange the confinement along traditional female lines. She was able to consider options that would not be available to most women, such as giving birth in one home versus another, and she had at her command the people and services she desired.

Yet another change came to women who delivered their children after the middle of the nineteenth century, and this was anesthesia. Beginning in 1847, physicians could, with the use of powerful pain blockers, alleviate much of the discomfort of labor and delivery. Still applied within the traditional confines of women's homes and the female birth environment created there, anesthesia added to the tools at the command of the medical birth attendants and increased, ultimately, the control they could exercise. Parturient women learned that they could determine portions of the birth experience by asking for drugged and instrument deliveries, and physicians learned that they could pattern labor and delivery with their interventions. Both physicians and women developed the perceptions that birth events were not fated but could be shaped in large part by planning and making use of medical advances.

The American woman first to take advantage of the new age of anesthetized childbirth was Fannie Appleton Longfellow, who adopted ether to obliterate the pain of labor in 1847, and who was followed by thousands of women similarly seeking to control one of the worst parts of the ordeal. Thus during the second half of the nineteenth century, some women had wide latitude in determining their confinement experiences. Other women, circumscribed by limited resources or cultural prohibitions against male attendants, continued to deliver their babies without any medical aids. But increasing numbers of women could set the atmosphere of the birthing room in the traditional ways of selecting attendants and location, and they could add to these choices physician attendants and the incorporation of the specific medical interventions.

The command women held over their parturient experiences, despite its latitude, remained constrained by factors outside their control. Even upper- and middle-class women, who had wider options than other women and who, in the nineteenth century, were most successful at limiting the size of their families, were at the mercy of physical forces that could not be overcome. These women may have been enduring labor and delivery less frequently than their foremothers, but they shared with their ancestors the fears and reality of maternal mortality. The experiences of Mary Ann Ditmar illustrate the limitations of women's choice. Mary Ann delivered her child in 1846 with the comforting support of her friends and with the help, it appears, of a physician. But, despite all of her choices and the presence of the experts, Mary Ann died—not because she had limited choice, but because at midcentury neither women nor medicine could control all of the forces of birth.

Bessie Rudd's childbirth experiences further illustrate the limitations of the middle nineteenth century. Rudd delivered her first child in 1860, at her childhood home to which she returned for the event. She put herself under the care of a physician early in her pregnancy; she engaged the services of a nurse to accompany her through her childbirth period. She made sure her mother and sisters could be with her. But Bessie suffered from tuberculosis, and its effects on the safety of the confinement added greatly to the fears for her survival. "Uncertain are all things," she wrote to her husband, meanwhile doing her best to counteract the potential dangers by walking outdoors and being "very very careful" of her activities. She surrounded herself with family and support and planned the experience in all particulars. Bessie survived her confinement, but her general condition weakened. Her postpartum recovery was very slow, and the following year she entered a tuberculosis sanitorium. Her second confinement, in 1862, preceded her death by only three months. Thus Bessie Rudd's experience teaches us again that some women, even with all available services at their command, fell victim to forces outside their control.[3]

To conclude from these examples that because women faced physical dangers of death from childbirth they had no choices would be a mistake. Individual women had many choices and made many decisions that did affect the nature of their experiences. Advantaged women determined who would attend them, where they would deliver, and what techniques would be used to aid the delivery. Less fortunate women determined who would help them through their ordeal. Women experienced these decisions as real and meaningful, and indeed they were. The power to plan the circumstances under which a stressful event would occur is significant; and women's holding on to this power during the entire home birth period indicates that they retained important elements of control and personal satisfaction.

The possibility of death followed all women and was not in itself determined by class or culture. Some groups were at greater risk for pregnancy or delivery-related complications—the malnourished, the rickets sufferers, the tubercular—but all women feared it. Childbirth-related death was anticipated and experienced by women of all classes, cultures, and time periods. In the sense that it threatened all parturients, death was an almost constant factor pushing those women who could afford it to modify and improve their birth experience by seeking medical advances. The modifications themselves were more related to the financial ability and cultural desires of women, and these factors must be integrated into our interactional analysis to understand the fuller meaning of choices available to parturient women. At any given point in American history, women with smaller financial resources had fewer decisions to make about their confinements than their cohorts among the more advantaged classes were able to make.

The specific importance of socioeconomic class to understanding childbearing experiences varied with time. The gap between the birth experiences of rich and poor women widened during the late eighteenth and the nineteenth century as medical obstetrical services became more available. Once financially secure women were able to choose physicians to attend them, the lack of such choice among working class and poor women meant that their experiences remained set in the traditional patterns. While some of the poorest women received the ministrations of some of the finest doctors in medical training centers, most women who had limited resources remained by necessity outside of the medical mainstream until the twentieth century. Middle- and upper-class women first invited physicians to attend them in childbirth; the interactions between these women and their medical attendants led to changes in the procedures and ultimately in the location of birth, and the changes instituted by these groups in turn altered most dramatically the childbirth experiences of all American women. Class and financial ability thus played a major role in determining women's childbirth experiences.

The cultural values and mores of the community in which women lived also helped determine the particulars of childbirth experiences. Cultural variations were more evident in the home birth period, before the 1930s, than they are today, because women giving birth in their own homes could maintain the traditions of their grandmothers without the restraint of homogenizing institutional routines. Some traditional practices might have been consciously chosen by parturient women wanting to connect themselves to their own pasts; others might have been practiced because of the expectations of the women attendants and not recognized by the participants as out of the ordinary or particular to their group. Cultural proscriptions might have determined very significant parts of the confinement: the common insistence, for example, on all female attendants. They may have determined the atmosphere of the room, the handling and aftercare of the newborn, or the conversation with the parturient.

A comparison of the 1890 confinements of Anita McCormick Blaine, whose upper class status and urban location allowed her maximum options in planning for her delivery, and Nannie Jackson, whose impoverished rural Arkansas life severely constrained her choices, illustrates some of the differences in childbirth experiences brought about by class considerations. Anita anticipated all the parts of her coming confinement and made decisions about how to have the safest and most comfortable experience. She returned to her parents' home, selected its most comfortable room, solicited the advice of her mother and friends, and arranged for medical and nursing attendance. Anita seemed most concerned about creating a comfortable atmosphere in which her friends and relatives could provide the support she would need. Assured she had done all she could, Anita Blaine prepared to deliver her child with the help of a physician and in the presence of her trusted friend, who came to Chicago from Virginia to be with her.

Nannie Jackson, whose delivery corresponded in time to Blaine's, could manage fewer parts of her confinement. Severe economic hardship limited her attendants to available friends and neighbors and kept her in her own small and already crowded home for the delivery. Nannie made sure her best friend Fannie and other women with birthing room experience were there to help out. The childbirths of these two women were different in almost every respect: one had all that money could provide; the other had none of the material advantages. One relied heavily on medical attention and interventions; the other minimally utilized such aids. But both women did have what they emphasized they most needed: trusted women friends to help them get through the event. For both women, close friends provided needed support and encouragement beyond the particulars of the circumstances of the deliveries. The comfort provided by the common experiences of women formed the basis upon which the women built their confinements.

Gender, in fact, was of enormous influence in establishing birth patterns in American obstetric history. The presence of women in birthing rooms influenced events in particular ways that went beyond the changing state of medical knowledge or practice. Women wanted people of their own sex with them when they performed the female job of childbirth, and the kind of help they wanted from these women emerged from the common biological and social bonds between them. The experiences of other women could be learning tools for birthing women, the success of previous births could be applied to the birth at hand, and the trust that developed across the childbirth bed could be relied upon in difficult times. In the words of one writer, women could do what had to be done "without telling." Women knew from their own confinements and from witnessing the births of others what to do, and they could be trusted to do it. The importance of this sex-shared experience cannot be overstated in understanding women's childbirth experiences. This female influence on the childbirth experience is vital to understanding some of the decisions women made and some of the changes that occurred.

The importance of other women was so great that the presence of men in this female environment—the male physicians who came to attend women and bring medical interventions or the husbands who were frequently called in to attend to specific tasks—did little to change the essentially female nature of the experience as long as birth remained a home-based event. The psychologically vital presence of trusted women friends, despite the influence of male medicine, continued to shape much of the childbirth experience for individual women. Men could be asked to do some things, restrained from doing others; they could be argued with and agreed with; but rarely were they allowed to make decisions on their own. Thus medicine changed the birth experience, but changed it only within the limits set by women's birthing-room culture. The gender-based context in which women gave birth continued in this country until birth moved to the hospital, until it physically was no longer part of women's world.

By the turn of the twentieth century, many women had what they perceived to be the best of both worlds of traditional female practices and useful medical interventions. Increasing numbers of women invited physicians to attend their deliveries, and they used the skills of medical attendants to shape the birth experiences in ways they desired. Accompanied by trusted female friends and relatives and strengthened by the familiar female atmosphere, birthing women could maintain the social traditions of birth at the same time they incorporated medical practices, even though, as we have seen, the obstetrical skill level of physicians varied greatly through this period.

Calling in a medical doctor did not necessarily mean that a woman would receive all the benefits that medicine could provide. There were enormous differences in training and ability among physicians. Moreover, a disconnection between medical theory and practice usually existed. This was especially evident in the bacteriological era, when physicians who accepted the germ theory still had difficulty controlling infection in their parturient patients. Knowledge about the ways infection spread did not mean that infection stopped spreading. Physicians coming to parturient women from other patients suffering from infectious diseases, despite their hand washing and clothes changing (which only some followed scrupulously), found that their parturient patients still developed puerperal fever. The advances in medical theory could not be guaranteed to have immediate application in the practices of physicians around the country.

Women in the generation of Blaine and Jackson, despite the many positive aspects of their confinements, continued to feel vulnerable because of a host of delivery and postpartum problems still associated with their medically attended confinements, and in their efforts to make birth safer, they helped to push medical participation in new directions. To these women and others that followed them, the hospital, promising added safety, looked attractive. Physicians felt they were unable to make birth safe as long as it remained in women's homes, where they did not have sufficient control over procedures. Increasingly frustrated by the conditions under which they attended parturient women, physicians became more assertive in their responses to birthing women's concerns. Especially as knowledge about germ transmission grew, and not incidentally concurrent with the expansion of professional consciousness, physicians realized that alone they could not do in women's homes what they might do together in hospitals. In homes they had to convince the women's friends about each intervention as it became indicated; in hospitals they could make the decisions without constant lay consultation. In homes they had to adjust techniques to meet the particular environment; in hospitals techniques became routine. In homes they found it difficult to achieve sterile conditions; in hospitals staff nurses provided the necessary aid. In short, with the growing technical nature of obstetric practice in the bacteriological era, physicians found medical and safety reasons to add to their personal and professional concerns for attempting to increase their controls over the process of parturition. Instead of acceding to the demands of their patients relatively easily, physicians at the beginning of the twentieth century increased their own demands.

The debates over the value of scopolamine illustrated the growing tensions between birthing women and the medical profession. Mrs. Francis X. Carmody, who helped to spearhead the drive for twilight sleep in 1914 and 1915, encountered a new kind of obstacle to her decision making. Having made up her mind to receive scopolamine for her childbirth, Carmody was faced with the same sort of situation that many women had faced at the middle of the nineteenth century when they chose ether or chloroform as an anesthetic and then had to convince their doctors to administer it. However, the first transition to anesthetic agents had been smoother. Physicians, largely at the insistence of their patients, tried anesthesia and incorporated it into their obstetric practices. In 1914 and 1915, however, many physicians simply refused to accommodate the women who wanted twilight sleep, and others turned the demands around and insisted that women had to enter the hospital to receive the drug. Carmody, and a few other women who sought to determine their own confinement procedures, was forced to travel to Germany (later the War made this impossible) to find a doctor willing to deliver her child the way she wanted. Women's response to the doctors' refusals was to build a movement of women to pressure doctors to change their ways; instead of negotiating across the birthing bed, women launched a campaign in the public sector. Carmody still made the basic choices about her birth experience, but she collided with some of the choices physicians were beginning to make about optimal conditions for the administration of obstetric technology. Negotiations between upper- and middle-class birthing women and their physicians that had once been possible only across the individual confinement beds now erupted into a public power confrontation.

However much physicians and twilight-sleep advocates might have disagreed with each other about use of a specific drug, both sides agreed that childbirth could best be monitored in well-equipped hospitals. The lure of the hospital grew in the years between the world wars. Physicians increasingly urged their parturient patients to join them in the hospital, where every convenience could be put at their disposal. Women believed, too, that medicine had been practiced imperfectly around the home birthing bed and that it promised more scientific application in the hospital setting. Both women and their physicians, realizing the variable state of obstetric practice and the decline in women's support networks at home, supported the move to the hospital. By 1938, half of American births occurred within medical institutions.[4]

But twentieth-century women giving birth within hospitals found their capacity to determine events in the birthing of their children severely limited by the hospital environment. More than any generation before them, mid-twentieth century women felt impotent and alone during the moments of their great physical task of bearing children. Katherine S. Egan underwent a "nightmare of impersonality" during her labor and delivery, feeling like "a pawn in a strange game." She entered the hospital in active labor in 1935, "kissed my husband goodbye in the lobby and went upstairs to face it, exhilarated but frightened and lonely." She found the labor routines of receiving an enema, being shaved with what felt like a "dull, rusty razor blade," and being put to bed in a room with six other "groaning and screaming women" extremely unpleasant.

The nurses were "only in the room part of the time. . . . I heard one say to a young Greek woman who was doing a lot of screaming: 'You had your fun, now you have to pay for it.' " In the delivery room, doctors administered an anesthetic: "I said I didn't want it, didn't need it, but they gave it to me anyway and against my protests." During her fourth confinement in 1944 the doctor insisted on strapping her down on the delivery table although she heartily resisted. "They fastened heavy leather straps on my wrists and ankles anyway. I was so angry and humiliated and helpless. It was totally unnecessary. It seemed to me an act of sadism."[5]

Marilyn Clohessy delivered her first child in 1953 under equally alienating circumstances. Arriving at the hospital after eleven hours of labor at home, she was prepped, given an enema, and "told that the bathroom was down the hall. I made it there but the trip back was agony and the nurse was no where in sight." All during her painful labor, "imploring someone to help me," this woman felt alone and scared. "I remember seeing 8 o'clock on the large clock and screaming out Mary, Jesus and Joseph over and over. . . . All of a sudden they crossed my legs and transfer[ed] me to something with wheels. There was a lot of rushing around and talking but all I could hear were my own screams echoing in my ears. Then I heard some one say 'For God's sake put her under.' Silence." Marilyn Clohessy believed she was treated as if she were "an inanimate object," and her inability to sleep for months afterward without remembering the horrors of her labor experience complicated her postpartum recovery.[6]

In their own homes, women could command much of the confinement situation. They could surround themselves with companions of their choice; they could gain sustenance from familiar sounds and smells, and they could participate in shaping their birth experiences. Birth was women's event in large part because it took place within women's sphere of influence, and the choices women made about their confinements were limited only by their resources and the availability of the services and people they desired. Even the women for whom choices were severely circumscribed because of their finances felt free to have their friends help them to make whatever choices were available to them.[7] This situation in which choice, however limited, existed for individual women changed radically when birth moved into medical institutions. In hospitals, control moved to the profession, and birthing women found themselves "alone among strangers" and unable to determine any parts of their birth experience.

Women at the middle of the twentieth century were bound in a medicalized system of birth that had evolved over the course of American history. Although they had participated in bringing about the changes, including the move to the hospital, women had not anticipated the full meaning of this last most crucial alteration. While physicians were aware of the importance of shifting locations of power, because they had been frustrated by their lack of power in women's homes, women, it seems from their own writings, were less in touch with what they were leaving behind by moving to the hospital. They did not realize that in gaining what they had hoped would be safer controls over the previously uncontrollable parts of home confinements, they were giving up their ability to determine the environment of their labor.

Changes throughout childbirth history were the result of long-term negotiations between upper- and middle-class birthing women and their physicians. Both believed they had something to gain by changing childbirth procedures at each historical juncture. Neither group could determine all parts of childbirth practices at any given time, but until the middle of the twentieth century both groups had enough power to negotiate their interests as they saw them. Many of the practices that evolved were gradual and piecemeal in their conception and adoption. For example, physicians in certain locales learned that bleeding might be more acceptable than forceps for their patients, and in these areas the use of bleeding predominated. Likewise, anesthesia use varied according to its local acceptability. In order to understand the birth practices of a particular time and place, it is essential to consider the convergence of all the relevant social, economic, and medical factors.

Throughout childbirth history, complete choice among the wide alternatives in practices was open only to a few. Most women were constrained by their finances, cultural proscriptions, and the availability of services. Most doctors were constrained in their practices by their training, the availability of support services, and the expectations of the parturient and attending women. But women and doctors did make choices, even if limited ones, and these are significant for understanding what was important to these groups at various historical periods.

For each generation that negotiated their available choices the next generation became victim to those choices. As more women chose physicians, fewer midwives had viable practices; as more women chose hospitals, fewer physicians would visit women at home. With the middle and upper class in the vanguard of changing procedures, the other groups in the population were molded into patterns not of their own creation. The limited kinds of childbirth options at the end of the twentieth century reflect the evolution of changing practices and, most important, the choices both women and their medical attendants made in previous generations.

The ideological and social context in which birth took place influenced priorities and adds to the complexity of our analysis. We have seen that women through American history felt strongly about the importance of having other women with them during their confinements. But this itself is subject to qualification. Women were able, even willing, to give up being with other women when hospitals promised the safety they had sought for generations. The importance of women companions shrank, too, in relation to husbands' increasing companionate role in the late nineteenth- and twentieth-century marriages. As husbands became confidants of intimacy in the way only women used to be, women had more desire to have their husbands accompany them through their confinement trials. This transition corresponded to the decline of women's culture and the loosening of gender bonds. Confinements could be times when women strongly felt the power of their own bodies and the power of womanhood in general, when they felt connected to other women; birth likewise could engender strong family bonds that were not necessarily sex linked.

Much of childbirth history reflects a debate between tradition, defined culturally, socially, and temporally, and a slowly developing rational model of science. Women frequently found themselves at odds with impersonal science as represented by the medical birth attendant, but at the same time they were attracted by the promises of science. They wanted what both worlds had to offer. Similarly, physicians practiced medicine within a cultural world and showed some of the same ambivalence of being pulled in two opposing directions. Medical science, especially before the twentieth century when it assumed a sterile, white-coated image of Progress, promised to answer some of the demands that both physicians and women brought to it, but it could not always achieve its potential.

The birth place was, in some respects, a battleground upon which medicine met tradition and vied for supremacy. The lure of science's promises allowed medicine to find its place in America's birth rooms; the cultural conditions under which birth traditionally occurred explained the context in which medicine maneuvered; and the constant interaction between traditional and medical forces and values ultimately determined the evolution of childbirth practices. Childbirth as practiced during the late twentieth century, now more than ever before heavily influenced by medical decision-making, is the result of shifting balances among the forces competing for supremacy in the birthing room. Change is not something that happened to women and doctors, but something they together created.

Historical analysis shows that women's biology or the strict biological experience of childbearing did not determine women's historical path. Throughout American history women responded to their biological experiences within a cultural and temporal context, and in ways that rejected passivity. They actively created the environment at birth that they needed; they significantly influenced the development of changing birth procedures; and they gained control of their bodies with the knowledge that they had power over their life courses. While changes over time did not always improve the childbirth experience for American women, women helped to determine the direction of those changes.

Women's ability to control confinement practices for most of American history, which has been the focus of this book, is unique in the annals of relationships between women and medicine. The more usual pattern of interactions between patients and doctors reveals a significant degree of dependence of the sick on the expertise and power of the medical profession. But women in the act of childbirth did not feel or act dependent. They negotiated procedures with their medical attendants from a position of strength originating in their historic dominance over confinement room practices. For millennia women had saved this event and, most important, knowledge about this event, for themselves. Although physicians acquired theoretical knowledge about parturition quite early in the profession's history, the male practitioners did not themselves possess the experiential secrets of the birthing room. Because women exclusively had attended confinements, they knew certain things that men did not. When physicians developed an interest in gaining their own expertise in childbirth, in part because they came to understand it could profitably expand their medical practices, they started at a disadvantage with respect to women's own position. Although medicine in the twentieth century won control over childbearing practices, it was not an easy battle. As physicians learned over the course of American history, women's expertise in this one area has been solid and longlasting.

Because women had a knowledge base that physicians only slowly acquired as their practical education and birthing-room experience expanded, women retained their ability to make decisions about what interventions they would require or accept from their birth attendants. The knowledge differential between birthing women and their female companions, who had birth experience, and physicians, who had little actual experience beyond their textbooks, helped women retain their own traditions despite medicine's growing privilege and power. Until well into the twentieth century, the medical profession did not provide its initiates with enough experience for individual practitioners to conquer the longstanding female traditions of birth. Because physicians' knowledge base was circumscribed, and because birth remained within women's homes, women could retain significant control over their own deliveries.

Women's authority over birth practices was never absolute. Despite all the comforts that birthing women derived from being within their own homes attended by the people they wanted, birth continued for most of American history to hold uncontrollable dangers. Many times the women in attendance watched helplessly as birthing women suffered through slow and painful labors, fell victim to difficult fetal presentations, or died from postpartum complications. Women's call for help from physicians, who devised treatments and instrument interventions for rescuing ill-fated deliveries, indicated that they did not feel in complete control. But until the twentieth century, women were able to keep a strong element of decision-making in their own hands. They called in the experts to perform needed interventions, but they decided themselves which procedures were acceptable. Childbirth remained women's business as long as it remained in women's homes.

Childbirth, through its often repeated reminders of how important women were to one another, was a very significant part of women's world. Childbirth customs and rituals formed a cornerstone of women's group identity. By attending confinements, women strengthened their life-long mutual bonds. Women could afford to ask medical experts to take care of some of the technical aspects of childbirth precisely because they had their support group in place to take care of the crucial emotional bonds associated with sharing the experience of giving birth to the next generation. The support network that women gathered around them at the time of their confinements provided the necessary base for women's ability to resist some medical practices and to keep considerable control in their own hands.

But physicians did not feel comfortable in this prescribed role as birth's technical advisers. Individually, and ultimately collectively, they struggled to expand their advice-giving to more thorough control over birthing events. Within women's homes, old patterns had persevered, and doctors repeatedly became frustrated in their attempts to determine how to manage labor and delivery. Moving childbirth into the hospital gave physicians the advantage they sought. Within medical institutions, women were cut off from their traditions and from their knowledge base: they became the dependent receivers of medical care. Whereas physicians had been in a sense alone among strangers in the female environment at home deliveries, women became the alienated party during hospital deliveries. Just as support had helped women keep control of childbirth earlier, the professional support in the hospital provided an important power base and allowed medicine to supersede, at last, women's traditions. Although physicians during the first third of the twentieth century still found there was much about birth they could not control, such as infection rates, they did succeed in taking decision making out of the hands of the birthing women and putting it into their own hands.

Today in the United States medical institutions and the physicians who work in them maintain significant control over childbirth practices. Most American women give birth in hospitals, under conditions set by the institutions. In recent years, however, there have been new rounds of negotiations and conflicts between birthing women and their physicians, and some of these have resulted in increasing the women's ability to determine what will happen to them within the hospitals.[8] In many respects the current situation mirrors the historical patterns described in this book. Small groups of middle- and upper-class women have managed to achieve some of the birthing practices they want, and they have opened the door again for change in birth practices for all women. Current interest emphasizes the psychological support aspects of the birthing procedures, the precise area that women lost so completely when childbirth first entered the hospital. Women are fighting to have husbands, lovers, mothers, sisters, and friends accompany and support them through labor and delivery, and they indicate a strong preference for introducing homelike environments into their hospital labor rooms. They also want to make decisions about interventions, such as episiotomies, anesthetic use, and fetal monitors. The specific demands trigger the bigger issues of choice and decision making and again raise the question of birthing-room authority. While ultimate decision-making powers within hospitals rest today with the medical professionals, the challenges now in progress may eventually affect wider areas of obstetric practices. Women are learning to influence events in the hospital, to bring birth back at least in part under their control. Hospital birthing rooms, alternative birth centers, and home births mark substantial movement in that direction.

History teaches us that medical authority over childbirth is new to the twentieth century. For most of American history women bore children under conditions they set themselves. Because of the complex of reasons analyzed in this book, women's authority was eroded by the promises of safety offered through applying medical answers to birth's traditional uncertainties. This is not an example of a medical conspiracy at work—at least initially, women participated equally with physicians in changing childbirth practices. But the result of the decisions made, however collectively, has been to increase women's dependence on physicians, to add childbirth to the other areas in which medicine increases its dominance over all of our lives.

Because medical jurisdiction over childbirth is relatively new, it may be more mutable than other areas under medical control. The traditions of women's strength and dominance over childbirth practices may resurface. The interactions between physicians and birthing women today indicate that both are struggling to find a resting place for the pendulum that has swung with such variation throughout American history. If childbirth in the twenty-first century is to reflect its own history, it must somehow meld the two traditions of women's birthing practices and medical contributions into a unified standard that acknowledges the possibilities of options and shared authority. The challenge is to use our knowledge about the past to plan the agenda for the future.

Epilogue

Recent events in American obstetrics indicate that women today have retained the commitment, traced in this book historically, to keep childbirth as their own event. Through their participation in local and national grassroot movements, many women have informed the medical profession that the hospitalized childbirth experiences common today do not meet their childbirth needs. Put to sleep or made partially insensible with a variety of drugs, many women fear they are missing one of the most exciting and important events of their lives. They feel distanced from their own bodies at the very moments their bodies are performing olympian feats. Women miss the ability to initiate decisions about what medical procedures will be applied during their labors and deliveries. They miss, too, the comforting atmosphere created by the presence of close friends and relatives. The activity of so many women in addressing these issues today, when childbirth for many years has been a medical event, indicates that women still feel connected to their own history and to the powers they once wielded over their own confinements.[1]

There are three forms of women's responses to medicalized and hospitalized childbirth, the birth experience of most Americans in the 1980s. A few women reject current medical practices altogether; some work to change existing medicalized delivery to shape it more to their needs; others find current practices altogether acceptable. The first represents the smallest, but in some ways the loudest, faction. A small but significant group of mostly middle- and upper-class American women are launching a direct challenge to medical management and are voicing an outright rejection of medical authority. These women feel that childbirth should return to its roots altogether, to be directed by women within their own cultural world. They want to dispense altogether with physician-directed and hospital-based practices, and they believe that medicine and hospitalization have created new problems for birthing women while not contributing sufficient benefits to outweigh the burdens. The reliance on lay midwife birth attendants by a small number of women throughout the country and the concomitant emphasis on home deliveries represent efforts to return to the values and practices of an earlier time, when women themselves presided over childbirth. Lay midwives, who in most states practice outside the law, attend women in their own homes and participate as one member of a team of friends and relatives who support the parturient through her labor. The challenge to hospitalization and medicalization that is voiced in the movement for lay-attended home deliveries is reminiscent of earlier times and an attempt to recapture some traditionally female-based practices.

Some women experience home and lay-attended deliveries not by choice but out of a lack of choice. In some American communities poor women lack access to medical attendance or cannot afford hospitalization, and they perforce continue to give birth along traditional patterns. Many of these women would not continue in these ways if other opportunities opened for them.

Physicians respond to the birthing women who reject their services with predictable negativism. Most physicians are very reluctant to attend confinements outside the hospital or maternity center. They believe that hospitals offer the only safe birth experience. They see nothing to gain by reverting to old practices that do not allow the full range of medical options and that put restraints on medical activity. They also fear legal repercussions and claim that malpractice insurance rates, already skyrocketing, would become even more prohibitive if they were to practice in home environments. Even while they might acknowledge that home births offer a unique degree of comfort to the parturient, most members of the medical profession believe that the risks of the situation outweigh the benefits.

A greater proportion of the attack on medicalized childbirth comes from a second group of women who do not reject medicine or its contribution to confinement practices. Ever since birth moved out of women's homes and into the hospital, birthing women individually and collectively have been trying to recapture some of what they lost, at the same time maintaining what they have won. Beginning with the publication of *Childbirth Without Fear* by Grantley Dick-Read in 1944 and accelerating with the psychoprophylactic methods of Ferdinand Lamaze, which became popular in the United States after the publication of Marjorie Karmel's *Thank You, Dr. Lamaze* in 1959, groups of women have tried to combat routine drugging and interventions during labor and delivery. The "natural" childbirth movement represented in part women's attempts to reexperience labor and delivery the way they had been before medicine intervened. The popularity especially of Lamaze techniques indicated women's desire to regain control over major aspects of their labors.

The women active in this effort to reform practices may find medicine in its hospitalized form insensitive, they may agree that many medical interventions can be harmful, but they unite in not wanting to turn back the clock to the period before medicine provided aid for parturient women. They seek to use medicine within a more female- and family-oriented context, but they want to continue to have medical help for women whose labor and deliveries put them in danger for their lives and health. However, they do not want medicine to assume all the decision-making authority over childbirth. They prefer decision making to occur in a negotiation between physicians, birthing women, and family members.

The reforms advocated by the second group of women who are dissatisfied with medicalized childbirth vary widely. They seek safe options that can be responsive to birthing women's interests and concerns. Birthing rooms within hospitals, in which family centered childbirth can occur with minimal interventions, are advocated by this group, because they can be places where the homelike atmosphere adds to the possibilities of making united decisions. Similarly, these critics want to do away with certain routine interventions, such as episiotomies, the use of fetal monitors, and automatic repeat cesarean sections, and substitute individual assessment and judgment in each case, so that women can play a more significant part in determining what procedures will be used on their bodies. Many women prefer to use the services of nurse-midwives, who, viewed as supportive, noninterventionist attendants, are popular among women who seek to participate actively in decision making during the course of labor and delivery.

The options for women who have enough financial flexibility to allow them to choose and to pressure for the birth experiences they want have been in one sense expanding and in another way contracting during the last decades of the twentieth century. That a prime-time television show in 1985 can make a passing reference to a LeBoyer style birth and to fathers preparing themselves to coach their wives through labor indicates a general knowledge on the part of the viewing public of these birthing alternatives.[2] Knowledge about birthing options has diffused through the culture, and these options have become acceptable to large groups of people.

When faced individually with parturient patients who want to decide what medical interventions will be used, many obstetricians cooperatively work out acceptable plans for labor management that incorporate the wishes of the women and the concerns of the physicians. Hospitals have responded too in establishing homelike birthing rooms and in allowing parturients to be accompanied by labor coaches and family members of their choice. But often the advance planning has proved untenable during the labor itself, either because of some unanticipated difficulty or because the physician who made the agreement was not personally available to carry it out. Thus some mothers today seeking to implement their chosen option still may be thwarted in their attempts, and may not be able to accomplish successfully the specific procedures they may desire.

The situation can be exacerbated by class and ethnicity factors. When the poor women of Chicago's inner city, many of whom were Hispanic and Black, tried to organize to save the home birth service of the Chicago Maternity Center, they were not successful in presenting their case about the importance of birth options. The closing of the Center in 1974, despite public protests from the women who had utilized or who wanted to utilize the service that Joseph DeLee had started in 1895, indicates that women, even when acting in unison, cannot always win their way. The collective presence of the profession within hospitals and the power and authority wielded by the institution lead many women individually and together to feel that, despite the accommodations, they remain unequal partners in their own deliveries.

Despite frequent frustrations, birthing women as health care consumers have made a significant impact on shaping their birth experiences in recent years. The rapid expansion in vaginal births after cesarean sections (VBACs) is a recent indication that birthing women have been able to affect routine obstetrical practices. Overturning within the last decade the universal acceptance of the necessity to repeat cesareans ("once a cesarean always a cesarean"), women have impressed upon the medical profession their needs and desires and have triumphed in their ability to engage actively in obstetrical decision making. The medical change was bolstered by clinical studies, and the motive for those studies derived in no small part from the culture and politics of the society at large.

Perhaps even more exciting within the context of what we have learned from history, recent research by Marshall Klaus, John Kennell, and their colleagues reveals that the presence of a supportive woman during labor and delivery significantly shortens labor and may reduce complications (including the need for cesarean sections) for the parturient and the baby. Women who have argued that they need to bring into the hospital people whom they can rely upon—women, in other words, who seek to repeat the collective experience of their foremothers—find that controlled research is reinforcing their position by showing that such support improves the course and outcome of labor. The age-old practice of cooperative behavior around the birthing bed has found a modern day scientific reason for its long lasting practice; women's traditions are finding their way into medical hospital based obstetrics.[3]

Many of birthing women's successes in increasing their powers over childbirth procedures have depended upon women reeducating themselves about childbirth. The enormous proliferation in recent decades of popular literature about giving birth, much of which advocates decreasing routine medical interventions, is evidence of women's attempts to reclaim knowledge previously more commonly held within women's world. When birth moved to the hospital and became dominated by technical interventions, women lost their understanding and familiarity with the processes of labor and delivery. Many women, realizing that their lack of knowledge distances them from their own bodies, are trying to recover some of that lost knowledge through self-education in normal physical functions. Some of the popular books are extremely thorough technical manuals; all of them stress education in birth processes as a way to help birthing women, whether they desire home or hospital deliveries, to participate more fully in their own confinement experiences.

In addition to the women who completely challenge medical authority and those who want to find ways to work in cooperation with it, there is a third group of American women today who find medical control of childbirth as practiced in most hospitals perfectly acceptable. They find the prospect of delivering babies frightening or uninteresting, and they wish to experience as little of it as possible. They want to be assured of a healthy outcome, but they do not feel the need to participate actively in bringing it about. They, like many women of the 1920s and 1930s, eagerly turn over their decision-making power to their doctors, who, in turn, readily accept it. The women hope that medicine can provide a streamlined and easy experience and that they will not have to suffer too much either in the process of labor and delivery or in its aftermath. Many women enter the hospital and emerge from it with their babies without having given the experience itself very much thought.

Many poor women accept what happens to them in the hospital without questioning it because they feel they have very few choices in the kind of labors and deliveries they have. These women, because they have few financial options or because they are single, rely on whatever services are available to them within their own communities free of charge. They have extremely limited choices; they may deliver their babies in public hospitals or they may deliver at home with midwife attendants. Poor women receive the care that society chooses for them.

Childbirth practices are still in flux in the United States. As throughout history, some women have many options when they plan for their confinements; others feel constrained by finances, availability, and the restraints of third-party payments to utilize the closest or least expensive alternatives. Significant numbers of women believe that society does not yet offer them the birth experiences they desire, and the agitation to increase the available safe options for birthing women continues. In part because of the decisions previous generations of birthing women have made and in part because of the authority and power of the medical profession, birthing women today are still constrained by a limited number of birth options.

The diversity of opinion about childbirth management evident at the end of the twentieth century reflects the cultural diversity of our nation. Throughout American history, women have wanted and have worked to achieve their own ideals of childbirth, ideals that have developed and been nurtured within their own communities in conjunction with the rest of their life experiences. Childbirth remains as it has always been, a cultural event as much as a biological one. Problems emerged during the middle of the twentieth century because the hospital acted to homogenize the birth experience and make it similar for all women. But childbirth cannot successfully be reduced to one kind of experience and at the same time satisfy the wide range of expectations women bring to it. The diversity that women seek will continue to reflect the differences of the women themselves.

Notes

Introduction

1. I use the phrases "feminist impulse" and "feminist inclinations" to differentiate this analysis from publicly political feminism as manifested by those women who were active in the suffrage movement or in any public advocacy for women's rights and emancipation. I stop short of labeling the birthing women as feminist, and refer instead to impulses and inclinations, because I think their actions were not consciously creating a new world as much as they were supporting an autonomous women's dimension within the existing one. For historians' debates on these issues, see Ellen DuBois, Mari Jo Buhle, Temma Kaplan, Gerda Lerner, and Carroll Smith-Rosenberg, "Politics and Culture in Women's History: A Symposium," *Feminist Studies* 6 (Spring 1980): 26–64.

2. My book builds on the previous work of other historians of childbirth. See, for example, Nancy Schrom Dye, "Review Essay on the History of Childbirth," *Signs* 6 (1980): 97–108; Catherine Scholten, " 'On the Importance of the Obstetrick Art': Changing Customs of Childbirth in America," *William and Mary Quarterly* 34 (1977): 426–45; and Richard W. Wertz and Dorothy C. Wertz, *Lying-In: A History of Childbirth in America* (New York: Free Press, 1977). My conclusions are often at variance with those of Edward Shorter, *A History of Women's Bodies* (New York: Basic Books, 1982), who maintains that twentieth-century medicine saved women from the burdens of their bodies and does not recognize women's own role in influencing their destiny. Traditional histories of obstetrics include Harvey Graham, *Eternal Eve: The History of Gynaecology and Obstetrics* (Garden City, N. Y.: Doubleday, 1951); Herbert Thoms, *Classical Contributions to Obstetrics and Gynecology* (Springfield, Ill.: Charles C Thomas, 1935); Palmer Findlay, *Priests of Lucina: The Story of Obstetrics* (Boston, 1939); Irving S. Cutter and Henry R. Viets, *A Short History of Midwifery* (Philadelphia: W. B. Saunders Company, 1964); Theodore Cianfrani, *A Short History of Obstetrics and Gynecology* (Springfield, Ill.: Charles C Thomas, 1960); Harold Speert, *Obstetric*

and Gynecologic Milestones: Essays in Eponymy (New York: Macmillan, 1958); and Speert's *Iconographia Gyniatrica: A Pictoral History of Gynecology and Obstetrics* (Philadelphia: F. A. Davis, 1973).

3. See for example, Jane B. Donegan, *Women and Men Midwives: Medicine, Morality, and Misogyny in Early America* (Westport, Conn.: Greenwood Press, 1978); Judy Litoff, *American Midwives, 1860 to the Present* (Westport, Conn.: Greenwood Press, 1978). Charlotte Borst is writing her Ph.D. dissertation, "The Transition from Midwife to Physician Attended Childbirth in Four Counties in Wisconsin, 1870–1930," at the University of Wisconsin, analyzing the conditions under which certain communities switched to physician attendants in the early twentieth century.

4. In focusing on the full-term birthing experiences of American women, I do not mean to suggest that these are the only or the most important parts of women's reproductive experiences with a history. Countless women became pregnant and did not carry to term, either by willfully aborting, by spontaneous abortion, or by very premature delivery. Some women had these events interspersed in their lives in between full-term deliveries; others never could or did carry to term. Still other women chose not to have children at all. Some who wanted to conceive and bear children found they could not. All these patterns were evident throughout American history and carried meaning for women as dimensions of possible reproductive patterns. But I had to limit the focus of this study, and this book concentrates on full-term confinement experiences.

Chapter 1. "Under the Shadow of Maternity": Childbirth and Women's Lives in America

1. Elizabeth Gordon Correspondence, Wisconsin State Historical Society Archives, letters from Jane Savine (?) of Warren, Pa., to Elizabeth Gordon of Cleveland, Ohio, quotation from letter of Feb. 26, 1846. See also letter of March 10, 1846.

The evidence in this chapter comes in large part from women themselves. I have searched out women's diaries, letters, and autobiographies to find birth accounts in women's voices; I have also relied on the accounts of family members, including husbands, fathers, brothers, sisters, cousins, and aunts, and the writings of the birth attendants, physicians, midwives, and friends, to uncover accounts relating what happened at confinements. Although I have been wide-reaching in my searches, I do not try to quantify my findings, nor can I suggest that these women whose accounts I have found represent all women. I do believe after all my research that my findings illustrate the general trends in feelings and activities describing American childbirth experiences.

2. See, for example, Augustin Caldwell, *The Rich Legacy: Memories of Hannah Tobey Farmer, Wife of Moses Gerrish Farmer* (Boston: Privately printed, 1890), 97.

3. For the history of birth control and fertility patterns in America, consult Linda Gordon, *Woman's Body, Woman's Right: A Social History of Birth Control in America* (New York: Viking, 1976); James Reed, *From Private Vice to Public*

Virtue: Birth Control in America (New York: Basic Books, 1978); Robert V. Wells, *Revolutions in Americans' Lives: A Demographic Perspective on the History of Americans, Their Families, and Their Society* (Westport, Conn.: Greenwood Press, 1982). On the history of childbirth, consult Janet Bogdan, "Care or Cure: Childbirth Practices in 19th Century America," *Feminist Studies* 4 (1978): 92–99; Nancy Schrom Dye, "Review Essay: History of Childbirth in America," *Signs* 6 (1980): 97–108; Richard W. and Dorothy C. Wertz, *Lying-In: A History of Childbirth in America* (New York: Free Press, 1977); Jane B. Donegan, *Women and Men Midwives: Medicine, Morality, and Misogyny in Early America* (Westport, Conn.: Greenwood Press, 1978); Judy Barrett Litoff, *American Midwives 1860 to the Present* (Westport, Conn.: Greenwood Press, 1978). For the history of women's health generally, consult the articles in Judith Walzer Leavitt, ed., *Women and Health in America: Historical Readings* (Madison: University of Wisconsin Press, 1984).

4. George Francis Dow, ed., *The Holyoke Diaries 1709–1856* (Salem, Mass.: The Essex Institute, 1911).

5. *Ibid.*, 62–64; Mary Beth Norton, *Liberty's Daughters: The Revolutionary Experience of American Women, 1750–1800* (Boston: Little, Brown, 1980), 73.

6. I am grateful to Patricia Barber Holland for leading me to Sarah Hale's letters and diaries and for sharing with me her 1972 seminar paper "The Obstetrical Biography of Mrs. Sarah Everett Hale." This quotation is from Sarah Preston Everett Hale's commonplace book, 1827–1850, entry for Sept. 5, 1841, Box 10, Hale Family Papers, Sophia Smith Collection, Smith College.

7. Warren C. Sanderson, "Quantitative Aspects of Marriage, Fertility and Family Limitation in Nineteenth Century America: Another Application of the Coale Specifications," *Demography* 11 (3) (Aug. 1979): 339–58; Ansley J. Coale and Melvin Zelnik, *New Estimates of Fertility and Population in the United States: A Study of Annual White Births from 1855 to 1960 and of Completeness of Enumeration in the Censuses from 1880 to 1960* (Princeton: Princeton University Press, 1963).

8. Stewart E. Tolnay, Stephen N. Graham, and Avery M. Guest, "Own-Child Estimates of U.S. White Fertility, 1886–99," *Historical Methods* 15 (Summer 1982): 127–38; Phillips Cutright and Edward Shorter, "The Effects of Health on the Completed Fertility of Nonwhite and White U.S. Women Born Between 1867 and 1935," *Journal of Social History* 13 (Winter 1979): 191–217. See also Joseph A. McFalls, Jr., and George S. Masnick, "Birth Control and the Fertility of the U.S. Black Population, 1880–1980," *Journal of Family History* 6 (Spring 1981): 89–106. It is important to keep in mind that active fertility control measures such as birth control or abortion are only part of the explanation for fertility variations. Poor nutrition and certain diseases, including venereal diseases, can curtail birth rates. See Jane Menken, James Trussell, and Susan Watkins, "The Nutrition Fertility Link: An Evaluation of the Evidence," *Journal of Interdisciplinary History* 11 (Winter 1981): 425–41.

9. Michael R. Haines, "Fertility and Marriage in a Nineteenth-Century Industrial City: Philadelphia, 1850–1880," *Journal of Economic History* 40 (March 1980): 151–58. See also Jerry Wilcox and Hilda H. Golden, "Prolific Immigrants and Dwindling Natives?: Fertility Patterns in Western Massachusetts, 1850 and 1880," *Journal of Family History* 7 (Fall 1982): 265–88, which concludes that declining fertility among native-born Americans was "especially noteworthy."

10. Susan Hooker to Alcesta Huntington, Aug. 19, 1872, Huntington-Hooker Papers, University of Rochester, quoted by Harvey Green, *The Light of the Home: An Intimate View of the Lives of Women in Victorian America* (New York: Pantheon Books, 1983), 33; Ellen Whitehead to Nellie Whitehead, Jan. 28, 1877, Whitehead Family Collection, Michigan Historical Collection, Bentley Historical Library, University of Michigan. Ellen envied Nell's being at the family home for the winter while pregnant, sent a recipe, and inquired, "who will you have with you when you are sick." The study that led me to the Michigan Historical Collection is Marilyn Ferris Motz, *True Sisterhood: Michigan Women and Their Kin* (Albany: State University of New York Press, 1983).

11. Cotton Mather, *The Angel of Bethesda*, chapter 53: "Retired Elizabeth: A long tho' no Very Hard, Chapter for, A Woman whose Travail approaches with Remedies to Abate the Sorrows of Child-bearing" (1710), (Barre, Mass.: American Antiquarian Society, 1972), 235–48; quotation, 237.

12. Margaret Jones Bolsterli, ed., *Vinegar Pie and Chicken Bread: A Woman's Diary of Life in the Rural South, 1890–1891* (Fayetteville: University of Arkansas Press, 1982), entry for July 1, 1890, p. 38.

13. Clara Clough Lenroot, Journals and Diaries, Part I, 1891 to 1929, edited by her daughter, Katharine F. Lenroot, typescript (May 1969) in family hands. My thanks to Katherine Vila, who shared copies of this diary with my class, "Women and Health in America," during the spring semester 1983.

14. Ellen Regal to Isaac Demmon, May 13, 1872, Regal Family Collection, Michigan Historical Collection, Bentley Historical Library, University of Michigan; Gro Nilsdatter Swendsen to Mother, Feb. 11, 1877 (translated), Ole Nilsen, Jr. and Family Papers, P1229, Archives/Manuscripts Division, Minnesota Historical Society. Lizzie Cabot and Sarah Ripley Stearns are quoted in Carl N. Degler, *At Odds: Women and the Family in America from the Revolution to the Present* (New York: Oxford University Press, 1980), 60. For similar eighteenth-century concerns, see Norton, *Liberty's Daughters*, 77–82.

15. E. S. Gunnell, Greenfield, Mass. to Weltha Brown, Hartford, Conn., May 9, 1821, Hooker Collection, Schlesinger Library, Radcliffe College, Cambridge, Mass., Box 1, Folder 15; Nettie Fowler McCormick Diary, Box 2, Vol. 19, entry for May 1, 1872, Wisconsin State Historical Society Archives. See also, for example, a physician's report: "October 2 I was called to attend Mrs. R. in confinement and found myself confronted with a number of unpleasant conditions, not the least of which was a morbid fear on my patient's part that she would not be able to give birth to her child . . . that she would not live through another confinement." L. W. Pence, letter to the editor, *Journal of the American Medical Association* 31 (Oct. 29, 1898): 1063. (Hereafter cited as *JAMA*.)

16. Georgiana Bruce Kirby journal, in Erna Olafson Hellerstein, Leslie Parker Hume, and Karen Offen, eds., *Victorian Women: A Documentary Account of Women's Lives in Nineteenth-Century England, France, and the United States* (Stanford: Stanford University Press, 1981), 211.

17. Bessie Huntting Rudd to her husband, Edward Payson Rudd, [Sag] Harbor, May 27[?], 1860, May 9, 1860; May 15, 1860, Huntting-Rudd Family Papers, Box 6, Folder 110, Schlesinger Library, Radcliffe College, Cambridge, Mass. Quoted with permission.

18. A. Dornberg, M.D., to Sarah Jane Stevens, March 9, 1880, Box 8,

James Christie and Family Papers, P1281, Archives/Manuscripts Division, Minnesota Historical Society; Alex Christie to Sarah Jane Stevens, Jan. 9, 1885, *ibid.*, Box 10.

19. Albina Wight Diary, William Wight Papers, Wisconsin State Historical Society. Volumes 11–15 are the diaries of William's wife, Albina Wight, 1869–76. Quotations are from Vol. 11, entries for April 14, 17, 1870. See also entry for May 13, 1870. Mary E. Cooley to Katy Cooley, April 10, 1875, Thomas M. Cooley Collection, Michigan Historical Collections, Bentley Historical Library, University of Michigan.

20. James S. Bailey, "Cases Illustrating Some of the Causes of Death Occurring Soon after Childbirth," *New York State Medical Society Transactions*, 1872, pp. 121–29; quotation, p. 121. For more on physicians' experiences with sudden puerperal death, see James L. Taylor, "What Killed the Woman?" *JAMA* 14 (June 14, 1890): 876–77; Fayette Dunlap, "Sudden Death in Labor and Childbed," *ibid.*, 9 (1887): 330–34; and Edward W. Jenks, "The Causes of Sudden Death of Puerperal Women," *Transactions of the American Medical Association* 29 (1878): 373–91.

21. William Thompson Lusk, "On Sudden Death in Labor and Childbed," *JAMA* 3 (1884): 427–31.

22. H. V. Sweringen, "Laceration of the Female Perineum," *Transactions of the Indiana State Medical Society* 32 (1882): 135. I am grateful to Ann Carmichael for this reference.

23. Haven Emerson and Harriet E. Hughes, *Populations, Notifiable Diseases and Deaths, Assembled for New York City, New York* (New York: DeLamar Institute of Public Health, College of Physicians and Surgeons, 1941) and *Supplement 1936–1953* (Jan. 1955). I would like to thank Gretchen Condran and Morris Vogel for bringing these volumes to my attention, and Evelyn Fine for compiling them and drawing the graph. The trend shown in these figures was probably similar outside the city, but specific dates may differ. Massachusetts statistics, which are also available for this period of time, mirror those of New York presented here. For a lengthy discussion of maternal mortality in New York City, see Janet Bogdan, "Maternal Mortality in New York," paper delivered at the Sixth Berkshire Conference on Women's History, Smith College, June 1983. See also Robert D. Retherford, *The Changing Sex Differential in Mortality* (Westport, Conn.: Greenwood Press, 1975), 57–69. I would like to thank George Alter for his reminder about increasing maternal mortality between 1910 and 1930. In 1980, maternal mortality rates in the United States approached one per 10,000 live births.

24. For a discussion of the relationship between tuberculosis and pregnancy and labor, consult, for example, Charles Sumner Bacon, "Pulmonary Tuberculosis as an Obstetrical Complication," *JAMA* 45 (Oct. 7, 1905): 1067–70; John O. Polak, "Tuberculosis and Pregnancy," *ibid.* 52 (March 20, 1909): 989–90; and Alice Weld Tallant, "Pulmonary Tuberculosis as a Complication of Pregnancy, with a Report of Three Cases," *Woman's Medical Journal* 22 (March 1912): 53–57. See also *The Crusader* (journal of the Wisconsin Anti-Tuberculosis Association) for the 1920s, and the numerous articles analyzing maternal mortality in the *American Journal of Obstetrics and Gynecology, JAMA,* and other medical journals in the decades between 1910 and 1940. Probably the best of

these is William Travis Howard, Jr., "The Real Risk-Rate of Death to Mothers from Causes Connected with Childbirth," *American Journal of Hygiene* 1 (1921): 197–233. See also state studies, for example, Lillian Richardson Smith, "Maternal Mortality in Michigan," *Medical Woman's Journal* 36 (Feb. 1929): 34–36.

25. Edward P. Davis, "Scientific Obstetrics in Private Practice," *JAMA* 22 (Feb. 24, 1894): 275.

26. The figure five births per married woman in the United States may in fact be low. Given the specific studies we have of immigrant and black fertility, five seems a realistic number for calculations. The chances of death are 1/150 for five pregnancies; so survival equals $(149/150)^5$; or the death risk is 1-$(149/150)^5$. I would like to thank Lewis Leavitt and Charlotte Borst for helping me with this calculation and for their warning that time changes in risk level over a woman's fertile years and parity could alter this figure slightly.

27. The Northwestern Mutual Life Insurance Company recorded that of 10,000 applicants for life insurance, "one man in every 17.3 who applied for insurance had a mother or sister or both who died from the immediate effects of childbirth." *The Crusader* noted, "It is believed that a considerable percentage of these deaths from childbirth were recorded on the death certificate as being due to tuberculosis, heart disease, etc., and that the applicant for insurance remembered the associated childbirth and not the cause of death given on the death certificate. Our present mortality records do not show the frequency with which childbirth is a contributing cause of death" (May 1920, p. 5). See also C. W. Earle's comments during a Chicago Medical-Legal Society discussion of J. H. Etheridge, "The Medico-Legal Aspects of Utterances Made in Medical Societies," *JAMA* 10 (May 5, 1888): 570.

28. Ellen Regal to Isaac Demmon, June 16, 1872, Regal Family Collection, Michigan Historical Collections, Bentley Historical Library, University of Michigan; S. L. Chatfield to A. G. Chatfield, July 21, 1837, Andrew G. Chatfield Papers, A .C492, Archives/Manuscripts Division, Minnesota Historical Society.

29. Ella Reeve Bloor, *We Are Many* (New York: International Publications, 1940), 33; *Memoirs of Paul Henry Kendricksen* (Boston: Privately printed, 1910), 302; Theressa Gay, *Life and Letters of Mrs. Jason Lee* (Portland, Ore.: Metropolitan Press, 1936), 84; Anne Lesley, in Susan Inches Lesley, *Recollections of My Mother* (Boston: Press of George H. Ellis, 1889), 306; Ebenezer Pettigrew journal entry, in Hellerstein et al., *Victorian Women,* 220; Welcolm Briggs to Mrs. Chapin, Dec. 13, 1861, Melissa and Welcolm Briggs Papers, P1056, Archives/ Manuscripts Division, Minnesota Historical Society. See also the U.S. Children's Bureau reports, for example, Florence Brown Sherbon and Elizabeth Moore, *Maternity and Infant Care in Two Rural Counties in Wisconsin,* Bureau Publication No. 46 (Washington: Government Printing Office, 1919); and Viola I. Paradise, *Maternity Care and the Welfare of Young Children in a Homesteading County in Montana,* Bureau Publication No. 34 (Washington: Government Printing Office, 1919).

30. For an interesting discussion of the relationship between demographic trends and mentalities, see Daniel Scott Smith, "A Perspective on Demographic Methods and Effects in Social History," *William and Mary Quarterly* 39 (July 1982): 442–68.

31. International comparisons of maternal mortality can be found in Grace

C. Meigs, *Maternal Mortality from All Conditions Connected with Childbirth in the United States and Certain Other Countries,* Children's Bureau Publication No. 6 (Washington, D.C.: Government Printing Office, 1917). Women became aware of continuing high maternal deaths in part from their own experience and in part from articles appearing in popular health journals such as *The Crusader* and in women's journals. See, for example, S. Josephine Baker, "Why Do Our Mothers and Babies Die?" *Ladies' Home Journal* 39 (April 1922): 32, 174.

32. See, for example, James A. Harrar, "The Causes of Death in Childbirth: Maternal Mortalities in 100,000 Confinements at the New York Lying-In Hospital," *American Journal of Obstetrics and Diseases of Women and Children* 77 (1918): 38–41; and Frederick S. Crum, "Deaths in Childbirth," *Medical Record* 78 (1910): 491–92.

33. Beatrice E. Tucker, "What Price Painless Childbirth?" *Ladies' Home Journal* 65 (June 1948): 36.

34. Henry Parker Newman, "Prolapse of the Female Pelvic Organs," *JAMA* 21 (Sept. 2, 1893): 335.

35. S. D. Gross, "Lacerations of the Female Sexual Organs Consequent upon Parturition:—Their Causes and Their Prevention," *JAMA* 3 (1884): 337–38. See also, for example, Dr. Belle Craver's description of "one of the most fearful perineal lacerations I ever saw," following a difficult labor and delivery. She revealed that the woman "being of a retiring and sensitive disposition, and not having the courage to undergo an operation," refused the aid available to her. S. Belle Craver, "The Management of Labor with Reference to the Prevention of Subsequent Uterine Disease," *Woman's Medical Journal* 4 (July 1895): 167–68. See also Marie J. Mergler, "Incontinence of Urine in Women, Due to Traumatism; with a Report of Two Cases," *ibid.* 10 (Jan. 1900): 2; Sara A. Janson, "Lacerations of the Pelvic Floor and Their Effects," *ibid.* 11 (Oct. 1901): 359–63; and Rose Talbott Bullard, "Vaginal and Cervical Lacerations," *ibid.* 11 (Nov. 1901): 389–91.

36. On J. Marion Sims and his contribution to gynecological surgery, consult J. Marion Sims, *The Story of My Life* (New York: D. Appleton, 1889); Seale Harris, *Woman's Surgeon: The Life Story of J. Marion Sims* (New York: Macmillan, 1950); Irwin H. Kaiser, "Reappraisals of J. Marion Sims," *American Journal of Obstetrics and Gynecology* 132 (Dec. 15, 1978): 878–84; and Lawrence D. Longo, "The Rise and Fall of Battey's Operation: A Fashion in Surgery," *Bulletin of the History of Medicine* 53 (1979): 244–67. Historians cannot assume that once the operation for the vesico-vaginal fistula was perfected that all women has access to it or even wanted to undergo the operation. See, for example, the case reported in which a woman refused the procedure: S. Belle Craver, "The Management of Labor with Reference to the Prevention of Subsequent Uterine Disease," *Woman's Medical Journal* 4 (July 1895): 167.

37. On postpartum lacerations, see, for example, Charles P. Noble, "The Causation of Diseases of Women," *JAMA* 21 (Sept. 16, 1893): 410–14; John C. Da Costa, "An Easy Method of Repairing the Perineum," *ibid.* 13 (Nov. 2, 1889): 645–47; Henry T. Byford, "The Production and Prevention of Perineal Lacerations During Labor, with Description of an Unrecognized Form," *ibid.* 6 (March 6, 1886): 253–57, 271; and H. V. Sweringen, "Laceration of the Female Perineum," *ibid.* 5 (Aug. 15, 1885): 173–77. See also the discussion of this last paper in the

Transactions of the Indiana State Medical Society 32 (1882): 258–64, during which Dr. Woolen of Indianapolis blamed physicians' interventions for the increased rate of perineal tears in women: "the frequent use of forceps is filling the country full of cases for our gynecologists, and it does seem to me that we are making a mistake" (p. 263). Physicians, frequently anxious to clear themselves of possible blame, more frequently named the baby's hard head rather than the hard forceps as the principal agent. See Chapter 6 for more discussion of perineal lacerations.

38. J. O. Malsbery, "Advice to the Prospective Mother, Assistance During Her Confinement and Care for a Few Days Following," *JAMA* 28 (May 15, 1897): 932.

39. Augustus K. Gardner, "On the Use of Pessaries," *Transactions of the Americal Medical Association* 15 (1865): 110.

40. Albina Wight Diary, 1869–76. Quotations are from vol. 11, entries of Aug. 20, Oct. 6, 19, 1873; Jan. 18, 1874. In the past, uterine prolapse commonly followed childbirth. Difficult labors and deliveries, unsutured perineal tears, prolonged bedrest, and corset use exacerbated this problem for nineteenth-century women. Physicians still report the condition, but today it is most frequently identified with aging women and is rarely found immediately postpartum. Surgical repairs predominate in current treatment of prolapsed uterus, but pessary-like uterine supports are still found to be helpful. Eliza's sister's treatment with calomel, a mercury compound that acts as a purgative, was more typical earlier in the nineteenth century, when doctors routinely bled and purged patients to relieve them of their ills.

41. Gardner, "On the Use of Pessaries," 113. See also, Rose Willard, "Pessary Worn over Thirty Years, " *Woman's Medical Journal* 6 (June 1897): 165–67.

42. Homer O. Hitchcock, "A Modified Ring Pessary for the Treatment and Cure of Anteflexion and Anteversion of the Uterus," *Transactions of the American Medical Association* 15 (1865): 103–6. See also, Kate Campbell Mead, "Non-Operative Treatment of Prolapsus Uteri. The Schatz Pessary, etc.," *Woman's Medical Journal* 16 (Jan. 1906): 1–4.

43. Reported in "Midwifery" section, *Transactions of the American Medical Association* 6 (1851): 361. The debate about physicians' blame for women's postpartum problems I address in Chapters 2 and 6 and in " 'Science' Enters the Birthing Room: Obstetrics in America Since the Eighteenth Century," *Journal of American History* 70 (Sept. 1983): 281–304. For some contemporary comment, see Hiram Corson, "On the Statistics of 3,036 Cases of Labor," *JAMA* 7 (July 31, 1886): 138–39.

44. Persis Sibley Andrew diary, in Hellerstein et al., *Victorian Women*, 218–19.

45. Agnes Just Reid, *Letters of Long Ago* (Caldwell, Idaho: Caxton Printers, 1936), 24–25. Daughter wrote these letters based on mother's actual experiences and mother edited them, 1871 birth.

46. Augustin Caldwell, *The Rich Legacy: Memories of Hannah Tobey Farmer, Wife of Moses Gerrish Farmer* (Boston: Privately printed, 1892), 97.

47. Mary Kincaid to Mamie Goodwater, Feb. 28, 1896. Correspondence reprinted in Elizabeth Hampsten, comp., *To All Inquiring Friends: Letters, Diaries, and Essays in North Dakota 1880–1910* (Grand Forks: University of North Dakota, Department of English, 1979), 18.

48. Elizabeth H. Emerson, *Glimpses of a Life* (Burlington, N.C.: J. S. Sargent, 1960), 4–5.

49. Lillie M. Jackson, *Fanning the Embers* (Boston: Christopher Publishing House, 1966), 90–91.

50. Hallie F. Nelson, *South of the Cottonwood Tree* (Broken Bow, Nebr.: Purcells, 1977), 173.

51. Harriet Connor Brown, *Grandmother Brown's Hundred Years, 1827–1927* (Boston: Little, Brown, 1929), 158; Susanna Corder, *Life of Elizabeth Fry, Compiled from Her Journal* (Philadelphia: J. Longstreth, 1855), 109–10; Evalyn Walsh McLean, *Father Struck It Rich* (Boston: Little, Brown, 1936), 161; Mrs. Hal Russell, "Memories of Marian Russell," *Colorado Magazine* 21 (1944): 35–36; Elizabeth G. Stern [Leah Morton, pseud.], *I Am a Woman—and a Jew* (New York: Arno, 1960; orig. pub. 1926), 90; Elsa Rosenberg, letter to the author in response to author's query in the *New York Times Book Review,* July 30, 1983.

52. Mary Hallock Foote letter of May, 1877 to Helena DeKay Gilder, Mary Hallock Foote Letters, Stanford University Library, Department of Special Collections, M115, M305. Quoted with permission.

53. Josephine Preston Peabody, *Diary and Letters of Josephine Preston Peabody,* ed. by Christina Hopkinson Baker (Boston: Houghton Mifflin, 1925), 214–15; 226–29.

54. Caroline Gardner Cary Curtis, ed., *The Cary Letters* (Cambridge: Harvard University Press, 1968), 60.

55. Marjorie Housepian Dobkin, ed., *The Making of a Feminist: Early Journals and Letters of M. Carey Thomas* (Kent State, Ohio: Kent State University Press, 1979). Hannah Smith's diary entry was dated Dec. 20, 1852, and Carey Thomas copied it on Sept. 1, 1878 (p. 149).

56. M. Carey Thomas, who never married or had children, went on to become the president of Bryn Mawr College and represented female emancipation for generations of women.

57. Mathilde Shillock to Marie (?), Dec. 8, 1859, Mathilde Shillock Papers, P613, Archives/Manuscript Division, Minnesota Historical Society.

Chapter 2. "Science" Enters the Birthing Room: The Impact of Physician Obstetrics

1. Cecil K. Drinker, *Not So Long Ago: A Chronicle of Medicine and Doctors in Colonial Philadelphia* (New York: Oxford University Press, 1937), 50–62; Jane B. Donegan, *Women and Men Midwives: Medicine, Morality, and Misogyny in Early America* (Westport, Conn.: Greenwood Press, 1978): and Catherine M. Scholten, " 'On the Importance of the Obstetrick Art': Changing Customs of Childbirth in America, 1760 to 1825," *William and Mary Quarterly* 34 (July 1977): 429–31.

2. Louis B. Wright and Marion Tinling, eds., *The Secret Diary of William Byrd of Westover, 1709–1792* (Richmond, 1941), 79. The phrase "called her women together" is common in early childbirth accounts. See, for example, the diary of midwife Martha Moore Ballard of Augusta, Maine, Nov. 21, 1785—"Mrs. Cowen called her women together this evening; was safely delivered of a daughter about the middle of the night and is comfortable"—and Feb. 18, 1786—"Mrs. Fletcher called her women again this morn, and was safely de-

livered of a daughter." Charles Elventon Nash, *The History of Augusta: First Settlements and Early Days as a Town, including the Diary of Mrs. Martha Moore Ballard* (1785 to 1812) (Augusta, Maine: Charles E. Nash, 1904), 243, 246.

3. "Diary of Ebenezer Parkman 1729–1738," *Proceedings of the American Antiquarian Society* 71 (1961): 447–48; Samuel Sewall, *Diary of Samuel Sewall 1674–1729,* Vol. 1, reprint edition (New York: Arno, 1972), entries for April, 1677; Charles E. Nash, *The History of Augusta: First Settlements and Early Days as a Town,* 235–464; Carroll Smith-Rosenberg, "The Female World of Love and Ritual: Relations between Women in Nineteenth-Century America," *Signs* 1 (Autumn 1975), 1–29. See also Ann Hulton, *Letters of a Loyalist Lady* (Cambridge: Harvard University Press, 1927), 33. For a discussion of social childbirth, see Richard W. Wertz and Dorothy C. Wertz, *Lying-In: A History of Childbirth in America* (New York: Free Press, 1977), 1–26; and Laurel Thatcher Ulrich, *Good Wives* (New York: Alfred A. Knopf, 1982); and "Perelous Siens," in *Maine at Statehood: The Forgotten Years 1783–1820,* eds. Charles Clark and James Leamer, forthcoming.

4. On midwives' practices, see Donegan, *Women and Men Midwives,* 9–11, 25, 127; Scholten, " 'On the Importance of the Obstetrick Art,' " 429–31; Janet Bogdan, "Care or Cure? Childbirth Practices in Nineteenth Century America," *Feminist Studies* 4 (June 1978): 94; and Claire E. Fox, "Pregnancy, Childbirth and Early Infancy in Anglo-American Culture: 1675–1830," Ph.D. dissertation, University of Pennsylvania, 1966, pp. 122–27.

5. Drinker, *Not So Long Ago,* 60–61; Lewis C. Scheffey, "The Earlier History and the Transition Period of Obstetrics and Gynecology in Philadelphia," *Annals of Medical History* 2 (May 1940): 215–16. The particulars of why midwives did not attend Shippen's classes are not clear from the extant records.

6. Scholten, " 'On the Importance of the Obstetrick Art,' " 434–36.

7. Bogdan, "Care or Cure?" 96–97; Donegan, *Women and Men Midwives,* 141–57.

8. Drinker, *Not So Long Ago,* 51–53, 58–61.

9. Jane B. Donegan argues that William Shippen practiced conservative obstetrics when compared with the "meddlesome midwifery" of others. Donegan, *Women and Men Midwives,* 118–19. For more on Shippen, see Betsy Copping Corner, *William Shippen, Jr.: Pioneer in American Medical Education: A Biographical Essay* (Philadelphia: American Philosophical Society, 1951).

10. Lawrence D. Longo, "Obstetrics and Gynecology," in *The Education of American Physicians: Historical Essays,* ed. Ronald L. Numbers (Berkeley: University of California Press, 1980), 205–8.

11. *Autobiography of Samuel D. Gross, M.D., with Sketches of His Contemporaries,* ed. Samuel Weissel Gross and Albert Haller Gross (2 vols., Philadelphia: George Barrie, 1887), II: 240.

12. *Ibid.,* 247.

13. William P. Dewees, *A Compendious System of Midwifery, Chiefly Designed To Facilitate the Inquiries of Those Who May Be Pursuing This Branch of Study* (Philadelphia: Carey & Lea, 1830), 295. See also Irving S. Cutter and Henry R. Viets, *A Short History of Midwifery* (Philadelphia: W. B. Saunders, 1964), 156–57.

14. Quoted in Longo, "Obstetrics and Gynecology," 210.

15. Quoted in Wertz and Wertz, *Lying-In,* 50.

16. Walter Channing, *A Treatise on Etherization in Childbirth, Illustrated by Five-Hundred and Eighty-One Cases* (Boston: William D. Ticknor, 1848), 229.

17. Dewees, *Compendious System*, 359; 361–62.

18. A. Clair Siddall, "Bloodletting in American Obstetric Practice, 1800–1945," *Bulletin of the History of Medicine* 54 (1980): 101–10.

19. Bogdan, "Care or Cure?" 96–98; Scholten, " 'On the Importance of the Obstetrick Art,' " 437–39. The crochet and other penetrating and crushing implements were used to destroy the fetus in utero and permit extraction to save the mother's life in extremely difficult labors.

20. Drinker, *Not So Long Ago*, 60–61.

21. Robert P. Harris, "History of a Pair of Obstetrical Forceps Sixty Years Old," *American Journal of Obstetrics and Diseases of Women and Children* 4 (May 1871): 55–59.

22. Dewees, *Compendious System*, 296.

23. *Ibid.*, 287.

24. Frank H. Hamilton, "A Few Practical Remarks on Rupture of the Perineum," reported in *JAMA* 5 (July 4, 1885): 26.

25. *Ibid.*, 291.

26. H. B. Willard Obstetrical Journal, June 29, 1854, p. 23, H. B. Willard Papers (State Historical Society of Wisconsin, Madison); ibid., Feb. 4, 1856, p. 29. I am grateful to Evelyn Fine for calling my attention to Willard's obstetrics journal. For a woman's perceptions of physicians' interventions, see Harriet Connor Brown, *Grandmother Brown's Hundred Years, 1827–1927* (Boston: Little, Brown, 1930), 93.

27. See, for example, Willard Obstetrical Journal, Oct. 27, 1849, p. 3; *ibid.*, Dec. 25, 1849, p. 2; *ibid.*, May 7, 1850, p. 4.

28. Dewees, *Compendious System*, 286*n*, 359; Harris, "History of a Pair of Obstetrical Forceps," 57. For more on women's power within the birthing room, see Chapter 4. Laurel Ulrich explores the compatibility of midwives and physicians in the birthing room and their sharing of patients in "Perelous Siens."

29. A. B. Spach, "A New Obstetric Forceps," *JAMA* 27 (1896): 1358.

30. Henry D. Fry, "The Application of Forceps to Transverse and Oblique Positions of the Head. Description of a New Forceps," *JAMA* 13 (Nov. 9, 1889): 651.

31. Quoted in *JAMA* 31 (1898): 862.

32. E. S. Mead, during discussion of Wallace A. Briggs, "The Functions and the Form of the Obstetric Forceps," *JAMA* 23 (Aug. 18, 1894): 277. The sensitivity in the first sentence in this quotation of this woman physician to the notion that the parturient, not the attendant, delivers the baby raises the question of the influence of the sex of the attendant, which is explored in Chapter 5.

33. "Four Cases of Uterine Traumatism, Produced by the Untimely Application of the Forceps," *Woman's Medical Journal* 4 (Dec. 1895): 326; W. P. Manton, "The Aftermath of Childbirth," *Boston Medical and Surgical Journal* 162 (March 3, 1910): 278. The question of a sexual division of forceps use still needs further examination by historians. On the differential treatments of obstetrical patients by male and female physicians, see Regina Markell Mor-

antz and Sue Zschoche, "Professionalism, Feminism, and Gender Roles: A Comparative Study of Nineteenth-Century Medical Therapeutics," in Judith Walzer Leavitt, ed., *Women and Health in America: Historical Readings* (Madison: University of Wisconsin Press, 1984), 406–21.

34. J. K. Bartlett, "Address of the Chairman of the Section of Obstetrics and Diseases of Women, of the American Medical Association, Read June, 1883," *JAMA* 1 (Aug. 4, 1883): 104.

35. H. H. Whitcomb, "A Report of 616 Cases of Labor in Private Practice," *JAMA* 8 (Feb. 5, 1887): 156.

36. Hiram Corson, "On the Statistics of 3,036 Cases of Labor," reported in *JAMA* 7 (July 31, 1886): 138; "Are Our Obstetrical Principles Unscientific?" *ibid.* (Aug. 7, 1886): 155.

37. George C. Mosher, "The Management of Lingering Labor," *JAMA* 19 (July 9, 1892): 35; Bert Hansen, "Medical Education in New York City in 1866–67: A Student's Notebook of Professor Budd's Lectures on Obstetrics at New York University," *New York State Journal of Medicine* 85 (Aug. and Sept. 1985). The citation is from the unpublished paper, 19, 49. I am grateful to Bert Hansen for sending me this paper and for allowing me to cite it.

38. Joseph Hoffman, "A Plea for the General Adoption of the Axis-Traction Forceps," *JAMA* 15 (Oct. 11, 1890): 528.

39. William S. Stewart, "When Should the Obstetric Forceps be Used? And What Form of Instrument Is Required?" *JAMA* 13 (Nov. 30, 1889): 770.

40. Dan Millikin, "Report of a Case in Which the Child's Arm Became Engaged in the Fenestrum of the Obstetric Forceps," *JAMA* 16 (June 27, 1891): 906–8.

41. H. C. Coe, "The Immediate Application of the Forceps to the After-Coming Head in Cases of Version with Partial Dilatation of the Os," *JAMA* 12 (Jan. 19, 1889): 101.

42. "Complete Dilatation of the Cervix Uteri, an Essential Condition to the Typical Forceps Operation," *JAMA* 5 (Aug. 29, 1885): 238–40.

43. Henry Davidson Fry, "Some Remarks on the Management of Protracted First Stage of Labor," *JAMA* 6 (Feb. 13, 1886): 171.

44. William H. Taylor, "The Consideration of Some Points Connected with Protracted Labor," *JAMA* 3 (Oct. 25, 1884): 449. Thirty-one cases of forceps delivery in the private practice of Boston-area physician Alfred Worcester illustrates what indications led physicians to use forceps, what kind of operation they represented, and the outcomes. Dr. Worcester indicated that approximately 15 percent of his obstetrical cases required forceps operations. Of the 31 reported in 1889, 18 needed high forceps and 13 low forceps. He rated only six operations as "hard." He used ether in 18 of the 31; 17 women experienced lacerations, ranging from "slight" to "torn through sphincter." In the practice of this physician, the reasons for forceps use were most commonly "head arrested," "no progress," or "poor pains." In only four instances did he operate because he perceived the patient to be exhausted. Alfred Worcester, "A Series of Two Hundred Consecutive Cases of Midwifery, in Private Practice," *Boston Medical and Surgical Journal* 120 (1889): 427–33; chart of forceps deliveries, 429.

45. Quoted in "Early Use of Obstetrical Forceps," *Woman's Medical Journal* 10 (Nov. 1900): 484–85.

46. Agnes Eichelberger, "Prophylaxis in Obstetrics," *Woman's Medical Journal* 11 (July 1901): 257–58.

47. Reported in *JAMA* 36 (June 1, 1901): 1580.

48. Dorothy Reed Mendenhall, "Prenatal and Natal Conditions in Wisconsin," *Wisconsin Medical Journal* 15 (March 1917): 353. See also the comments of Dorothy Reed Mendenhall and Florence Sherbon, in American Association for Study and Prevention of Infant Mortality, *Transactions of the Seventh Annual Meeting,* Milwaukee, Oct. 19–21, 1916 (Baltimore, 1917), 67–68, 63–64. It is difficult to compare midwife and physician statistics because of the incomplete record. Furthermore, conclusions might be skewed because physicians were more likely to be called in complicated cases, and their rates would have to be adjusted to acknowledge their role in difficult cases where outcomes were risky.

49. H. H. Whitcomb, "A Report of 616 Cases of Labor in Private Practice," *Medical and Surgical Reporter* 56 (Feb. 12, 1887): 201. See also the American Association for the Study and Prevention of Infant Mortality, *Transactions of the Seventh Annual Meeting,* 67.

50. See, for example, Dorothy I. Lansing, W. Robert Penman, and Dorland J. Davis, "Puerperal Fever and the Group B Beta Hemolytic Streptococcus," *Bulletin of the History of Medicine* 57 (1983): 70–80.

51. Russell Kelso Carter, *The Sleeping Car "Twilight"; or, Motherhood without Pain* (Boston: Chapple, 1915), 10–11.

52. Nettie Fowler McCormick to Anita McCormick Blaine, Aug. 1890, Series 1E, Box 459, Nancy Fowler McCormick Papers (Wisconsin State Historical Society); Anita McCormick Blaine to Nettie Fowler McCormick, Aug. 24, 1890, Series 2B, Box 46, *ibid.*

53. Leon Herman, *A Surgeon Thinks It Over* (Philadelphia: University of Pennsylvania Press, 1962), 60; Morris Fishbein, *An Autobiography* (Garden City, N.Y.: Doubleday, 1969), 25; Helen MacKnight Doyle, *A Child Went Forth: The Autobiography of Dr. Helen MacKnight Doyle* (New York: Gotham House, 1934), 322; Charles Fox Gardiner, *Doctor at Timberline* (Caldwell, Idaho: Caxton Printers, 1938), 211–12.

54. William B. Dewees, "Relaxation and Management of the Perineum During Parturition," *JAMA* 13 (Dec. 14, 1889): 845–46.

55. *Ibid.*, 847. The pressures physicians felt in home birthing rooms did not abate as long as birth remained at home. Dr. Samuel X. Radbill, who delivered babies in the 1930s before limiting his practice to pediatrics, related working under the close observation of female relatives and friends. In one delivery he attended, the parturient's mother, who, after two days of labor, was anxious for her daughter's welfare, and "came rushing in in a rage, brandishing the [kitchen] knife and yelling: 'Doctor, if my daughter dies, I kill you!' " Radbill reported with great relief: "About five minutes later the baby was safely delivered and everybody was as delirious with joy as they had been frantic with terror before." Under such conditions physicians had to keep a cool head as well as a steady hand. The physician was relieved when a nearby hospital opened its maternity ward, and he could deliver his patients there. Letter from Samuel X. Radbill, June 24, 1985, in response to Author's Query for birth accounts, in the *New York Times Book Review,* July 1983.

56. George S. King, *Doctor on a Bicycle* (New York: Rinehart 1958), 61–63. See also Marcus Bossard, *Eighty-one Years of Living* (Minneapolis: Midwest Printing Co., 1946), 39–40; and Mary Bennett Ritter, *More than Gold in California 1849–1933* (Berkeley: Professional Press, 1933), 219.

57. S. H. Landrum, Altus, Okla., letter to the editor, *JAMA* 58 (1912): 576. I would like to thank Carolyn Hackler for calling this letter to my attention.

58. William M. Gregory to editor, *JAMA* 58 (Feb. 24, 1912): 577; J. H. Guinn to editor, *ibid.* (March 23, 1912): 880; J. H. Mackay to editor, *ibid.* (March 9, 1912): 720. For more evidence of the "negotiations" between birthing women and their physicians, consult Chapters 4, 5, and 6.

59. "Management of Normal Labor," *JAMA* 58 (Jan. 27, 1912): 274; F. W. MacManus to editor, *ibid.* (March 9, 1912): 720; and Landrum to editor, *ibid.* (Feb. 24, 1912): 576. The Kelly pad was the invention of Howard Kelly, gynecologist at the Johns Hopkins University Medical School. It consisted of a rubber cushion with an inflatable rim and was designed to allow blood and discharges to fall into a bucket at the bedside and to keep the bed clean, thereby reducing the woman's chance of infection. See Harold Speert, *Obstetrics and Gynecology in America: A History* (Baltimore: Waverly, 1980), 209. On the question of digital examination without sight, it is interesting to note that policy at the New England Hospital for Women and Children, where all the physicians were women, continued Dewees's practice. As Emma Call, a physician at the hospital, wrote: "It was considered most indelicate to uncover a woman's genitals except at the end of the labor, when supporting the perineum. A student was held to be very awkward, who could not pass a catheter by touch, without seeing the urethra." In this case, respect for women's bodies replaced the earlier tradition of modesty. Emma L. Call, "The Evolution of Modern Maternity Technic," *American Journal of Obstetrics* 58 (1908): 394.

60. Edward P. Davis, "Scientific Obstetrics in Private Practice," *JAMA* 22 (Feb. 24, 1894): 273.

61. A. H. Halberstadt, "Advances in Obstetrics During the Last Half Century," *JAMA* 36 (April 27, 1901): 1167.

62. Florence Sherbon, "Discussion," 63–64.

63. Francis A. Long, *A Prairie Doctor of the Eighties: Some Personal Recollections and Some Early Medical and Social History of a Prairie State* (Norfolk, Nebr.: Huse, 1937), 29. See also Longo, "Obstetrics and Gynecology," 211–14; Virginia G. Drachman, "The Loomis Trial: Social Mores and Obstetrics in the Mid-Nineteenth Century," in *Health Care in America: Essays in Social History*, ed. Susan Reverby and David Rosner (Philadelphia: Temple University Press, 1979), 67–83; American Association for Study and Prevention of Infant Mortality, *Transactions of the Seventh Annual Meeting*, 63–64; and Edward C. Atwater, " 'Making Fewer Mistakes': A History of Students and Patients," *Bulletin of the History of Medicine* 57 (1983): 165–87. For other physician experiences, see James Westaway McCue, *Cape Cod Doctor* (Plymouth County, Mass.: New England Book Co., 1945), 6–7; and Leon Herman, *A Surgeon Thinks It Over* (Philadelphia: University of Pennsylvania Press, 1962).

64. J. Whitridge Williams, "Medical Education and the Midwife Problem in the United States," *JAMA* 58 (Jan. 6, 1912): 1, 2, 5; R. H. Riley, "The Public Health Aspect of the Teaching of Obstetrics in Undergraduate Medical Schools,"

ibid. 106 (April 25, 1936): 1438. See also Lawrence D. Longo, "John Whitridge Williams and Academic Obstetrics in America," *Transactions and Studies of the College of Physicians of Philadelphia* 3 (Dec. 1981): 221–54.

Chapter 3. "Overcivilization and Maternity": Differences in Women's Childbirth Experiences

1. Franklin S. Newell, "The Effect of Overcivilization on Maternity," *American Journal of the Medical Sciences* 136 (1908): 533–41. The negative response to the suggestion of cesarean sections on women who did not manifest "mechanical obstruction" is evident in, for example, William Gillespie, "The Advance or Decay of Obstetric Knowledge and Practice," *The Lancet–Clinic* 100 (1908): 488–92.

2. Catharine Beecher, *Letters to the People on Health and Happiness* (New York, 1856; Arno Reprint, 1972), 124. See also Joy Curtis and Bruce Curtis, "Illness and the Victorian Lady: The Case of Jeannie Sumner," *International Journal of Woman's Studies* 4 (Nov.–Dec. 1981): 527–43.

3. Quoted from the *Water Cure Journal* 26 (1858), 96, by Regina Markell Morantz, "Making Women Modern: Middle Class Women and Health Reform in 19th Century America," *Journal of Social History* 10 (1977): 490–507. The ideology of the "lady" that permeated nineteenth-century society may have little reality in describing women's actual lives, but it was no doubt important in some women's emphasis of their languorous behavior. It may have greatly contributed, for example, to women's portrayal of themselves as sickly, regardless of the actual nature of their health. See Barbara Sicherman, "Review Essay: American History," *Signs* 1 (Winter 1975): 461–85, for an analysis of the true woman ideology.

4. Edward H. Clarke, *Sex in Education, or, A Fair Chance for the Girls* (Boston, 1873; reprint edition, New York: Arno, 1972), 63.

5. George Engelmann quoted in Carroll Smith-Rosenberg and Charles Rosenberg, "The Female Animal: Medical and Biological Views of Woman and Her Role in Nineteenth-Century America," *Journal of American History* 60 (Sept. 1973): 332–56.

6. Cyrus Edson, "American Life and Physical Deterioration," *The North American Review* 157 (Oct. 1893): 442. Edson told the story of his friend, whose only son was engaged to marry a woman from Germany. A third friend observed that "the prospective bridegroom had shown a lack of patriotism in his choice." Edson's friend retorted: "I should like to have more than one grandchild, for there is money enough, and I do not want my son to bear the sorrow I have borne. It means a good deal to a man to be forced to watch the person who is dearest to him a hopeless invalid." This man and many like him feared that American women could not be trusted to bear healthy children or themselves remain healthy through adulthood (pp. 449–50).

7. "The Health of American Women," *JAMA* 21 (Oct. 21, 1893): 622.

8. Edmund Andrews, "Are American Women Physically Degenerated?" *JAMA* 21 (Oct. 21, 1893): 613–14.

9. James D. Morgan, letter to the editor, *JAMA* 21 (Nov. 4, 1893): 710.

10. See for example, C. E. Ruth, "Female Weakness," *JAMA* 23 (Sept. 8, 1894): 389–90.

11. Newell, "Overcivilization," 535.

12. Azel Ames, Jr., *Sex in Industry: A Plea for the Working-Girl* (Boston: James R. Osgood, 1875), 31.

13. Elizabeth Stow Brown, "The Working-Women of New York: Their Health and Occupations," *Journal of Social Science* 25 (1889): 78–92.

14. For a discussion of the relative incidence of tuberculosis in men and women, see David E. Osler and Barbara Gutmann Rosenkrantz, "Phthisis and Puberty: Sex Differences in the Incidence of Consumption Among 19th Century Adolescents," unpublished paper presented to the American Association for the History of Medicine, May 1974; and S. Adolphus Knopf, "Tuberculosis Among Young Women," *JAMA* 90 (Feb. 18, 1928): 532–35. For the effects of tuberculosis on women's lives, see, for example, Sarah Pratt's Diary, 1844–47, Wisconsin State Historical Society Archives.

15. "Tuberculosis and Pregnancy," *JAMA* 42 (June 19, 1904): 775. See the debate about abortion following the discussion of Charles Sumner Bacon, "Pulmonary Tuberculosis as an Obstetrical Complication," *ibid.* 45 (Oct. 7, 1905): 1069–70.

16. Charles Sumner Bacon, *ibid.*, 1067–68.

17. Alice Weld Tallant, "Pulmonary Tuberculosis as a Complication of Pregnancy, with a Report of Three Cases," *Woman's Medical Journal* 22 (March 1912): 56.

18. Huntting Rudd Family papers, Schlesinger Library, Radcliffe College, Cambridge, Mass.

19. J. Whitridge Williams, *Obstetrics: A Textbook for the Use of Students and Practitioners*, 3rd edition (New York: Appleton, 1916), 724. See also, Effa V. Davis, "A Study of the Bony Pelvis in One Hundred and Fifty Cases," *JAMA* 45 (Dec. 2, 1905): 1709–10.

20. See for example Effa V. Davis, *ibid.*

21. Phillips Cutright and Edward Shorter, "The Effects of Health on the Completed Fertility of Nonwhite and White Women Born Between 1867 and 1935," *Journal of Social History* 13 (Winter 1979): 191–217; Mark Thomas Connelly, *The Response to Prostitution in the Progressive Era* (Chapel Hill: University of North Carolina Press, 1980). See also Allan M. Brandt, *No Magic Bullet: A Social History of Venereal Disease in the United States Since 1880* (New York: Oxford University Press, 1985).

22. Charlotte B. Brown, "Rest Therapy in Gynaecology," *Woman's Medical Journal* 4 (Aug. 1895): 213.

23. Joseph B. DeLee, "Obstetrics Versus Midwifery," *JAMA* 103 (Aug. 4, 1934): 310; Mary Kincaid to Mamie Goodwater, June 28, 1896, in Elizabeth Hampsten, comp., *To All Inquiring Friends: Letters, Diaries, and Essays in North Dakota 1880–1910* (Grand Forks: University of North Dakota, Department of English, 1979), 19; quoted by Mary A. Dixon-Jones, "A Talk on Subjects Relating to Parturition," *Woman's Medical Journal* 4 (Nov. 1895): 282.

24. Paul Starr, *The Social Transformation of American Medicine* (New York: Basic Books, 1983), 65–71.

25. Margaret Jarman Hagood, *Mothers of the South: Portraiture of the White Tenant Farm Women* (New York: W. W. Norton, 1977), 109.

26. Michael M. Davis, Jr., *Immigrant Health and the Community* (New York: Harper & Bros., 1921), 189. On health differentials, see, for example, Judith Walzer Leavitt, *The Healthiest City: Milwaukee and the Politics of Health Reform* (Princeton: Princeton University Press, 1982), chapter 1; and John Duffy, *A History of Public Health in New York City*, 2 vols. (New York: Russell Sage Foundation, 1968, 1974).

27. Virginia Drachman, "The Loomis Trial: Social Mores and Obstetrics in Mid-Nineteenth Century America," in Judith Walzer Leavitt, *Women and Health in America: Historical Readings* (Madison: University of Wisconsin Press, 1984), 166–74. See also, for example, the journal of Martha E. (Hutchings) Griffith, 1863–81, a record of her obstetrical training at a Boston area hospital, Indiana University Lilly Library. I am grateful to Ann Carmichael for leading me to this journal.

28. Morris Fishbein, *An Autobiography* (Garden City, N.Y.: Doubleday, 1969), 25; Charles W. Mayo, *Mayo. The Story of My Family and My Career* (Garden City, N.Y.: Doubleday, 1968), 64; Franklin H. Martin, *The Joy of Living: An Autobiography* (Garden City, N.Y.: Doubleday, Doran, 1933), Vol. 1, pp. 178, 214–16; Mary Bennett Ritter, *More Than Gold in California 1849–1933* (Berkeley: Professional Press, 1933), 162.

29. Adele Comandini, *Doctor Kate, Angel on Snowshoes: The Story of Kate Pelham Newcomb, M.D.* (New York: Rinehart, 1956), 43–44, 50–58.

30. Margaret R. Stewart, *From Dugout to Hilltop* (Culver City, California: Murray & Gee, 1951), 78–79.

31. Leon Herman, *A Surgeon Thinks It Over* (Philadelphia: University of Pennsylvania Press, 1962), 60.

32. "Rats in the Hospitals," *Harper's Weekly* 4 (1860): 273.

33. Davis, *Immigrant Health*, 191–94.

34. Grace Meigs, "Rural Obstetrics," *Transactions of the Seventh Annual Meeting of the American Association for the Study and Prevention of Infant Mortality* (Baltimore: Franklin Printing Co., 1917), 52. See also, Elizabeth C. Forrest, "Stork Expected at Point Barrow," *Atlantic Monthly* 157 (Feb. 1936): 129–37.

35. Susan Cayleff, " 'Wash and Be Healed': The Nineteenth Century Water-Cure Movement, 1840–1900: Simple Medicine and Women's Retreat," paper presented at the American Association for the History of Medicine, Durham, N.C., May 17, 1985; and Ronald L. Numbers, "Do-It-Yourself the Sectarian Way," in *Sickness and Health in America: Readings in the History of Medicine and Public Health*, eds. Judith Walzer Leavitt and Ronald L. Numbers, (Madison: University of Wisconsin Press, 1978), 87–96. I am grateful to Susan Cayleff for sending me a copy of her unpublished paper, which is based on her Brown University Ph.D. dissertation. See also Jane B. Donegan, *"Hydropathic Highway to Health": Women and Water-Cure in Antebellum America* (New York: Greenwood Press, 1986).

36. The variations in the skills of the regular profession are discussed at greater length in Chapters 2, 5, and 6.

37. See, for example, Beatrice E. Tucker, "Maternal Mortality of the Chicago Maternity Center," *American Journal of Public Health* 27 (1937): 33–36.

38. Hagood, *Mothers of the South*, 111.

39. Nancy Schrom Dye, "Scientific Obstetrics and Working-Class Women:

The New York Midwifery Dispensary," paper delivered at the American Historical Association, San Francisco, Dec. 1983, pp. 4–7.

40. Philadelphia County Almshouse Hospital, Bureau of Charities, Maternity Cases, 1894–98, (City of Philadelphia Department of Records, City Archives, Microfilm 976940). I am grateful to Morris Vogel for suggesting this source and for making it possible for me to see the microfilmed records.

41. There was yet another element of female control that physicians had to acknowledge if they wanted women to continue to ask them to attend childbirth. The wishes of the middle-class women who, in their charity work, established institutions to meet the needs of poor women in their communities became an important determinant of doctor-patient interactions in the nineteenth century. Historian Virginia Quiroga has studied several New York City charity and public institutions and concluded that "until the early twentieth century, physicians held little authority in the traditional female world of childbirth and child care, and even less in the helping institutions which were founded in the 19th century." While Quiroga found that the values of the middle-class ladies' clubs and individual reformers might not have matched the values of the women they tried to help, their "maternalistic vision" was important in setting the environment into which physicians had to fit. The women transferred the values developed within their own confinement rooms into the institutionalized rooms they helped to found. This created yet another common bond among different classes of women who in other ways discussed above were different. See Virginia Anne Metaxas Quiroga, "Poor Mothers and Babies: A Social History of Childbirth and Child Care Institutions in Nineteenth Century New York City," Ph.D. dissertation, Department of History, State University of New York at Stony Brook, May 1984, pp. v, 51.

Chapter 4. "Only a Woman Can Know": The Role of Gender in the Birthing Room

1. Catherine Scholten, " 'On the Importance of the Obstetrick Art,' " in *Women and Health in America: Historical Readings*, ed. Judith Walzer Leavitt (Madison: University of Wisconsin Press, 1984), 150. See also her *Childbearing in American Society 1650–1850* (New York: New York University Press, 1985).

2. Ebenezer Parkman, *The Diary of Ebenezer Parkman 1703–1782*, ed. Francis G. Walett (Worcester, Mass.: American Antiquarian Society, 1974), entry for Feb. 16, 1747, p. 150.

3. Mary Louise Fowler to Nettie Fowler McCormick, Oct. 25, 1863, McCormick Family Papers, Incoming Correspondence, 1860–64, Wisconsin State Historical Society Archives. See also, letter from Mary (Mildred) Sullivan to Nettie, Nov. 2, 1874.

4. Albina Wight Diary, Wisconsin State Historical Society, Vol. 11, April 14, 1870.

5. Malinda Jenkins, *Gambler's Wife: The Life of Malinda Jenkins*, as told in conversations to Jessie Lilienthal (Boston: Houghton Mifflin, 1933), 48. For evidence of this practice of neighboring women attending confinements along with physicians, see, for example, Price County Department of Public Welfare

Papers, Wisconsin State Historical Society, Series 25, Box 1, Folder 71; Box 2, Folder 22.

6. Elizabeth Elton Smith, *The Three Eras of Woman's Life* (New York: Harper & Bros., 1836), 85. That birth was most commonly perceived and experienced as women's province does not mean that the historical record omits instances of male attendance. Husbands, for example, did find themselves in attendance at their wives' confinements, sometimes in the absence of other help. Frances Evelyn Prince Cahoon, for example, wrote in her diary about her 1888 confinement, during which she was aided by a physician, a neighbor woman, and her husband. She had sent her 15-year-old sister, who had been helping with household chores, out of the house, presumably because she was too young. Of her husband's participation, Cahoon wrote, "When the child was first born my husband stood at the head of the bed with his arm around me, I looked up at him, and saw every tooth in his head, and his eyes were fixed in perfect delight on the place where he could see the movements of his child." Diary, vol. 105 [1888], entry, "First Two Months Her Birthday," Josiah B. Chaney Papers, P1331, Archives/Manuscript Division, Minnesota Historical Society. See also Jill Suitor, "Husband's Participation in Childbirth: A Nineteenth Century Phenomenon," *Journal of Family History* 6 (1981): 278–93.

7. Anita McCormick Blaine to Nettie Fowler McCormick, Aug. 1890, McCormick Papers, Wisconsin State Historical Society.

8. Nettie Fowler McCormick to Anita McCormick Blaine, *ibid.*, 1E, Box 459.

9. Georgiana Bruce Kirby journal, in Erna Olafson Hellerstein, Leslie Parker Hume, and Karen Offen, eds., *Victorian Women: A Documentary Account of Women's Lives in Nineteenth–Century England, France, and the United States* (Stanford: Stanford University Press, 1981), 211–13; Martha Slayton to Mrs. Slayton and Gussie Slayton, July 31, 1917, Slayton Family Collection, Michigan Historical Collection, Bentley Historical Library, University of Michigan.

10. Mary Hallock Foote Letters, Stanford University Library, transcripts of letters to Helena DeKay Gilder 1874–86, Department of Special Collections, M115, M305. Quoted with permission.

11. Elizabeth G. Stern [Leah Morton, pseud.], *I Am a Woman—and a Jew* (New York: Arno, 1969; originally published 1926), 87.

12. Hannah Bingham to Maria Seymour, April 10, 1844, Bingham Family Collection, Michigan Historical Collections, Bentley Historical Library, University of Michigan; Dorothy Lawson McCall, *The Copper King's Daughter: From Cape Cod to Crooked River* (Portland, Ore.: Binfords & Mort, 1972).

13. Gladys Brooks, *Boston and Return* (New York: Atheneum, 1962).

14. Malcolm R. Lovell, *Two Quaker Sisters: From the Original Diaries of Elizabeth Buffum Chase and Lucy Buffum Lovell* (New York: Liverright, 1937), 1–2. See also, for example, Forest W. NcNeir, *Forest McNeir of Texas* (San Antonio: Naylor, 1956); Elsa Maxwell, *R.S.V.P.: Elsa Maxwell's Own Story* (Boston: Little, Brown, 1954); and Susan Allison, *A Pioneer Gentlewoman in British Columbia: The Recollections of Susan Allison*, ed. Margaret A. Ormsby (Vancouver: University of British Columbia Press, 1976).

15. Mattie White Briscoe, *Dun-Movin: The Memoirs of a Minister's Wife* (New York: Exposition Press, 1963).

16. Willie Elmore Glass, *Miss Willie: Happenings of a Happy Family, 1816–1926* (Essington, Pa.: Huntingdon Press, 1976), 12; Diary of Julia Gage Carpenter, 1882–1904, in Elizabeth Hampsten, comp., *To All Inquiring Friends: Letters, Diaries, and Essays in North Dakota 1880–1910* (Grand Forks: University of North Dakota, Department of English, 1980), 234–36.

17. Emily McCorkee Fitzgerald, *Army Doctor's Wife on the Frontier: Letters from Alaska and the Far West 1874–1878*, ed. Abe Laufe (Pittsburgh: University of Pittsburgh Press, 1962).

18. Letter from Sarah Hale to Edward Everett Hale and Emily Hale, Nov. 30, 1853, Box 11, Folder 315, Hale Family Papers, Sophia Smith Collection, Smith College.

19. Letter from Sarah Hale to her daughters, *ibid.*, Oct. 24, 1853.

20. Bolsterli, *Vinegar Pie*, entries for Aug. 15, 16, 17, 1890, pp. 60–61.

21. William P. Preston to his daughter, May, on her fifteenth birthday, May 19, 1864, from the collection of the McKeldin Library Archives and Manuscripts, University of Maryland, College Park. I would like to thank Virginia Beauchamp for sending me this reference from her forthcoming book, *The Language of Silence: Madge Preston's Story*.

22. Abbie Field to Flora (?), May 25, 1864, Field Family Collection, Michigan Historical Collection, Bentley Historical Library, University of Michigan; Laura B. Gaye, *Laugh on Friday, Weep on Sunday: One Woman's Reminiscence* (Calabasas, Calif.: Loma Palaga Press, 1968), 55.

23. Hagood, *Mothers of the South*, 112.

24. Agnes Just Reid, *Letters of Long Ago* (Caldwell, Idaho: Caxton Printers, 1936), 24. The birth occurred Oct. 26, 1871.

25. Christiana Holmes Tillson, *A Woman's Story of Pioneer Illinois*, ed. Milo Milton Quaife (Chicago: Lakeside Press, 1919), 128.

26. *The Life of Mrs. Robert Clay, Afterwards Mrs. Robert Bolton (Née Ann Curtis), 1690–1738* (Philadelphia, 1928), 154.

27. May Hartley [Mary's granddaughter], *Whither Shall I Go?: A Story of an Itinerant Circuit Rider's Wife* (Southold, N.Y.: Academy Printing Services, 1975), 89. See also L. F. Smith to Elmire M. Bunce, March 9, 1851, Henry A. Smith Papers, A .S649, Archives/Manuscripts Division, Minnesota Historical Society.

28. Mathilde Shillock to Marie (?), Oct. 25, 1856, typed and translated from the German, in the Mathilde Shillock Papers, P613, Archives/Manuscripts Division, Minnesota Historical Society; Mary Kincaid to Mamie Goodwater, June 28, 1896, in Elizabeth Hampsten, comp., *Read This Only to Yourself*, 106; Fay Noe, *All in a Lifetime* (Chicago: Adams Press, 1965), 79. See also Melissa and Welcolm Briggs Papers, P1056, Minnesota Historical Society.

29. David S. Kellogg, *A Doctor at All Hours. The Private Journal of a Small-Town Doctor's Varied Life 1886–1909* (Brattleboro, Vt.: Stephen Greene Press, 1970), 154.

30. Frances Jacobs Alberts, ed., *Sod House Memories* (Hastings, Nebr.: Sod House Society, 1972), memoir of C.O. and Ann Almquist of Nebraska, 7.

31. Marguerite Wallace Kennedy, *My Home on the Range* (Boston: Little, Brown, 1951), 274–75.

32. Patricia Cooper and Norman Bradley Buferd, *The Quilters: Women and*

Domestic Art (Garden City, N.Y.: Doubleday, 1977), 154. The quotation is from oral history interviews with women in the Southwest.

33. Gaye, *Laugh on Friday, Weep on Sunday*, 55; Hartley, *Whither Shall I Go?*, 76.

34. Anna Maria Thornton, "Diary of Mrs. William Thornton, 1800–1863," *Records of the Columbia Historical Society* 10 (1907): 100.

35. Esther Burr, *Esther Burr's Journal* (Washington, D.C.: Howard University Print, 1903).

36. Susan Allison, *A Pioneer Gentlewoman in British Columbia: The Recollections of Susan Allison*, ed. Margaret A. Ormsby (Vancouver: University of British Columbia Press, 1976), 28. Allison went on to have thirteen more children, all with the help of Indian women.

37. Letter from Sarah Hale to Edward Everett and Emily, Nov. 30, 1853, Box 11, Folder 315, Hale Family Papers, Sophia Smith Collection, Smith College.

38. Stella B. Gowan, *Wildwood: A Story of Pioneer Life* (New York: Vantage, 1959), 27–29. See also, for example, (?) To Brother and Sister, April 20, 1874, Samuel D. Carrell and Family Papers, A .C314, Archives/Manuscripts Division, Minnesota Historical Society.

39. Jane Reid to Sarah Jane Stevens, March 8, 1885, Box 10, James Christie and Family Papers, P 1281, Archives/Manuscripts Division, Minnesota Historical Society.

40. Laura Lenoir Norwood letter, in Hellerstein et al., *Victorian Women*, 218.

41. Elizabeth Y. Atkinson Richmond, Papers, 1851–98, Wisconsin State Historical Society, Letter from Elizabeth to her mother, Dec. 11, 1851. See also Stella B. Gowan, *Wildwood: A Story of Pioneer Life* (New York: Vantage, 1959).

42. Mrs. A. Graves, *Girlhood and Womanhood . . . Sketches of My Schoolmates* (Boston: Carier, 1844).

43. Grace Lumpkin, *To Make My Bread* (New York: Macaulay, 1932). My thanks to Mari Jo Buhle for calling this reference to my attention.

44. Mrs. Carrie W. Keeley correspondence, 1905–11, Wisconsin State Historical Society, letter from S. M. Thatcher to Carrie Keeley, March 15, 1910. See also, for example, Susan Allison, *A Pioneer Gentlewoman*, 28; Elizabeth Avery Meriwether, *Recollections of Ninety-two Years, 1824–1916* (Nashville: Tennessee Historical Commission, 1958), 109–10. The women's sphere that is operating in these examples gave way in the late nineteenth century and early twentieth century as women developed closer relationships with their husbands. So-called "companionate" marriages, in which men and women shared intimacies that earlier generations usually did not tolerate, eroded the power of women's emotional ties to one another.

45. Mrs. W. H. Maxwell, M.D., *A Female Physician to the Ladies of the United States, Being a Familiar and Practical Treatise on Matters of Utmost Importance Peculiar to Women; Adapted for Every Woman's Own Private Use* (New York: published by Mrs. W. H. Maxwell, 1860), 3.

46. Letter to the author, Sept. 9, 1983, in response to Author's Query in the *New York Times Book Review*, July 1983.

47. Bolsterli, *Vinegar Pie*, entry of June 27, 1890, p. 35.

48. Laurel Thatcher Ulrich, *Good Wives: Image and Reality in the Lives of Women in Northern New England 1650–1750* (New York: Alfred A. Knopf, 1982), 133.

49. Fleetwood Churchill, *The Diseases of Females: Including Those of Pregnancy and Childbed*, 4th American edition (Philadelphia: Lea and Blanchard, 1847), 340.

50. John G. Meachem, Sr., autobiography, papers, 1823–96, State Historical Society of Wisconsin, Box 1, p. 6. See also Carl Binger, *Revolutionary Doctor: Benjamin Rush, 1746–1813* (New York: W. W. Norton, 1966), 77.

51. Ellen Regal to Isaac Demmon, May 13, 1872, Michigan Historical Collection, Bentley Historical Library, University of Michigan.

52. Franklin H. Martin, *The Joy of Living. An Autobiography* (2 vols., Garden City, N.Y.: Doubleday, Doran, 1933), I: 214.

53. William Allen Pusey, *A Doctor of the 1870s and 80s* (Springfield, Ill.: Charles C Thomas, 1932), 106.

54. Mable Hobson Draper, *Through the Long Trail* (New York: Rinehart & Co., 1946), 278–79. This is a fictionalized first person account of Draper's mother's experiences, written "in homely words and phrases Mother would have used at the time of the experience" (p. x).

55. Dairy of Dr. Daniel Cameron, entry of May 25, 1853, p. 53, Wisconsin State Historical Society.

56. Jane B. Kelly Diaries, 7 vols., 1866–98, Wisconsin State Historical Society, Vol. 4, entries for July 4, 6, 1886. See also Dorothy Rood's diary, March 3–15, 1912, March 11–29, 1914, Box o, Vol. 3, Dorothy Atkinson Rood and Family Papers, P11, Archives/Manuscripts Division, Minnesota Historical Society.

57. Harriet Connor Brown, *Grandmother Brown's Hundred Years, 1827–1927* (Boston: Little, Brown, 1929), 158.

58. Theressa Gay, *Life and Letters of Mrs. Jason Lee* (Portland, Ore.: Metropolitan Press, 1936), 84.

59. Letter from Dr. Thomas Steel to his father, December 12, 1844, in the Steel Collection, Wisconsin State Historical Society. I am grateful to Peter Harstad for calling my attention to Steel's obstetrical cases.

60. Fay Noe, *All in a Lifetime* (Chicago: Adams Press, 1965), 79.

61. William Potts Dewees, *Compendious System of Midwifery* (1832), 189.

62. Alexander Hamilton, *A Treatise on the Management of Female Complaints and of Children in Early Infancy*, new edition (New York: Printed and sold by Samuel Campbell, 1792), 174.

63. Edward Henry Dixon, *Woman and Her Diseases from the Cradle to the Grave*, 10th edition (New York: A. Ranney, 1857), 261–62.

64. Frederick Hollick, *The Matron's Manual of Midwifery and the Diseases of Women During Pregnancy and in Childbed*, 47th edition, (New York: T. W. Strong, 1849), 226. See also M. Chailly, *Practical Treatise on Midwifery*, trans. Gunning S. Bedford (New York: Harper & Bros., 1844), 207–8.

65. Thomas Bull, *Hints to Mothers, for the Management of Health During the Period of Pregnancy, and in the Lying-in Room* (New York: Wiley & Putnam, 1842), 125–26.

66. *Ibid.*, 126.

67. Mrs. P. B. Saur, M.D., *Maternity: A Book for Every Wife and Mother* (Chicago: L. P. Miller, 1891), 226. Dr. John Buchanan believed that no women friends or relatives should be allowed to be in the labor room. *A Practical Treatise on Midwifery, and Diseases of Women and Children* (Philadelphia: John Buchanan, 1868), 136.

68. John Milton Duff, "Parturition as a Factor in Gynecologic Practice," *JAMA* 35 (Aug. 25, 1900): 465; Price's comment came during the discussion of this paper, 467.

69. Bert Hansen located a student's transcriptions of Budd's lectures at New York University, and he presents segments of them in "Medical Education in New York City in 1866–67: A Student's Notebook of Professor Budd's Lectures on Obstetrics at New York University," *New York State Journal of Medicine* 85 (Aug. and Sept., 1985). The citation here is from excerpt 53, p. 68 of Hansen's unpublished manuscript. I am grateful to Professor Hansen for his permission to quote from the paper and to Morris Vogel for originally calling it to my attention. The transcriptions are very valuable for helping scholars to understand many aspects of medical practices in the birthing rooms at mid-century.

70. E. L. Larkins, "Care and Repair of the Female Perineum," *JAMA* 32 (Feb. 11, 1899): 284; L. A. Harcourt, during a discussion at the Chicago Medical Society, reported in *ibid.* 1 (Dec. 1883): 629.

71. Reported in James A. Harrar, *The Story of the Lying-In Hospital of the City of New York* (New York: Society of the Lying-In Hospital, 1938), 34. On the point of rebellion of women inside the hospital as well as outside, see Nancy Schrom Dye, "Scientific Obstetrics and Working-Class Women: The New York Midwifery Dispensary," paper delivered at the American Historical Association, San Francisco, Dec. 1983.

72. J. H. Mackay, letter to the Editor, *JAMA* 58 (1912): 720. For an analysis of physicians' need to educate birthing women to recognize medical authority, see Agnes Eichelberger, "Prophylaxis in Obstetrics," *Woman's Medical Journal* 11 (July 1901): 255–58.

73. Dixon, *Woman and Her Diseases*, 262; E. K. Brown, "A Plea for Stricter Prophylaxis and More Scientific Management of Obstetrical Cases in Tenement House Practice," *Medical Record* 73 (May 16, 1908): 810–16.

74. Recent research has revealed that the presence of "supportive women" actually decreases the length of labor and improves its course, a finding that is corroborated in the historical literature. R. Sosa, J. Kennell, M. Klaus, S. Robertson, and J. Urrutia, "The Effect of a Supportive Companion on Perinatal Problems, Length of Labor and Mother-Infant Interaction," *New England Journal of Medicine,* 303 (Sept. 11, 1980): 597–600. See Chapter 2 for more examples of physicians' lack of control in home deliveries.

75. Marilyn Clohessy, letter to author, Sept. 9, 1983, in response to Author's Query in the *New York Times Book Review,* July 1983.

76. Carroll Smith-Rosenberg, "The Female World of Love and Ritual: Relations between Women in Nineteenth-Century America," *Signs* 1 (1975): 1–29.

77. Drinker, *Not So Long Ago,* 60. An unmarried man, unfamiliar with women's habits and thus not sympathetic, might also be more likely to be seeking (sexual?) excitement.

78. Maxwell, *A Female Physician* (1860), 40.

79. S. Josephine Baker, *Fighting for Life* (New York: Macmillan, 1939), 113; "The Function of the Midwife," *Woman's Medical Journal* 23 (Sept. 1913): 197.

80. Mary Roth Walsh, *"Doctors Wanted, No Women Need Apply": Sexual Barriers to Women in the Medical Profession* (New Haven: Yale University Press, 1978); and Regina Morantz-Sanchez, *Sympathy and Science: Women in American Medicine* (New York: Oxford University Press, 1985). The question of why women physicians declined in numbers in the early twentieth century, especially in light of the demand that existed for their services, is a complex one, and both of these historians analyze this question.

81. Helen MacKnight Doyle, *A Child Went Forth: The Autobiography of Dr. Helen MacKnight Doyle* (New York: Gotham House, 1934), 277. See also Charlotte Blake Brown, "Obstetric Practice Among the Chinese in San Francisco," *Pacific Medical and Surgical Journal* 26 (July 1883): 15–21.

82. Alfred M. Rehwinkel, *Dr. Bessie* (St. Louis: Concordia, 1963), 68.

83. Baker, *Fighting for Life*, 52.

84. Lilian Welsh, *Reminiscences of Thirty Years in Baltimore* (Baltimore: Norman, Remington Co., 1925), 42.

85. Morantz-Sanchez, *Sympathy and Science*. See especially Chapter 6.

86. Maxwell, *A Female Physician*, 46.

87. *Ibid.*, 45.

88. Margaret E. Colby, "Pregnancy and Parturition from a Woman's Point of View," *Woman's Medical Journal* 12 (Dec. 1902): 272–75; editorial, *ibid.* 29 (Nov. 1922): 299.

89. Mary A. Dixon-Jones, "A Talk on Subjects Relating to Parturition," *Woman's Medical Journal* 4 (Nov. 1895): 286; Inez C. Philbrick, "Women, Let us Be Loyal to Women," *Medical Woman's Journal* 36 (Feb. 1929): 41.

90. Eliza M. Mosher, "The Human in Medicine, Surgery and Nursing," *Woman's Medical Journal* 20 (April 1910): 72. For an analysis of women's use of this argument see Regina Markell Morantz, "The Connecting Link: The Case for the Woman Doctor in 19th-Century America," in Judith Walzer Leavitt and Ronald L. Numbers, *Sickness and Health in America: Readings in the History of Medicine and Public Health* (Madison: University of Wisconsin Press, 1978), 117–28.

91. For historians' debates on this issue, consult Regina Markell Morantz and Sue Zschoche, "Professionalism, Feminism, and Gender Roles: A Comparative Study of Nineteenth-Century Medical Therapeutics," in Judith Walzer Leavitt, ed., *Women and Health in America: Historical Readings* (Madison: University of Wisconsin Press, 1984), 406–421; and Laurie Crumpacker, "Female Patients in Four Boston Hospitals of the 1890s," paper presented at the 1974 Berkshire Conference of Women Historians (copy in the Schlesinger Library, Radcliffe College).

92. Margaret R. Stewart, *From Dugout to Hilltop* (Culver City, Calif.: Murray & Gee, 1951), 96.

93. See, for example, Rachelle S. Yarros, "From Obstetrics to Social Hygiene," *Medical Woman's Journal* 33 (Nov. 1926): 305–9.

94. Samuel Gregory, *Letters to Ladies, in Favor of Female Physicians for Their Own Sex*, 2nd edition (Boston: Female Medical Education Society, 1854), 21.

95. See, for example Baker, *Fighting for Life,* 113.; and Elizabeth Blackwell, *Opening the Medical Profession to Women* (New York: Schocken, 1977, reprint of the 1895 edition).

96. Welsh, *Reminiscences of Thirty Years,* 58–59.

97. See, for example, Virginia G. Drachman, *Hospital with a Heart* (Ithaca, N.Y.: Cornell University Press, 1983); "Female Solidarity and Professional Success: The Dilemma of Women Doctors in Late Nineteenth-Century America," *Journal of Social History* 15 (Summer 1982): 607–19; and Regina Markell Morantz and Sue Zschoche, "Professionalization, Feminism, and Gender Roles: A Comparative Study of Nineteenth-Century Medical Therapeutics," *Journal of American History* 67 (Dec. 1980): 568–88.

Chapter 5. "The Great Blessing of This Age": Pain Relief in Obstetrics

1. Edward Wagenknecht, ed., *Mrs. Longfellow: Selected Letters and Journals of Fanny Appleton Longfellow (1817–1861)* (New York: Longmans, Green & Co., 1956), 129–30. I would like to thank Elizabeth Black for calling this account to my attention. Ether's anesthetic qualities were first discovered by a Boston dentist, William T. G. Morton in 1846; by 1848 nitrous oxide and chloroform had been added to the list of painkilling drugs. James Y. Simpson pioneered the use of chloroform in obstetrics in the British Isles and was instrumental in introducing the drug to the United States. For an excellent account of the early uses of anesthesia in America, consult Martin S. Pernick, *A Calculus of Suffering: Pain, Professionalism, and Anesthesia in Nineteenth-Century America* (New York: Columbia University Press, 1985).

2. Mrs. Hal Russell, "Memoirs of Marian Russell," *Colorado Magazine* 21 (Jan. 1944): 35–36; Walter Channing, *Treatise on Etherization,* 165.

3. "Dr. Meigs' Reply to Professor Simpson's Letter," *Medical Examiner and Record of Medical Science* 11 (March 1848), 148–51. See also John Duffy, "Anglo-American Reaction to Obstetrical Anesthesia," *Bulletin of the History of Medicine* 38 (Jan.–Feb. 1964): 32–44.

4. Channing, *Treatise on Etherization,* 300. Walter Channing did not report what proportion of all physician-attended births surveyed used anesthesia.

5. *Ibid.,* 334–35. The woman was 43 years old and had had five children prior to this delivery.

6. *Ibid.,* 335.

7. *Ibid.,* 347, 348, 356.

8. *Ibid.,* 348–49.

9. B. E. Cotting, "Anesthetics in Midwifery," *Boston Medical and Surgical Journal* 59 (Dec. 9, 1858): 369; Bedford Brown, "The Therapeutic Action of Chloroform in Parturition," *JAMA* 25 (Aug. 31, 1895): 355.

10. A. D. Bundy, "Obstetrics in the Country," *Medical and Surgical Reporter* 56 (Feb. 12, 1887): 201; D. M. Barr, "Anaesthesia in Labor," *ibid.* 42 (March 13, 1880): 221.

11. Brown, "Therapeutic Action," 356; Barr, "Anesthesia in Labor," 228. Barr did admit there may be a few cases "where absolute counterindications existed," but he did not tell what they were.

12. D. W. Young, "Chloroform in Parturition," *Medical and Surgical Reporter* 3 (1859): 291; Cotting, "Anaesthetics in Midwifery," 372–73.

13. "Report of the Committee on Obstetrics," *Transactions of the American Medical Association* 2 (1849): 233–52.

14. Charles Fox Gardiner, *Doctor at Timberline* (Caldwell, Idaho: Caxton Printers, 1938), 211. See also Barr, "Anaesthesia in Labor," 227.

15. J. F. Ford, "Use of Drugs in Labor," *Wisconsin Medical Journal* 3 (Oct. 1904): 257–65, quote from 258; Florence Sherbon, from discussion following Grace Meigs, "Rural Obstetrics," American Association for the Study and Prevention of Infant Mortality, *Transactions of the Seventh Annual Meeting*, 1916, pp. 63–64. See also Edward D. and Lucinda Holton, Family Diary, 1845–83, Wisconsin State Historical Society Archives; and Gladys Brooks, *Boston and Return* (New York: Atheneum, 1962), 143–45.

16. Brown, "Therapeutic Action," 354; Charles W. Mooney, *Doctor in Belle Starr Country* (Oklahoma City: Century Press, 1975), 126; Duffy, "Anglo-American Reaction," 38. See also Ford, "Use of Drugs in Labor."

17. Ford, "Use of Drugs in Labor," 257–58; Bundy, "Obstetrics in the Country," 200–201. In 91,000 births in Iowa physicians used forceps in 7 percent of cases. E. D. Plass and H. J. Alvis, "A Statistical Study of 129,539 Births in Iowa, with Special Reference to the Method of Delivery and the Stillbirth Rate," *American Journal of Obstetrics and Gynecology* 28 (Aug. 1934): 297.

18. Barr, "Anaesthesia in Labor," 226–27. In the twentieth century, obstetricians appear to have used anesthesia with the intent to produce unconsciousness, and forceps use consequently increased.

19. J. Herbert Claiborne, "Use of Chloroform in Labor," *JAMA* 3 (Oct. 1884): 402.

20. H. C. Ghent of Texas during discussion of Claiborne, "Use of Chloroform in Labor," 405.

21. "Report of the Committee on Obstetrics," *Transactions of the American Medical Association* 1 (1848): 227.

22. *Ibid.*, 230–31.

23. "What is the Safest Anaesthetic?" *JAMA* 8 (May 7, 1887): 520–21.

24. "Chloroform in Obstetrics," *JAMA* 13 (Aug. 10, 1889): 204.

25. J. F. Baldwin, "The More Frequent Use of Chloroform in Obstetrics," reported in *JAMA* 15 (July 12, 1890): 75.

26. E. Chenery, letter to the editor, *JAMA* 28 (Jan. 16, 1897): 133–34.

27. W. S. Caldwell, letter to the editor, *JAMA* 28 (Feb. 6, 1897): 279–80.

28. I tried to find a pattern to the obstetrical use of ether or chloroform, historians having suggested that the region of the country may have governed physicians' choices between the two. Having been able to identify no such regional variation (for example, ether in the North; chloroform in the South), I am forced to conclude that either serendipity played its part in physician choice or that teachers' and mentors' selection initially governed physicians in deciding whether ether or chloroform should predominate in childbirth. Individual experience with the agents ultimately led physicians to their favorites.

29. See, for example, "Comparative Study of Ether and Chloroform in Parturition," *JAMA* 30 (April 16, 1898): 922.

30. W. B. Ulrich, "Address on Obstetrics," *JAMA* 26 (March 7, 1896): 449–52.

31. I. N. Love, "Relief from Pain in Labor," *JAMA* 21 (Aug. 26, 1893): 311–12.

32. Bedford Brown, "The Therapeutic Action of Chloroform in Parturition," *JAMA* 25 (Aug. 31, 1895): 354–58.

33. Laura H. Branson, "Anesthesia in Obstetrical Practice," *Woman's Medical Journal* 18 (May 1908): 95. See Pernick, *A Calculus of Suffering*, for a discussion of perceptions of women's particular pain sensitivity.

34. Testimony quoted in Marguerite Tracy and Mary Boyd, *Painless Childbirth* (New York: Frederick A. Stokes Co., 1915), 188–89. For a complete account of the twilight sleep controversy in America, see Lawrence G. Miller, "Pain, Parturition, and the Profession: The Twilight Sleep in America," in *Health Care in America: Essays in Social History*, ed. Susan Reverby and David Rosner (Philadelphia: Temple University Press, 1979), 19–44.

35. Tracy and Boyd, *Painless Childbirth*, 198.

36. Bertha Van Hoosen, "The New Movement in Obstetrics," *Woman's Medical Journal* 25 (June 1915): 122; and *Scopolamine-Morphine Anaesthesia* (Chicago: House of Manz, 1915), 101. Scopolamine is an alkaloid found in the leaves and seeds of solanaceous (nightshade) plants. It is an amnesiac, causing forgetfulness of pain rather than blocking the pain sensation. For obstetrical twilight sleep, scopolamine was administered with morphine—the most active alkaloid of opium—in the first dose, and alone for subsequent doses. I would like to thank Dr. Selma Calmes for correcting my classification of scopolamine.

37. *New York Times* (June 9, 1917), 13.

38. Van Hoosen, *Scopolamine-Morphine Anaesthesia*, 42; "New Movement," 121.

39. Marguerite Tracy and Constance Leupp, "Painless Childbirth," *McClure's Magazine* 43 (1914): 37–51. Scopolamine was used in surgery in the United States beginning with the new century, but Germany pioneered in its application to obstetrics.

40. *Ibid.*, 43. For the same sentiment among American physicians, see, for example, John O. Polak, "A Study of Scopolamin and Morphine Amnesia as Employed at Long Island College Hospital," *American Journal of Obstetrics* 71 (1915): 722; and Henry Smith Williams, *Painless Childbirth* (New York: Goodhue Co., 1914), 90–91. The classic descriptions of the ideal scopolamine delivery are Bernhard Kronig, "Painless Delivery in Dammerschlaf" (1908); and Carl J. Gauss, "Births in Artificial Dammerschlaf" (1906) and "Further Experiments in Dammerschlaf" (1911), all translated and reprinted in Tracy and Boyd, *Painless Childbirth*, 205–308.

41. Mary Boyd and Marguerite Tracy, "More about Painless Childbirth," *McClure's Magazine* 43 (1914): 57–58.

42. Hanna Rion, *Painless Childbirth in Twilight Sleep* (London: T. Werner Laurie Ltd., 1915), 239. See also her article, "The Painless Childbirth," *Ladies' Home Journal* 31 (1914): 9–10.

43. See, for example, "Is the Twilight Sleep Safe—for Me?" *Woman's Home Companion* 42 (1915): 10, 43; William Armstrong, "The 'Twilight Sleep' of Freiburg: A Visit to the Much Talked of Women's Clinic, *Woman's Home Companion* 41 (1914): 4, 69; *New York Times* (Sept. 17, 1914), 8; (Nov. 28, 1914), 2.

44. On women's clubs and clubwomen, see Mary P. Ryan, *Womanhood in America: From Colonial Times to the Present* (New York: New Viewpoints, 1975), 227–32; Edith Hoshino Altbach, *Women in America* (Lexington, Mass.: D.C. Heath, 1974), 114–21; William L. O'Neill, *Everyone Was Brave: A History of Feminism in America* (Chicago: Quadrangle, 1969), 107–68; Sheila M. Rothman, *Woman's Proper Place: A History of Changing Ideals and Practices, 1870 to the Present* (New York: Basic Books, 1978), 63–93; Gerda Lerner, *The Majority Finds Its Past* (New York, Oxford University Press, 1979); and Karen Blair, *The Clubwoman as Feminist: True Womanhood Redefined, 1868–1914* (New York: Holmes & Meier, 1980).

45. Russell Kelso Carter, *The Sleeping Car "Twilight" or Motherhood without Pain* (Boston: Chapple, 1915), 174–75.

46. Tracy and Boyd, *Painless Childbirth*, 145.

47. Eliza Taylor Ransom, "Twilight Sleep," *Massachusetts Club Women* 1 (1917): 5. I am grateful to Regina Markell Morantz-Sanchez for this reference.

48. The connections between clubwomen and suffrage or other women's issues are explored in Altbach, 114–15; O'Neill, 49–76, 146–68; Ryan, 230–49; and Eleanor Flexner, *Century of Struggle: The Woman's Rights Movement in the United States* (New York: Atheneum, 1970), 172–92.

49. Tracy and Boyd, *Painless Childbirth*, 145.

50. Quoted in the *New York Times* (Nov. 18, 1914), 18.

51. Tracy and Boyd, *Painless Childbirth*, 145.

52. Clara G. Stillman, "Painless Childbirth," *New York Call* (July 12, 1914), 15.

53. Sam Schmalhauser, "The Twilight Sleep for Women," *International Socialist Review* 15 (1914): 234–35. I am grateful to Mari Jo Buhle for this and the previous reference.

54. Bertha Van Hoosen, *Petticoat Surgeon* (Chicago: Pellegrini & Cudahy, 1947), 282–83.

55. See, for example, Bertha Van Hoosen, "A Fixed Dosage in Scopolamine-Morphine Anaesthesia," *Womans' Medical Journal* 26 (1916): 57–58; and "Twilight Sleep in the Home," *ibid.*, 132.

56. For early American trials, see William H. Wellington Knipe, " 'Twilight Sleep' from the Hospital Viewpoint," *Modern Hospital* 2 (1914): 250–51; A. M. Hilkowich, "Further Observations on Scopolamine-Narcophin Anesthesia during Labor with Report of Two Hundred (200) Cases," *American Medicine* 20 (1914): 786–94; William H. Wellington Knipe, "The Freiburg Method of Dammerschlaf or Twilight Sleep," *American Journal of Obstetrics* 70 (1914): 364–71; and James A. Harrar and Ross McPherson, "Scopolamine-Narcophin Seminarcosis in Labor," *Transactions of the American Association of Obstetricians and Gynecologists* 27 (1914): 372–89.

57. Quoted during the discussion of Rongy, Harrar, and McPherson papers, *Transactions of the American Association of Obstetricians and Gynecologists* 27 (1914): 389.

58. W. Francis B. Wakefield, "Scopolamine Amnesia in Labor," *American Journal of Obstetrics* 71 (1915): 428. For more of this kind of enthusiasm, see also Elizabeth R. Miner, "Letter and Report of Nineteen Cases in Which 'Twilight' Was Used," *Woman's Medical Journal* 26 (1916): 131.

59. Ralph M. Beach, "Twilight Sleep," *American Medicine* 21 (1915): 40–41.

60. Bertha Van Hoosen, *Scopolamine-Morphine Anaesthesia*, 101. Some physicians reported success using twilight sleep at home, but most thought the method best suited to hospital deliveries.

61. *JAMA* (June 6, 1914), quoted in " 'Twilight Sleep' and Medical Publicity," *Literary Digest* 49 (1914): 60.

62. Ralph M. Beach, "Twilight Sleep: Report of One Thousand Cases," *American Journal of Obstetrics* 71 (1915): 728.

63. Frederick A. Stratton, "Scopolamine Anesthesia," *Wisconsin Medical Journal* 8 (1908–9): 27.

64. Van Hoosen, *Scopolamine-Morphine Anaesthesia*, 101.

65. The breathing disorder, oligopnea, usually resolved after a few hours, but it was frightening to observe, especially for attendants who had no experience with it. See Gauss, "Further Experiments in Dammerschlaf," 302.

66. See discussion of the Polak paper in the *American Journal of Obstetrics* 7 (1915): 798; and Hilkowich, 793.

67. *American Medicine* 21 (Jan. 1915): 24–70.

68. See, for example, the discussion following Knipe's paper in the *American Journal of Obstetrics* 70 (1914): 1025. For articles with positive conclusions, see John Osborn Polock, "A Study of Twilight Sleep," *New York Medical Journal* 101 (1915): 293; Robert T. Gillmore, "Scopolamine and Morphine in Obstetrics and Surgery," *ibid.* 102 (1915): 298; William H. Wellington Knipe, " 'Twilight Sleep' from the Hospital Viewpoint," 250; W. Francis B. Wakefield, "Scopolamine Amnesia in Labor," 428; Samuel J. Druskin and Nathan Ratnoff, "Twilight Sleep in Obstetrics—with a Report of 200 Cases," *New York State Journal of Medicine* 15 (1915): 152; and Charles B. Reed, "A Contribution to the Study of 'Twilight Sleep,' " *Surgery, Gynecology and Obstetrics* 22 (1916): 656. For a negative conclusion, see Joseph Louis Baer, "Scopolamin-Morphin Treatment in Labor," *JAMA* 64 (1915): 1723–28. The actual dangers of the drug varied according to dosage and timing, and it is impossible for the historian to assess the events accurately without individual case records. Any drug can be dangerous if misused, and the variability in advice about scopolamine suggests that some disasters occurred with it.

69. See, for example, *New York Times*, Aug. 22, 1914, p. 9; and Sept. 10, 1914. Tracy and Boyd listed American hospitals that used scopolamine at the time their book, *Painless Childbirth*, was published.

70. Anna Steele Richardson's survey was reported in the *New York Times*, May 10, 1915, p. 24.

71. Litoff, *American Midwives*, 69–70. For more on the development of hospital obstetrics, consult Chapter 7.

72. Mary Boyd, "The Story of Dammerschlaf," *Survey* 33 (1914): 129. See the same statement in Boyd and Tracy, "More about Painless Childbirth," 69.

73. Constance Leupp and Burton J. Hendrick, "Twilight Sleep in America," *McClure's Magazine* 44 (1915): 172–73. The argument about expertise appeared repeatedly. See, for example, William H. W. Knipe, "The Truth about Twilight Sleep," *Delineator* 85 (1914): 4. Twilight-sleep women were aware that theirs was an expensive demand. They expected the cost of physician-attended childbirth to jump from $25 to $85. Tracy and Boyd, *Painless Childbirth*, 180.

74. Druskin and Ratnoff, 1520.

75. *New York Times*, April 30, 1915, p. 8.

76. Quoted from the *New Orleans Medical and Surgical Journal* in Miller, "Pain, Parturition, and the Profession," 24.

77. Van Hoosen, *Petticoat Surgeon*, 282.

78. Ford, "Use of Drugs in Labor," 257. The obstetrical use of ergot will be examined more fully in Chapter 6.

79. Dr. Francis Reder, during a discussion of Rongy, Harrar, and MacPherson papers, *Transactions of the American Association of Obstetricians and Gynecologists* 27 (1914): 386.

80. Tracy and Boyd, *Painless Childbirth*, 149.

81. For physicians' perceptions of "demanding" women, see, for example, the discussion following the Rongy and Harrar papers, *Transactions of the American Association of Obstetricians and Gynecologists* 27 (1914): 382-83. For more on social and medical perceptions of pain, consult Pernick, *A Calculus of Suffering*.

82. Other contributing factors included growing professionalization and specialization within medicine that produced tensions among groups of doctors that surfaced during this debate. Also the method's German origins invalidated it for many Americans during the war years. The importance of the issue of control is indicated by the intensity in the arguments of women and of physicians on this issue during the twilight-sleep controversy.

83. Letter from "Ex-Medicus" in *New York Times*, Nov. 28, 1914, p. 12.

84. Tracy and Boyd, *Painless Childbirth*, 147. Emphasis in original.

85. Rion, *Painless Childbirth in Twilight Sleep*, 47.

86. Tracy and Boyd claimed "four to five million" twilight-sleep followers, obviously an exaggeration (*Painless Childbirth*, p. 144).

87. See, for example, *New York Times*, Nov. 28, 1914, p. 12.

88. See especially Tracy and Boyd; Rion; Ransom; and Van Hoosen.

89. *New York Times*, Sept. 26, 1914, p. 10.

90. Quoted from *JAMA* in "Another 'Twilight Sleep,' " *Literary Digest* 50 (1915): 187; W. Gillespie, "Analgesics and Anesthetics in Labor, Their Indication and Contra-Indications," *Ohio Medical Journal* 11 (1915): 611; "Twilight Sleep Again," *American Medicine* 21 (1915): 149.

91. " 'Twilight Sleep' in the Light of Day," *Scientific American* 79, Supplement 2041 (1915): 112. See also the *New York Times* (Oct. 20, 1914), 12; (Nov. 28, 1914), 12; (Feb. 5, 1915), 10; (Feb. 11, 1915), 8.

92. Arthur J. Booker in his remarks defending Van Hoosen's use of scopolamine, quoted in Van Hoosen, *Scopolamine-Morphine Anaesthesia*, 12.

93. *New York Times*, April 24, 1915, p. 10; April 30, 1915, p. 8; May 29, 1915, p. 20; Aug. 25, 1915, p. 10; Aug. 16, 1916, p. 7.

94. Van Hoosen, "A Fixed Dosage," 57.

95. Beach, "Twilight Sleep," 43.

96. *New York Times*, Aug. 24, 1915, p. 7.

97. *Ibid.*, Aug. 31, 1915, p. 5.

98. See, for example, Frank W. Lynch, "Nitrous Oxide Gas Analgesia in Obstetrics," *JAMA* 64 (1915): 813.

99. See, for example, Henry Schwarz, "Painless Childbirth and the Safe

Conduct of Labor," *American Journal of Obstetrics and Diseases of Women and Children* 79 (1919): 46–63; and W. C. Danforth and C. Henry Davis, "Obstetric Analgesia and Anesthesia," *JAMA* 81 (1923): 1090–96.

100. See the assessment of anesthesia used in childbirth in New York Academy of Medicine Committee on Public Health Relations, *Maternal Mortality in New York City: A Study of All Puerperal Deaths 1930–1932* (New York: Commonwealth Fund, 1933), 113. See also Joyce Antler and Daniel M. Fox, "Movement toward a Safe Maternity: Physician Accountability in New York City, 1915–1940," *Bulletin of the History of Medicine* 50 (1976): 569–95.

101. Mabel E. Gardner, "The Ethics of Avoiding Pain in Labor," *Medical Woman's Journal* 37 (March 1930): 77, quoting from the *JAMA* and the *Ohio State Medical Journal*.

102. The legacy for the parent-infant bond and for subsequent child development is explored in M. H. Klaus and J. H. Kennell, *Maternal Infant Bonding: The Impact of Early Separation or Loss on Family Development* (St. Louis: C. V. Mosby, 1976). For a feminist perspective on women's missing their deliveries, see Adrienne Rich, *Of Woman Born: Motherhood as Experience and Institution* (New York: W. W. Norton, 1976).

Chapter 6. Why Women Suffer So: Meddlesome Midwifery and Scrupulous Cleanliness

1. S. Belle Craver, "The Management of Labor with Reference to the Prevention of Subsequent Uterine Disease," *Woman's Medical Journal* 4 (July 1895): 165.

2. Eugene P. Bernardy, "The Value of Biniodide of Mercury as an Antiseptic in Obstetrics," *JAMA* 6 (April 17, 1886): 423.

3. For example, Dr. H. C. White of Boston blamed a homeopathic doctor's lack of action during delivery for a recto-vaginal fistula that needed repair. Reported in *JAMA* 3 (Sept. 1884): 270.

4. Harriet Garrison, "The Uses and Abuses of Ergot in Obstetrical Practice," *Woman's Medical Journal* 6 (Feb. 1897): 32; Dr. Volger, during the discussion of Charles B. Noble, "A Case in Which Four Drachms of Squibbs' F. E. Ergot Was Administered Early in Labor," *JAMA* 12 (May 4, 1889): 640. The meaning of Volger's statement about hysterical women not being able "to regulate the pains" is not clear: what women could regulate contractions?

5. F. M. Johnson, "Address in Obstetrics and Gynecology," *JAMA* 9 (July 9, 1887): 34.

6. T. Ridgway Barker, "The Routine Practice of Administering Ergot after the Third Stage of Labor," *JAMA* 21 (Sept. 23, 1893): 455–57.

7. "The Place of Ergot in Obstetric Practice," *JAMA* 21 (Oct. 7, 1893): 543. See also George B. Wood and Franklin Bache, *The Dispensatory of the United States of America*, 14th edition (Philadelphia: J. B. Lippincott, 1879), 396–98.

8. Alex Christie to Sarah Jane Stevens, March 16, 1885, Box 10, James Christie and Family Papers, P1281, Archives/Manuscripts Division, Minnesota Historical Society.

9. E. Stuver, "Should Ergot Be Used During Parturition and the Subse-

quent Involution Period?" *JAMA* 23 (Sept. 15, 1894): 425–26. See also "Rupture of the Uterus," *ibid.* 17 (Dec. 12, 1891): 937.

10. "Queries and Minor Notes," *JAMA* 42 (May 7, 1904): 1233.

11. Eugene P. Bernardy, "Biniodide of Mercury, Its Antiseptic Use. Obstetrical Cases," *JAMA* 12 (April 20, 1889): 563.

12. Anna M. Fullerton, "Obstetric Surgery with the Report of a Porro Case," *Woman's Medical Journal* 1 (March 1893): 37.

13. Mary A. Whery, "The Prevention of Lacerations of the Perineum," *Woman's Medical Journal* 13 (Jan. 1903): 6.

14. Olga McNeile, "Sociological Aspects of Gynecology and Obstetrics," *Medical Woman's Journal* 29 (June 1922): 108.

15. Philip Adolphus, "On the Causes of Laceration of the Perinaeum during Parturition, and its Prevention," reported in *JAMA* 2 (May 1884): 524–27; "The 'English Method' of Perineal Protection," *ibid.* 3 (Aug. 1884): 159.

16. Thad. A. Reamy, "Address in Obstetrics and Diseases of Women," *JAMA* 3 (Sept. 1884): 316.

17. S. D. Gross, "Lacerations of the Female Sexual Organs Consequent upon Parturition:—Their Causes and Their Prevention," *JAMA* 3 (Sept. 27, 1884): 337–45, quotations from 343, 341.

18. Charles Meigs Wilson, "Observations from the Study of One Hundred and Forty-Two Cases of Hystero-Trachelorrhaphy," *JAMA* 3 (Nov. 1884): 495.

19. "A Craniotomy, Was it Justifiable?" *JAMA* 41 (Dec. 12, 1903): 1487.

20. Quoted from the New Jersey State Medical Society Proceedings, in *JAMA* 53 (Aug. 21, 1909): 649.

21. Statement made during the discussion of Daniel H. Craig, "Repair of Lacerations of the Cervix Uteri: An Investigation as to the Proper Time for the Operation," *JAMA* 41 (Oct. 31, 1903): 1072.

22. Letter to the editor, *JAMA* 5 (Aug. 29, 1885): 249; H.V. Sweringen, "Laceration of the Female Perineum," *ibid.* 5 (Aug. 15, 1885): 176; George B. Somers, during the discussion of his paper, "Repair of the Perineum," *ibid.* 45 (Nov. 11, 1905): 1416. See also Bedford Brown, "Abstract of a Paper on the Successful Treatment of Lacerations and Fissures of the Os Uteri of Long Standing Without Surgical Operation," *ibid.* (Oct. 10, 1885): 400–401; and James Hawley Burtenshaw, "Lacerations of the Pelvic Floor: The Principles Involved in Their Primary and Secondary Repair," *ibid.* 43 (Dec. 3, 1904): 1690–92; and B. C. Hirst, "Injuries to the Anterior Vaginal Wall in Labor: Their Primary, Intermediate and Secondary Repair," *ibid.* 43 (Nov. 12, 1904): 1431.

23. Reported in *JAMA* 6 (1886): 271.

24. "Letter from New York," *JAMA* 6 (June 19, 1886): 699.

25. See, for example, Henry T. Byford, "The Production and Prevention of Perineal Lacerations During Labor, with Description of an Unrecognized Form," *JAMA* 6 (March 6, 1886): 253–57; Thomas C. Smith, "A Case of Transverse Laceration of the Cervix Uteri," *ibid.* 9 (Nov. 10, 1888): 665–66; Henry Parker Newman, "Prolapse of the Female Pelvic Organs," *ibid.* 21 (Sept. 2, 1893): 334–36; and A. H. Tuttle, "The Injuries of Parturition, the Time, Method, and Reasons for Their Repair," *ibid.* 29 (Dec. 25, 1897): 1301–4. For an optimistic turn-of-the-century outlook, see Barton Cooke Hirst, "The Plastic Surgery in the University Maternity for the Year 1903," *JAMA* 42 (March 5, 1904): 646–47.

26. Anna Broomall, "The Operation of Episiotomy as a Prevention of Perineal Ruptures in Labor," *American Journal of Obstetrics and Diseases of Women and Children* 11 (1878): 517–27.

27. Frank A. Stahl, "Concerning the Principles and Practice of Episiotomy," *JAMA* 25 (Aug. 31, 1895): 353.

28. Reported in *JAMA* 33 (Dec. 16, 1899): 1553.

29. Mary A. Whery, "The Prevention of Lacerations of the Perineum," *Woman's Medical Journal* 13 (Jan. 1903): 6.

30. Emma Jewel Neal, "Sane Obstetrics," *Medical Woman's Journal* 30 (Oct. 1923): 292.

31. Gladys Brooks, *Boston and Return* (New York: Atheneum, 1962), 144.

32. Evaline Peo, "Report of Cases Occurring in a Maternity Practice—Retained Foetus, Unusual—Dystocia due to Youth of Mother—Twins, Birth of Different Sex. Both Breech Presentation—Neuritis in Twin Pregnancy," *Woman's Medical Journal* 14 (March 1904): 50.

33. Emma Jewel Neal, "Sane Obstetrics," 290.

34. J. H. MacKay, Letter to the Editor, *JAMA* 58 (March 9, 1912): 720.

35. George S. King, *Doctor on a Bicycle* (New York: Rinehart, 1958), 61.

36. See, for example, Grace L. Meigs, *Maternal Mortality from All Conditions Connected with Childbirth in the United States and Certain Other Countries* (Washington: Government Printing Office, 1917). This report concluded that of the 15,000 women dying in childbirth each year, 7,000 died from infection. "During the 13 years from 1900 to 1913 [death rates from chilbed fever] have shown no demonstrable decrease. . . . During that time the typhoid rate has been cut in half, the rate from tuberculosis markedly reduced, and the rate from diphtheria reduced to less than one-half" (p. 7).

37. Oliver Wendell Holmes, "On the Contagiousness of Puerperal Fever," in *Medical Essays 1842–1882* (Boston: Houghton Mifflin, 1887), 128–72; Ignaz Semmelweis, *The Etiology, Concept, and Prophylaxis of Childbed Fever*, trans. & ed., K. Codell Carter (Madison: University of Wisconsin Press, 1983).

38. Charles D. Meigs, *On the Nature, Signs, and Treatment of Childbed Fever in a Series of Letters Addressed to the Students of His Class* (Philadelphia, 1854).

39. Reported in *JAMA* 2 (June 1884): 689.

40. Madison Reece, "The Use of Antiseptics in Puerperal Cases," *JAMA* 3 (Aug. 1884): 120–21; Ida R. Gridley Case, "Asepsis in Midwifery," *Woman's Medical Journal* 4 (April, 1895): 83; Remark made during the discussion following Theophilus Parvin, "Puerperal Septicaemia," *JAMA* 3 (October 18, 1884): 426.

41. See, for example, Fanny C. Hutchins, "Hints Gathered While Taking a Course at the Lying-In Hospital of the City of New York," *Woman's Medical Journal* 10 (Nov. 1900): 464–65.

42. Theophilus Parvin, "Puerperal Septicaemia," 421.

43. During discussion of *ibid.*, 426. For a discussion of how long after exposure to infection a physician should resume obstetric practice, see George F. French, "How Soon After Exposure to Sepsis May the Accoucheur Resume Practice?" *JAMA* 5 (July 4, 1885): 5–8.

44. Reported in the Proceedings of the Medical Society of Virginia in *JAMA* 7 (Nov. 13, 1886): 552. An interesting part of the debate, which we cannot delve

into in this context but which fascinated the medical world of the 1880s, was whether or not a single germ caused puerperal fever. Parvin believed that a case would develop only if transmitted from another puerperal fever case. Other physicians thought scarlet fever, diphtheria, erysipelas and possibly other diseases, when transferred to a parturient woman, would produce puerperal fever. See the reaction to Parvin's remarks in *ibid.*, 554–56. See also A. Maclaren, "The Relation Between Erysipelas and Puerperal Fever, Considering Erysipelas Both as an Acute and a Latent Disease," *JAMA* 9 (Aug. 20, 1887): 231–35; the editorial "Relation of Erysipelas to Puerperal Sepsis," *ibid.*, 243–44.

45. A. B. Miller, during a discussion of John Milton Duff, "Parturition as a Factor in Gynecologic Practice," *JAMA* 35 (Aug. 25, 1900): 467.

46. J. S. Dukate, "Antiseptic Obstetrics," *Medical and Surgical Reporter* 70 (Jan. 20, 1894): 77–78.

47. J. H. Etheridge, "The Medico-Legal Aspect of Utterances Made in Medical Societies," reported in *JAMA* 10 (May 5, 1888): 567–68. See the entire discussion reported on 566–71, 599–600. See also the editorials, *ibid.* (May 12, 1888), 587–88; (May 19, 1888), 621–22; and (May 26, 1888), 656–57.

48. *Ibid.*, 569.

49. For an analysis of changing procedures with regard to the vaginal douche, see Frank A. Stahl, "The Douche: Its Rise and Decline, But Present Restoration," *JAMA* 33 (Sept. 23, 1899): 779–81. By 1902 physicians uncategorically condemned the use of the antepartum douche. See, for example, J. F. Baldwin, "The Prevention of Pelvic Diseases During and After Labor," *ibid.* 38 (Feb. 15, 1902): 437–40.

50. Reported from G. Frank Lydston, "Puerperal Septicaemia and Prophylaxis of Puerperal Inflammations," in *JAMA* 2 (June 1884): 665–68.

51. Chicago Medical Society Proceedings, *JAMA* 2 (June 1884): 667.

52. "How It Strikes the Country Practitioner," *JAMA* 10 (May 19, 1888): 633–34.

53. William Allen Pusey, *A Doctor of the 1870s and 80s* (Springfield, Ill.: Charles C Thomas, 1932), 105. See also Hiram Corson, "Antiseptics," *JAMA* 16 (May 30, 1891): 765–70. Corson concluded that "there is real danger to the woman from the use of antiseptics—more danger than there is in the practice of the physicians who do not use them" (p. 768). See also the editorial "Puerperal Poisons," *ibid.* 18 (Jan. 2, 1892): 13–14. See also J. K. Bartlett, "Address of the Chairman of the Section of Obstetrics and Diseases of Women, of the American Medical Association, Read June, 1883," *ibid.* 1 (Aug. 4, 1883): 106–9.

54. Gustav Zinke, "Puerperal Fever, and the Early Employment of Antiseptic Vaginal Injections," *JAMA* 7 (Nov. 13, 1886): 542.

55. Joseph Price, "A Year's Work in a Maternity Hospital," Reported in *JAMA* 12 (March 30, 1889): 460.

56. *Ibid.*, 462. Price refers to the dangers of "sewer gas," associated with bringing pathogenic bacteria into homes that could afford plumbing and modern conveniences. See, for example, Judith Walzer Leavitt, *The Healthiest City: Milwaukee and the Politics of Health Reform* (Princeton: Princeton University Press, 1982).

57. Munde, quoted from the *American Journal of Obstetrics* in *JAMA* 31 (Aug. 13, 1898): 370.

58. Bertha Van Hoosen, "Post-Partum Surgery," *Woman's Medical Journal* 11 (Dec. 1901): 420.

59. J. Suydam Knox, "The Use of the Curette and Intra-Uterine Douche after Labor at Term," *JAMA* 9 (Nov. 22, 1887): 614.

60. Ida R. Gridley Case, "Asepsis in Midwifery," *Woman's Medical Journal* 4 (April 1895): 83.

61. Olive Wilson, "Puerperal Sepsis," *Woman's Medical Journal* 13 (April 1903): 63. See also Marion Whitacre, "Puerperal Fever," *The Lancet-Clinic* 100 (1908): 142–47.

62. Frederick Holme Wiggin, "Diagnosis, Prevention and Treatment of Puerperal Infection," *JAMA* 38 (April 19, 1902): 1006.

63. J. F. Baldwin, "The Prevention of Pelvic Disease During and After Labor," *JAMA* 38 (Feb. 15, 1902): 437–40.

64. The original article was unsigned. "Management of Normal Labor," *JAMA* 58 (1912): 274–75. Comments to it appeared in the same volume, 428–29; 576–77; 649; 720; 880.

65. Emma Jewel Neal, "Sane Obstetrics," *Medical Woman's Journal* 30 (Oct. 1923): 291. See also Marcus Bossard, *Eighty-one Years of Living* (Minneapolis: Midwest Printing Company, 1946), 39–40.

66. Eliza H. Root, "Asepsis and Faulty Technique in the Practice of Obstetrics," *Woman's Medical Journal* 9 (June 1899): 207.

67. Edward Reynolds, "The Frequency of Puerperal Sepsis in Massachusetts: Its Diagnosis and Efficient Treatment," *Boston Medical and Surgical Journal* 131 (1894): 153.

68. "Puerperal Infection in Private Practice," *JAMA* 38 (April 19, 1902): 1008–9.

69. See letters to the editor, *JAMA* 38 (May 10, 1902): 1243–44.

70. See the Society report in *JAMA* 39 (July 5, 1902): 41.

71. M. Howard Fussell, "Obstetrics and the General Practitioner," *JAMA* 39 (Dec. 27, 1902): 1631. See also, R. E. Skeel, "Some Common Errors in Obstetric Practice," *ibid.* 43 (Nov. 19, 1904): 1571–72.

72. Frances Horton Lee, "An Unusual Cause of Fever in the Puerperium," *Woman's Medical Journal* 7 (Aug. 1898): 224.

73. S. H. Blakely, abstracted in *Woman's Medical Journal* 17 (Oct. 1907).

74. Albert H. Burr, "Gonorrhea in the Puerperium," *JAMA* 26 (Aug. 1, 1896): 236–39. See also Burr's "Gonorrhea as a Factor in Puerperal Fever," *ibid.* 31 (Sept. 3, 1898): 533–35. For a history of sexually transmitted diseases, see Allan M. Brandt, *No Magic Bullet: A Social History of Venereal Disease in the United States Since 1880* (New York: Oxford University Press, 1985).

75. Anna E. Blount, "Obstetrics in Relation to Chronic Gonorrhoea," *Medical Woman's Journal* 31 (June 1924): 150.

76. Their argument, originating in the Philadelphia area, attempts to vindicate the early nineteenth-century argument of Philadelphian Charles Meigs, who had vehemently debated Oliver Wendell Holmes over the extent of physician culpability. Dorothy I. Lansing, W. Robert Penman, and Dorland J. Davis, "Puerperal Fever and the Group B Beta Hemolytic Streptococcus," *Bulletin of the History of Medicine* 57 (1983): 70–80.

77. Madison Reece, "The Use of Antiseptics in Puerperal Cases," *JAMA*

3 (Aug. 1884): 120. At Bellevue Hospital Alonzo Clark developed the opium treatment for puerperal peritonitis. Narcotizing suffering women to "within an inch of their lives," Clark saved every one of the infected women he treated, according to Dr. Stephen Smith, who, reporting that the treatment continued at Bellevue for twenty years "with satisfactory results," began a lively discussion of opium-puerperal-fever therapy when he advocated its readoption in 1891. "Letter from New York," *JAMA* 16 (June 13, 1891): 863–64.

78. Charles P. Noble, "Celiotomy for Puerperal Septicemia and for Puerperal Inflammatory Conditions," *JAMA* 25 (Aug. 24, 1895): 312–15.

79. Reuben Peterson, "Hysterectomy for Puerperal Infection," *JAMA* 25 (Aug. 17, 1895): 268–72. Discussants of these papers agreed on the beneficial potential of abdominal surgery in infection cases that could not be otherwise controlled. See also Bayard Holmes, "When Shall Hysterectomy Be Performed in Puerperal Sepsis?" *ibid.* 25 (Nov. 23, 1895): 901–8.

80. R. R. Kime, "Is Hysterectomy for Puerperal Infection Justifiable?" *JAMA* 26 (April 11, 1896): 719–20; and his "Puerperal Infection: Its Pathology, Prevention and Treatment," *ibid.* 27 (Aug. 1, 1896): 234–39.

81. C. S. Bacon, "Treatment of Puerperal Fever," *JAMA* 40 (April 18, 1903): 1051.

82. See, for example, John B. Deaver, "Postpuerperal Sepsis: Indications for and Operative Treatment Thereof," *JAMA* 33 (Aug. 19, 1899): 447–49.

83. D. S. Fairchild, "The Use of the Curette in Acute Infection of Uterus with Adherent Placenta," *JAMA* 31 (Sept. 3, 1898): 527–28.

84. J. T. Priestley, during discussion at the AMA meeting in May, 1896, *JAMA* 27 (Aug. 1, 1896), 239.

85. Morcedai Price during discussion of John Milton Duff, "Parturition as a Factor in Gynecology Practice," *JAMA* 35 (Aug. 25, 1900): 466. See also Thomas J. Watkins, "The Treatment of Puerperal Infection," *ibid.* 53 (Oct. 23, 1909): 1386–89.

86. "Preparation of the Parturient Patient," *JAMA* 44 (Jan. 21, 1905): 230.

87. Ida R. Gridley Case, "Asepsis in Midwifery," *Woman's Medical Journal* 4 (April 1895): 84.

88. Reported in *JAMA* 45 (Nov. 25, 1905): 1676.

89. Eliza H. Root, "Asepsis and Faulty Technique in the Practice of Obstetrics," *Woman's Medical Journal* 9 (June 1899): 208.

90. Emma Jewel Neal, "Sane Obstetrics," *Medical Woman's Journal* 30 (Oct. 1923): 292.

91. Benjamin Earle Washburn, *A Country Doctor in the South Mountains* (Asheville, N.C.: Stephens Press, 1955), 14–15.

92. Olive Wilson, "Puerperal Sepsis," *Woman's Medical Journal* 13 (April 1903): 65.

93. W. A. Shannon, during a discussion of John A. McKenna, "Present Day Methods of Conducting Labor Cases and the Results Obtained," *JAMA* 45 (Dec. 16, 1905): 1854.

94. Baldwin, "Prevention of Pelvic Disease," 439.

95. "Puerperal Infection in Private Practice," letter to the editor of *JAMA* 38 (May 10, 1902): 1243.

Chapter 7. "Alone Among Strangers": Birth Moves to the Hospital

1. Betty MacDonald, *The Egg and I* (Philadelphia: Lippincott, 1945), 163.
2. Neal Devitt, "The Transition from Home to Hospital Birth in the United States, 1930–1960," *Birth and the Family Journal* 4 (1977): 47–58.
3. Jane B. Donegan, *Women & Men Midwives: Medicine, Morality, and Misogyny in Early America* (Westport, Conn.: Greenwood Press, 1978); Catherine M. Scholten, " 'On the Importance of the Obstetrick Art': Changing Customs of Childbirth in America, 1760–1825," *William and Mary Quarterly* 34 (1977): 426–45; Richard W. Wertz and Dorothy C. Wertz, *Lying-In: A History of Childbirth in America* (New York: Free Press, 1977); Janet Bogdan, "Care or Cure? Childbirth Practices in Nineteenth Century America," *Feminist Studies* 4 (1978): 92–99; Judy Barrett Litoff, *American Midwives 1860 to the Present* (Westport, Conn.: Greenwood Press, 1978); Nancy Schrom Dye, "History of Childbirth in America," *Signs* 6 (1980): 97–108; and Margaret Jarman Hagood, *Mothers of the South: Portraiture of the White Tenant Farm Woman* (New York: W. W. Norton, 1977), 108–27.
4. Nettie Fowler McCormick Papers, Wisconsin State Historical Society Archives. See letters of July and August 1890. See Chapter 5 for further analyses of women's home birth experiences. For hospital deliveries in the nineteenth century confined to "destitute women when they need both shelter and assistance," see, for example, Joseph Price, "Comparative Report of Hospital and Out-Door Obstetrical Cases," *JAMA* 10 (May 19, 1888): 629–30.
5. See, for example, Caroline Gardner Cary Curtis, ed., *The Cary Letters* (Cambridge: Riverside Press, 1891), 60. Paul Starr argues that the Progressive ideology at the turn of the century helped make medical expertise desirable to many Americans. See *The Social Transformation of American Medicine* (New York: Basic Books, 1983), 246.
6. See for example, Harvey Graham, *Eternal Eve: A History of Gynecology and Obstetrics* (Garden City, N.Y.: Doubleday, 1951); Alan Frank Guttmacher, *The Story of Human Birth* (New York: Blue Ribbon Books, 1937); Richard Harrison Shryock, *The Development of Modern Medicine* (New York: Hafner, 1969); and, most recently, Edward Shorter, *A History of Women's Bodies* (New York: Basic Books, 1982).
7. Starr, *The Social Transformation of American Medicine*, 18–19, 246.
8. Barbara Moench Florence, ed., *Lella Secor: A Diary in Letters, 1915–1922* (New York: Burt Franklin, 1978), 170.
9. Aldine R. Bird, "Progress of Obstetric Knowledge in America," *Hygeia* 11 (May, 1933): 439.
10. Josephine H. Kenyon, "Letter to Mothers of the Health and Happiness Club," *Good Housekeeping* 107 (Sept. 1938): 160. See also Kenyon's "A Message to Prospective Mothers: Take Good Care of Your Baby Before He Comes," *ibid.* 106 (May 1938): 83, 217; and "Medieval Thinking about Childbirth," editorial, *Ladies' Home Journal* 53 (Oct. 1936): 4.
11. Katherine Glover, "Making America Safe for Mothers," *Good Housekeeping* 88 (May 1926): 270.
12. Rose Wilder Lane, "Mother No. 22,999," *Good Housekeeping* 70 (May 1920): 28–29.

13. Hallie F. Nelson, *South of the Cottonwood Trees* (Broken Bow, Nebr.: Purcellow, 1977), 214; *Life History of Thomas A. and Ida C. Wolsey* (1978), 214. Typed copy in the Wisconsin State Historical Society.

14. See, for example, Pearl Wolfe Mockbee, *My Home in the Hills* (1977), 61; Elsa Maxwell, *R.S.V.P.: Elsa Maxwell's Own Story* (Boston: Little, Brown, 1954), 29; Laura B. Gaye, *Laugh on Friday, Weep on Sunday: One Woman's Reminiscence* (Calabasas, Calif.: Loma Palaga Press, 1968), 55–58; May Hartley, *Whither Shall I Go? A Story of an Itinerant Circuit Rider's Wife* (Southold, N.Y.: Academy Printing Services, 1975), 76, 89.

15. Quoted in "I Had a Baby Too: A Symposium," *Atlantic* 163 (June 1939): 764. See also Hagood, *Mothers of the South*, 111–19.

16. Women quoted in M. F. Ashley Montagu, "Babies Should Be Born at Home!" *Ladies' Home Journal* 72 (Aug. 1955): 52–53.

17. Gladys Denny Shultz, "Journal Mothers Report on Cruelty in Maternity Wards," *Ladies' Home Journal* 75 (May 1958): 44; M. F. Ashley Montagu, "Babies Should Be Born at Home!" 52.

18. Many factors converged to encourage women to move to the hospital, including the new anesthetic agent scopolamine, which was best monitored in the hospital (discussed in detail in Chapter 5), and the preference of the specialists, discussed later in this chapter. Other factors include federal subsidy of hospitalization, lowering hospital costs after 1935; the growth of the hospitals themselves; and the declining number of midwives in this period. See Morris J. Vogel, *The Invention of the Modern Hospital: Boston, 1870–1930* (Chicago: University of Chicago Press, 1980); David Rosner, *A Once Charitable Enterprise: Hospitals and Health Care in Brooklyn and New York, 1885–1915* (Cambridge: Cambridge University Press, 1982); Judy Barrett Litoff, *American Midwives 1860 to the Present* (Westport, Conn.: Greenwood Press, 1978); Frances E. Kobrin, "The American Midwife Controversy: A Crisis of Professionalization," *Bulletin of the History of Medicine* 40 (July-Aug. 1966): 350–63; Neal Devitt, "The Statistical Case for Elimination of the Midwife: Fact versus Prejudice, 1890–1935," *Women and Health* 4 (Spring 1979): 81–96; *ibid.* (Summer 1979): 169–86; and Paul Starr, *The Social Transformation of American Medicine.*

19. See, for example, Dorothy Reed Mendenhall, *Hygiene of Maternity and Childhood* (Washington, D.C.: The Children's Bureau, 1921).

20. E. Gustav Zinke, "The Practice of Obstetrics," *JAMA* 37 (Sept. 7, 1901): 612–13; Harris is quoted from the discussion following a series of papers of which Zinke's was one, p. 619. See also Zinke, "The Mortality and Morbidity of Child-Bearing Women Could Be Reduced to a Minimum if Maternity Hospitals Were More in Favor with the Profession and Laity," *Lancet-Clinic* Vol. C, No. 3 (July 18, 1908): 71–80, in which Zinke argues that "scenes in the confinement-chamber, charming because of the pleasant environments of the home and the presence of dear friends," are mere sentiment and should be replaced by the hospital where "the full benefit of what the science and art of midwifery can do for them" is available.

21. Charles Fox Gardiner, *Doctor at Timberline* (Caldwell, Idaho: Caxton Printers, 1938), 210–11.

22. Henry P. Newman, "Address of the Chairman Delivered at the Fifty-second Annual Meeting of the A.M.A.," *JAMA* 36 (June 22, 1901): 1758; Mabel

E. Gardner, "The Obstetrical Problem," *Medical Woman's Journal* 31 (Sept. 1924): 264; Alfred M. Rehwinkel, *Dr. Bessie* (St. Louis: Concordia, 1963), 90.

23. Joseph B. DeLee, "The Prophylactic Forceps Operation," *American Journal of Obstetrics and Gynecology* 1 (Oct. 1920): 40–41, 34–35, 44.

24. Williams and others quoted during the discussion of DeLee's paper in *ibid.*, 77–80; Williams on 77. DeLee himself immediately noted that he did not advise prophylactic forceps in every labor: "I have had in the last two years over 200 private cases, and of this number 85 were forceps applications, and 39 cases of prophylactic forceps. I do not do the operation in every case. Most of the cases of multiparae with large pelves do not need prophylactic forceps" (p. 80). For more reaction to prophylactic forceps, see J. Whitridge Williams, "A Criticism of Certain Tendencies in American Obstetrics," *New York State Journal of Medicine* 22 Nov. 1922): 493–99.

25. J. P. McEvoy, "Our Streamlined Baby," *Reader's Digest* 32 (May 1938): 15–16.

26. "I Had a Baby Too: A Symposium," *Atlantic Monthly* 163 (June 1939): 768. See also Lenore Pelham Friedrich, "I Had a Baby," *ibid.* (April 1939): 461–65. Clara Rust gave birth to five babies at home before going to the hospital to have her sixth in 1926. She was apprehensive about leaving home but went to the hospital on her doctor's advice. Jo Anne Wold, *This Old House: The Story of Clara Rust* (Anchorage: Alaska Northwest, 1976), 207–8.

27. Roy P. Finney, *The Story of Motherhood* (New York: Liverright, 1937), 6–7. See also Alan Frank Guttmacher, *Into This Universe: The Story of Human Birth* (New York: Blue Ribbon Books, 1937), 192–267.

28. Erva Slayton to Mrs. Slayton (mother), Jan. 1, 1919. Slayton Family Collection, Michigan Historical Collection, Bentley Historical Library, University of Michigan.

29. New York Academy of Medicine Committee on Public Health Relations, *Maternal Mortality in New York City: A Study of All Puerperal Deaths, 1930–1932* (New York: Commonwealth Fund, 1933), 213–15, 115–27.

30. *Ibid.*, 113–17, 126–27. An Iowa study found that 11.8 percent of all births and 23 percent of hospital births were operative statewide. Plass and Alvis, "Statistical Study," 293–305.

31. See Robert D. Retherford, *The Changing Sex Differential in Mortality* (Westport, Conn.: Greenwood Press, 1975), 57–69.

32. Joseph B. DeLee, "The Prophylactic Forceps Operation," *American Journal of Obstetrics and Gynecology* 1 (1920): 34–44.

33. Joseph B. DeLee, "The Maternity Ward of the General Hospital," *The Modern Hospital Yearbook* 6 (1926): 67–72.

34. These quotations are from Joseph B. DeLee and Heinz Siedentopf, "The Maternity Ward of the General Hospital," *JAMA* 100 (Jan. 7, 1933): 6–14. See also DeLee, "What Are the Special Needs of the Modern Maternity?" *The Modern Hospital* 28 (March 1927): 59–69; and "How Should the Maternity Be Isolated?" *ibid.* 29 (Sept. 1927): 65–72.

35. DeLee and Siedentopf, "The Maternity Ward of the General Hospital," 68. For reported epidemics see, for example, Frank L. Meleney et al., "Epidemiologic and Bacteriologic Investigation of the Sloane Hospital Epidemic of Hemolytic Streptococcus Puerperal Fever in 1927," *American Journal of Obstet-*

rics and Gynecology 16 (Aug. 1928): 180–94; B. P. Watson, "An Outbreak of Puerperal Sepsis in New York City," *ibid.*, 157–78.

36. J. Whitridge Williams, "Is an Architecturally Isolated Building Essential for a Lying-In Hospital?" *The Modern Hospital* 28 (April 1927): 58–61.

37. L. A. Sexton of Hartford Hospital, Hartford Conn., quoted in "The Open Forum: Separate Building or Department for the Maternity?" *The Modern Hospital* 28 (May 1927): 103–5, quotes from 105.

38. Florence Brown Sherbon, "Maternal Efficiency—A Field for Research," *Woman's Medical Journal* 27 (Feb. 1917): 36; New York Academy of Medicine Committee on Public Health Relations, *Maternal Mortality in New York City: A Study of All Puerperal Deaths, 1930–1932* (New York, 1933); Philadelphia County Medical Society Committee on Maternal Welfare, *Maternal Mortality in Philadelphia, 1931–1933* (Philadelphia, 1934); White House Conference on Child Health and Protection, *Fetal, Newborn, and Maternal Morbidity and Mortality: Report of the Subcommittee on Factors and Causes of Fetal, Newborn, and Maternal Morbidity and Mortality* (New York, 1933); Matthias Nicoll, Jr., "Maternity as a Public Health Problem," *American Journal of Public Health* 19 (Sept. 1929): 967; B. P. Watson, "Can Our Methods of Obstetric Practice Be Improved?" *Bulletin of the New York Academy of Medicine* 6 (Oct. 1930): 647–63. It is important to note, too, that in addition to increased infection rates, maternal deaths from instrument and operative causes also were prevalent in the hospital. Because hospital equipment and staff made interventions so easy, doctors became even more active interventionists than they had been in attending home deliveries. These increased interferences in labor and delivery, as the New York Academy of Medicine study documented, increased the dangers of hospital births over home births.

39. "Childbirth: Nature v. Drugs," *Time*, May 25, 1936, p. 36; Matthias Nicoll, Jr., "Maternity as a Public Health Problem," *American Journal of Public Health* 19 (Sept. 1929): 967. See also R. W. Holmes, R. D. Mussey, and F. L. Adair, "Factors and Causes of Maternal Mortality," *JAMA* 93 (Nov. 9, 1929): 1440–47.

40. Philadelphia County Medical Society, Committee on Maternal Welfare, *Maternal Mortality in Philadelphia, 1931–1933* (Philadelphia: County Medical Society, 1934), 130. See also New York Academy of Medicine, *Maternal Mortality*, 32–38.

41. White House Conference on Child Health and Protection, *Fetal, Newborn, and Maternal Morbidity and Mortality: Report of the Subcommittee on Factors and Causes of Fetal, Newborn, and Maternal Morbidity and Mortality* (New York: Appleton-Century, 1933), 14, 220. For information about the effects of instrumental deliveries on children, see Charles Edwin Galloway, "Prevention of Birth Injury and Its Resulting Mortality from the Standpoint of the Obstetrician," *JAMA* 106 (Feb. 15, 1936): 505–7.

42. Beatrice E. Tucker and Harry B. Benaron, "Maternal Mortality of the Chicago Maternity Center," *American Journal of Public Health* 27 (1937): 36.

43. Joyce Antler and Daniel M. Fox, "The Movement Toward a Safe Maternity: Physician Accountability in New York City, 1915–1940," in *Sickness and Health in America: Readings in the History of Medicine and Public Health*, ed. Judith Walzer Leavitt and Ronald L. Numbers (Madison: University of Wisconsin

Press, 1978), 386. Other factors converged with hospital regulations to cause the decrease in maternal mortality after 1935. The prenatal care movement, spearheaded by middle-class women, succeeded in gaining adherents and in educating the public about the importance of care during pregnancy. Probably most important in the decelerating death rates was the wide adoption of sulfonamides, blood transfusions, and, after World War II, antibiotics, which were successful in combating infection and hemorrhaging. With these two major causes of maternal death conquered, maternal mortality fell dramatically. Lawrence D. Longo and Christina M. Thomsen, "The Evolution of Prenatal Care in America," in *Proceedings of the Second Motherhood Symposium*, ed. Sophie Colleau (Madison: Women's Studies Research Center, 1982), 29–70. During the 1920s and 1930s, when increasing numbers of women moved to the hospital to have their babies, maternal mortality rates remained as high as they had been earlier in the century, approximately 60 deaths per 10,000 live births (over 100 per 10,000 for nonwhite women). See Sam Shapiro, Edward R. Schlesinger, and Robert E. L. Nesbitt, Jr., *Infant, Perinatal, Maternal, and Childhood Mortality in the United States* (Cambridge, Mass: Harvard University Press, 1968), 144–45. When maternal mortality rates started falling after 1935, the decrease was not due to the hospital per se but to measures such as antibiotics that could have been used at home.

44. Joseph B. DeLee, "Before the Baby Comes," *Delineator* 109 (Oct. 1926): 35, 84.

45. Joseph B. DeLee to Paul deKruif, quoted in Morris Fishbein, *Joseph Bolivar DeLee: Crusading Obstetrician* ([New York]: E. P. Dutton, 1949), 252, 253.

46. Tucker and Benaron, "Maternal Mortality of the Chicago Maternity Center," 36; Paul deKruif, "Forgotten Mothers," *Ladies' Home Journal* 53 (Dec. 1936): 12–13, 64–68; "Saver of Mothers," *ibid.* 49 (March 1932): 6–7, 124–25.

47. See, for example, Roy P. Finney, *The Story of Motherhood* (New York, 1937), 6–7; and Alan Frank Guttmacher, *Into This Universe: The Story of Human Birth* (New York, 1937), 192–267.

48. Margaret R. Budenz, *Streets* (Huntingdon, Ind.: Our Sunday Visitor, 1979), 266; Quoted in Gladys Denny Shultz, "Journal Mothers Report on Cruelty in Maternity Wards," *Ladies' Home Journal* 75 (May 1958): 44–45. See also M. P. M. Richards, "Aspects of Development in Contemporary Society," in *Changing Patterns of Childbearing and Child Rearing*, Proceedings of the 17th Annual Symposium of the Eugenics Society, London, 1980, eds. R. Chester, Peter Diggory, and Margaret B. Sutherland (London: Academic, 1981), 90.

49. Schultz, "Cruelty," 45.

50. Quotations are from personal communications to the author from women answering a *New York Times Book Review* Author's Query of July 1983. About two hundred responses have been received. Quotes here from Katherine S. Egan, Aug. 25, 1938; Marilyn Clohessy, Sept. 9, 1983; Elsa Rosenberg, July 30, 1983; and others from letters by women who wish to remain anonymous, July, Aug., and Sept., 1983. Marilyn Clohessy noted, too, that she had not been prepared for the pain that accompanied childbirth: "The severity of the pain was like nothing I had ever experienced before. A thrusting, ramming sensation never seeming to let up again and again and again. . . . I thought I would go to the hospital—they would knock me out & I would wake up a

mother no one told me about all *this pain*." The lack of empathy that women reported coming from nurses as well as doctors needs more investigation. Were nurses showing their identification with the medical system; were they all unmarried and unsympathetic or even jealous of the childbearing women; were there significant class differences between the nurses and the birthing women that stood in the way of empathetic gestures; were the women's reports of nurses' insensitivity overdrawn? These questions would prove fruitful areas for future research.

51. Lenore Pelham Friedrich, "I Had a Baby," 461–65. See also the response "I Had a Baby Too: A Symposium," 764–72.

52. Ann Rivington, "Motherhood—Third Class," *American Mercury* 31 (Feb. 1934): 160–65. See also Leotha B. Southmayd, "Motherhood—Third Class: A Reply," *ibid.* (April 1934): 509–10, who believed Rivington exaggerated the experience.

53. "I Had a Baby, Too," 768.

54. Margarete Sandelowski, *Pain, Pleasure, and American Childbirth: From the Twilight Sleep to the Read Method, 1914–1960* (Westport, Conn: Greenwood Press, 1984). Events during the 1950s should be seen within the context presented here of dissatisfied birthing women seeking to upgrade their hospital deliveries.

55. Julie Harris, as told to Betty Friedan, "I Was Afraid To Have a Baby," *McCalls*, Dec. 1956, pp. 68–74, quote from 74.

Chapter 8. Decision-Making and the Process of Change

1. George Francis Dow, ed., *The Holyoke Diaries 1709–1856*, 77, 75, 70.

2. Hale Family Papers, Box 12, Folder 321, letter from Sarah to Edward Everett Hale, May 28, 1859. Sophia Smith Collection, Smith College.

3. Huntting-Rudd Family Papers, Schlesinger Library, Radcliffe College.

4. Part of the interest obstetricians had in moving birth to the hospital was to concentrate it in the hands of specialists. Although usually characterized as a major move against midwives, and viewed in this book primarily as a response to the difficult conditions under which doctors had to manage deliveries in women's homes, the specialists were probably equally concerned with controlling the practices of their general colleagues. The Sheppard-Towner Act of 1921, which provided federal funds for maternal and child health, and the Social Security Act of 1935, which provided federal funding for hospitalization, hastened the twentieth-century medicalization of childbirth. While this book has not focused on public policy, it has documented the growth of a public conscience about women's risks during childbirth. As the public sector became aware of the social problem of maternal mortality and morbidity, funds to improve conditions became available, and public money was crucial in equalizing the childbirth experiences and expectations of rich and poor women.

5. Katherine S. Egan to JWL, Aug. 25, 1983, in response to Author's Query in the *New York Times Book Review*.

6. Marilyn Clohessy, Sept. 9, 1983, in response to Author's Query.

7. The relative value of the use of the word "choice" in this historical

context must be emphasized. Individual women felt and made choices within their specific contexts, although social pressures growing from traditional community practices and from their perceptions of medical authority may have circumscribed their actual choices. Thus, individuals made choices within the parameters set by the culture around them. Individual doctors also had choices at their disposal, but they, too, were limited by the pressures emanating from cultural and professional expectations.

8. Barbara Katz Rothman, "Awake and Aware, of False Consciousness: The Cooption of Childbirth Reform in America," in Shelly Romalis, ed., *Childbirth: Alternatives to Medical Control* (Austin: University of Texas Press, 1981), 150–80. Rothman believes that medicine has coopted just enough of traditional practices to silence women, but that physicians and hospitals do not show a commitment to giving women real decision-making authority within modern medicalized childbirth. She fears that current negotiations between birthing women and their physicians will add to physicians' ultimate authority. See also Barbara Katz Rothman, *In Labor: Women and Power in the Birthplace* (New York: W. W. Norton, 1982).

The issue of informed consent, by which women presumably accept or reject specific interventions, is not the same as decision-making powers that women traditionally held. Informed consent is, at best, a woman's ability to react to suggestions from the medical community. It does not insure her initiating powers or independent control over the events. For an interesting discussion of women's changing values about anesthesia use before, during, and after delivery, see Jay J. J. Christensen-Szalanski, "Discount Functions and the Measurement of Patients' Values," *Medical Decision Making* 4 (1984): 47–58.

Epilogue

1. See, for example, Shelly Romalis, ed., *Childbirth: Alternatives to Medical Control* (Austin: University of Texas Press, 1981); Adrienne Rich, *Of Woman Born: Motherhood as Experience and Institution* (New York: W. W. Norton, 1976); and Barbara Katz Rothman, *In Labor: Women and Power in the Birthplace* (New York: W. W. Norton, 1982).

2. Television show, "Cagney and Lacey," November 13, 1985.

3. R. Sosa, J. Kennell, M. Klaus, S. Robertson, and J. Urrutia, "The Effect of a Supportive Companion on Perinatal Problems, Length of Labor and Mother-Infant Interaction," *New England Journal of Medicine* 303 (Sept. 11, 1980): 597–600.

Chronology of Events in Childbirth History

ca. 1400
Middle English translation of Latin obstetrical and gynecological text largely taken from thirteenth-century sources. The first known obstetrical source available in the English language.

1500
Jacob Nufer, a Swiss peasant, performed the first successful cesarean section on his wife, saving her life and the life of her child. The operation remained extremely dangerous and rare until the end of the nineteenth century.

1540
The Byrth of Mankynde, an English translation from the Latin of Eucharius Rosslin's *Rosengarten,* an early book on midwifery.

1551
Ambroise Pare, the French physician known as the "father of surgery," published an obstetrical text describing podalic version—a reintroduction of the work of Soranus of Ephesus (second century A.D.), who taught midwives to turn the fetus under prescribed conditions.

1598
Approximate date when Peter Chamberlen the Elder is credited with developing the forceps. This unique obstetrical instrument was kept a secret by succeeding generations of Chamberlen family physicians until the death of Hugh Chamberlen, Jr., in 1728. In the eighteenth century, other physicians independently devised similar instruments to extract the fetus during difficult deliveries.

1668
François Mauriceau of Paris published his influential text, translated into English under the title *The Accomplisht Midwife,* reporting tubal pregnancy, describing brow presentation, advising the rupture of membranes to induce labor

to control hemorrhage for *placenta previa,* describing puerperal fever epidemics, and advising the substitution of the bed for the birth stool.

1671
Jane Sharp, an English midwife, published *The Midwives Book, or the Whole Art of Midwifery Discovered* (later titled *Compleat Midwife's Companion*).

1740s
William Smellie made the first precise measurements of the female pelvis and taught his students in London how to manage forceps deliveries with his unique curve-bladed instrument. He published *A Course of Lectures upon Midwifery* in 1742 and *Treatise on the Theory and Practice of Midwifery* in 1752.

1750s
Anatomist William Hunter, who studied with Smellie, taught anatomy and obstetrics in London; among his students was William Shippen, who brought medical obstetrics teaching to America.

1752
James Lloyd returned from study in London with William Smellie and William Hunter to Boston, where he practiced obstetrics, possibly the first such specialist in America.

1760
Elizabeth Nihell, a famous English midwife, published *A Treatise on the Art of Midwifery . . .*, in which she opposed the entrance of male physicians into the practice of midwifery.

1762
William Shippen returned from study in Europe and began, the following year, the first classes on midwifery in the colonies.

Forceps use became established in the colonies as physicians began regular attendance at birth.

1774
William Hunter published *Anatomy of the Human Gravid Uterus,* which, along with Smellie's contributions, made obstetrics more scientific.

1782
Fielding Ould, an obstetrician at the Rotunda Lying-In Hospital in Dublin, probably was the first to perform an episiotomy. The practice did not become popular in the United States until the late nineteenth century, and it was not in wide use until the twentieth century.

1800
Fertility rate in the United States was 7.04 for white married women.

Valentine Seaman published his series of obstetrics lectures, *The Midwives' Monitor and Mother's Mirror,* the first guide for midwifery published in the United States.

1807
John Stearns published an account of the obstetrical uses of ergot, which he had learned about from midwives.

Samuel Bard published the first American textbook of midwifery, *Compendium of the Theory and Practice of Midwifery*.

1809
Kentucky physician Ephraim McDowell performed the first ovariotomy, paving the way for abdominal surgery. The patient was Mrs. Jane Todd, age 47, who suffered from a rapidly growing ovarian tumor. The surgery was executed without the benefit of anesthesia.

1822
The stethoscope, discovered by René Théophile Laennec in 1819, was used to hear the fetal heartbeat through the abdomen of pregnant women.

1824
William Potts Dewees, professor of midwifery at the University of Pennsylvania, published his textbook, *A Compendious System of Midwifery*, which went through an influential twelve editions.

1827
John Lambert Richmond, M.D., performed the first successful cesarean section in the United States.

1843
American physician Oliver Wendell Holmes published "On the Contagiousness of Puerperal Fever," positing the contagious nature of postpartum infections and advising doctors not to attend confinements if they had been attending a case of puerperal fever or if they had assisted at a postmortem examination of such a case.

1847
Fanny Appleton Longfellow became the first American woman to use ether during childbirth. After this date physicians used anesthetic agents during approximately half of the births they attended.

Scottish physician James Young Simpson initiated the obstetrical use of chloroform, first discovered in 1831 by Justis von Liebig in Germany and Eugene Soubeiran in France. Charles Meigs in Philadelphia dissented to obstetrical anesthesia; the debates between Simpson and Meigs on the merits of anesthesia were widely reported.

Hungarian Ignaz Semmelweis instituted hand washing at the Vienna Lying-In Hospital to prevent puerperal fever.

The American Medical Association formed.

1848
Walter Channing, professor of obstetrics at Harvard and one of anesthesia's greatest advocates, published *Treatise on Etherization in Childbirth*.

1849
Elizabeth Blackwell graduated from Geneva (New York) Medical College, the first woman to receive a regular medical degree in the United States, opening the medical world to women.

1850
The Female Medical College of Philadelphia, later called the Woman's Medical College of Pennsylvania, opened. It became the primary medical college for training women physicians, although it was joined by sixteen other women's medical colleges, sectarian and regular, during the remainder of the nineteenth century. It outlasted all the rest, becoming coeducational and admitting male students in the 1970s.

James Platt White, professor of obstetrics at Buffalo Medical College, introduced "demonstrative midwifery," the practice of giving medical students practical knowledge of parturition, causing great controversy in the medical community. Some students benefited from this innovation during the second half of the nineteenth century, but many others continued to receive only didactic obstetric training.

1852
J. Marion Sims published his paper, "On the Treatment of Vesico-Vaginal Fistula," which set forth his methods of repairing this terrible postpartum condition.

1860
Etienne Stephane Tarnier, a French obstetrician, developed the axis-traction forceps, designed with a perineal curve to direct the head with the least amount of force.

1861
Ignaz Semmelweis published *On the Etiology, Concept, and Prophylaxis of Puerperal Fever,* outlining his work of preventing postpartum infections in maternity wards at the Vienna hospital and other European medical centers.

1867
Scottish surgeon Joseph Lister published a paper on surgical antisepsis, the first clinical application of bacteriological principles on the role of microorganisms in causing disease and infection.

1876
Eduardo Porro, an Italian surgeon, developed a cesarean section technique that involved amputating the body of uterus—thus removing the major source of infection—before suturing the abdomen, making the operation considerably safer.

1879
French chemist Louis Pasteur demonstrated that the streptococcus, which he had identified in 1860, was responsible for puerperal fever. Some physicians ignored or tried to refute bacteriological theories during the rest of the century, but most of the profession accepted them.

1882

Max Sanger published a treatise on the classical cesarean section suggesting that the upper part of the uterus be opened and, following delivery, sutured separately from the abdominal wall.

1895

Joseph DeLee opened the Maxwell Street Dispensary of the Chicago Lying-In Hospital (later called the Chicago Maternity Center) to serve the obstetric needs of the urban poor.

1898

X-ray pelvimetry was first used in the diagnosis of difficult obstetric cases; it was not in general obstetrics use until the 1930s.

1900

Fertility rate in the United States was 3.56 for white married women.

Midwives and physicians shared American births approximately equally—50 percent of reported births attended by midwives and 50 percent attended by physicians.

1901

The American Medical Association reorganized to represent physicians who were members of state and local medical associations, strengthening the national organization and helping it become the twentieth-century voice of the medical profession.

1910

One maternal death reported for every 154 live births in the United States. The comparable rate in Sweden was reported at one mother lost to every 430 live births.

Infant mortality reported at 124 deaths per 1,000 live births in the United States.

1911

Bellevue (Hospital) School for Midwives founded in New York, the first (and only) publicly funded midwifery school in the United States. It closed in 1938.

1912

U.S. Children's Bureau founded. Its studies revealing high maternal and infant mortality were crucial in increasing public support for improving prenatal and childbearing care of American women.

1914

Twilight sleep debates raged in the United States as women and physicians struggled with this controversial method of alleviating the pain of childbirth.

1915

Approximately 60 mothers (over 100 non-white) died for every 10,000 live births in the United States.

The low cervical cesarean section developed, a method popularized in the United States by Joseph B. DeLee and Alfred C. Beck. It significantly decreased the incidence of infection and uterine rupture.

1918
New York Maternity Center Association founded, a beginning step in the establishment of nurse-midwifery.

1920
Joseph DeLee published his influential article, "The Prophylactic Forceps Operation," which encouraged routine physician intervention during labor and delivery.

1921
The Sheppard-Towner Act passed, providing federal support for maternal and child care. In effect until 1929.

1925
Mary Breckinridge established the Frontier Nursing Service in Leslie County, Kentucky, staffed by nurse-midwives.

1926
Cecil I. B. Voge published a laboratory test for diagnosis of pregnancy.

1928
Scottish physician Alexander Fleming discovered penicillin and its antibiotic effect; the drug was purified in 1940 and became widely available to civilians at the end of World War II. It dramatically reduced mortality from postpartum infections, cesarean sections, and other obstetric dangers.

1930
Approximately 15 percent of all births in the United States attended by midwives, 80 percent of whom lived in the South.

Approximately 2.5 percent of all United States deliveries were performed by cesarean section.

Infant mortality in the United States reported at 65 deaths per 1,000 live births, reduced almost by half from the 1910 rates.

Maternal mortality in the United States reported at 70 deaths per 10,000 live births. There had been no decrease since the beginning of the century.

The American Board of Obstetrics and Gynecology established, regulating specialty practice.

1933
New York Academy of Medicine issued its report on maternal mortality, initiating a medical campaign against unnecessary instrument and drug intervention.

1935
The antibiotic action of sulphonamides discovered.

1936
Hospital blood banks established for blood typing and transfusions. Aids greatly in treatment of postpartum hemorrhages.

1938
Approximately half of all births in the United States occurred in hospitals, general and maternity. The remainder still took place in women's homes.

1955
Ninety-five percent of all births in the United States occurred in hospitals.

The American College of Nurse-Midwifery founded.

Glossary of Medical Terms

accoucheur
: birth attendant.

anesthesia
: loss of feeling or sensation.

anesthetic
: a substance which when ingested by inhalation or injection produces a loss of sense of touch or pain. See also *ether, chloroform, twilight sleep.*

antisepsis
: prevention of infection by destroying or inhibiting the growth of microorganisms. Following the empirical discoveries of Oliver Wendell Holmes and Ignaz Semmelweis in the 1840s, some physicians followed a regimen of washing their hands before examining women in labor, thus preventing infection. Not until the discoveries of Louis Pasteur and other early bacteriologists in the 1860s, 1870s, and 1880s, did scientists understand the role of microorganisms in causing infection. By the end of the nineteenth century, physicians routinely tried to use antiseptic techniques in the management of childbirth.

antiseptic
: a substance that will inhibit the growth and development of microorganisms. Scottish physician Joseph Lister, applying Pasteur's theories, discovered the effectiveness of antiseptics for preventing infection in surgery in the 1860s, and his techniques were incorporated into medical practice during the last third of the nineteenth century.

asepsis
: absence of infected matter; freedom from infection; the prevention of the access of microorganisms.

autogenesis
: self-generation; origination within the organism.

bacteria
one-celled microorganisms, many of which cause infectious diseases in humans.

bacteriology
the science of the study of bacteria. The beginnings of bacteriology are usually associated with the work of French chemist Louis Pasteur, whose investigations in the 1860s led to the identification of specific microorganisms and an understanding of their role in causing infection and disease.

bloodletting
see *venesection*.

cervix
the neck of the uterus. The cervix is said to be fully dilated when it opens to 10 cm.

cesarean section
delivery of the fetus by incision through the abdominal and uterine wall.

childbed fever
see *puerperal fever*.

chloroform
a clear, colorless, volatile liquid, $CHCl_3$, administered by inhalation as an anesthetic. Introduced into obstetrics in America by 1848.

confinement
the time period of labor and delivery; childbirth.

contraction
tension or contraction of the uterine muscle during labor.

craniotomy
the process of destruction of the fetal head in order to facilitate delivery.

crochet
a hook used in delivering the fetus after craniotomy.

douche
a stream of water, gas, or vapor directed against a part or into a cavity. In obstetrics, the washing out of the vagina.

eclampsia
convulsions sometimes followed by coma and death occurring in a pregnant or puerperal woman, associated with high blood pressure.

engagement
the entrance of the fetal head, or the presenting part, into the pelvis and beginning descent through the pelvic canal.

episiotomy
surgical incision in the perineal tissues to facilitate delivery.

ergot
a fungus-derived medication that contracts smooth muscle fibers. It is used to check hemorrhage after childbirth and to hasten labor.

ether
a colorless liquid, $C_4H_{10}O$, the vapor of which may be inhaled as a general anesthetic. First used in obstetrics in America in 1847.

fetus
the developing offspring in the human uterus after the end of the second month of gestation. Before 8 weeks, called an embryo.

fistula

a pathologic, tunnel-like connection or hole between two organs or from an internal hollow organ to the skin.

rectovaginal fistula an abnormal opening between the rectum and vagina, often associated with difficult labor and delivery.

vesicovaginal fistula an abnormal opening from the bladder into the vagina, often associated with difficult labor and delivery.

forceps

an instrument with two blades and handles for pulling; utilized to extract the fetus by the head from the maternal passages during delivery.

low forceps delivery the forceps is applied when the head reaches the perineal floor during contractions.

medium (mid) forceps delivery the forceps is applied after engagement has taken place but before the head meets the perineal floor.

high forceps delivery the forceps is applied to the head before engagement has taken place.

floating forceps delivery the forceps is applied to the head before the head has reached the pelvic rim.

axis-traction forceps obstetrical forceps so constructed that traction may be made in the line of the pelvic axis.

germ theory

the theory of disease based on bacteriological findings about the role of pathogenic microorganisms in causing disease.

iatrogenic

resulting from the activity of physicians.

Kelly pad

rolled rubber sheeting to carry the discharges off the bed during labor and delivery. Developed by Howard Kelly of the Johns Hopkins University Medical School, its use was encouraged to keep the bed clean and to reduce the possibility of postpartum infection.

labor

the process by which the fetus is expelled from the uterus through the vagina to the outside world. Also called accouchement, childbirth, confinement, parturition, and travail.

obstructed labor labor hindered by some mechanical obstruction, such as a tumor or a contraction in some part of the birth canal. Also referred to as *compacted labor*.

prolonged or protracted labor labor that is prolonged beyond the ordinary limits.

lacerations

wounds made by cutting or tearing of tissue. In obstetrics, tears in the perineal tissues during childbirth.

laudanum

tincture (alcoholic solution) of opium.

male midwives

male physicians who entered normal obstetrics beginning in the middle of the eighteenth century. The term was used throughout the nineteenth century.

meddlesome midwifery
nineteenth-century phrase referring to excessive medical interference in labor and delivery.

multigravida
a woman pregnant for the third (or more) time.

multipara
a woman who had had two or more pregnancies that resulted in viable offspring, whether or not the offspring were alive at birth.

opium
the dried juice of the opium poppy plant. Opium produces relaxation, sleep, and pain relief for birthing women.

os
the external opening to the uterus.

parturient
a woman in labor.

parturition
labor; the act or process of giving birth to a child.

pelvis
the basin-shaped ring of bone at the lower extremity of the trunk, supporting the spinal column, through which in women the fetus passes during a vaginal delivery. The upper extremity of the pelvic canal is known as the inlet or brim. The lower outlet of the pelvis is closed by the perineal muscles that form the floor of the pelvis. The fetus is said to be engaged when the head or presenting part has passed the brim and begun its descent through the pelvic canal.

perineum
the anatomical region at the lower end of the trunk between the thighs.

pessary
an instrument placed in the vagina to support the uterus or rectum.

placenta
a circular fleshy organ connected to the fetus by the umbilical cord. The placenta is attached to the uterus during pregnancy and is ejected from the uterus after the fetus is delivered. It is through the placenta that blood-borne nutrients are exchanged between mother and fetus.

postpartum
occurring after childbirth, or after delivery.

presentation
that part of the fetus that is touched by the examining finger through the cervix; the presenting part.
cephalic presentation presentation of any part of the fetal head in labor.
breech presentation presentation of the buttocks of the fetus in labor.
footling presentation presentation of the fetus in labor with one or both feet prolapsed into the vagina.
shoulder presentation presentation of the fetal shoulder in labor.

primigravida
a woman pregnant for the first time.

primipara
a woman who has had one pregnancy that resulted in a viable child,

regardless of whether the child was living at birth, and regardless of whether it was a single or multiple birth.

prolapsed uterus

see *uterus*, prolapsed.

puerperal

pertaining to the period or state of confinement after labor.

puerperal fever postpartum infection; developing a fever after childbirth.

puerperal convulsions spasm or eclampsia occurring just before, or just after, childbirth.

puerperium

the period after labor and delivery.

septic

infected.

septicemia

a widespread infection caused by the presence of microorganisms and their associated toxins in the blood. It is characterized by chills, fever, and great prostration; also called septic infection. Microorganisms gain access to the blood during childbirth via the cervix and the vaginal mucous membranes.

stages of labor

labor is designated as passing through four stages:

first stage lasts from the onset of labor contractions through the dilatation of the os.

second stage the period during which the fetus is expelled from the uterus.

third stage the period following birth of the infant and ending with the expulsion of the placenta and membranes from the uterus.

fourth stage the period intervening between the expulsion of the placenta and the occurrence of a satisfactory reaction of the mother to delivery.

symphysiotomy

surgical separation of the pubic bones, sometimes performed to allow a vaginal delivery when the fetal head can not pass through the mother's pelvis.

touch

nineteenth-century term describing how birth attendants were instructed to examine and deliver parturient women, without looking at the woman's genitals.

twilight sleep

semi-narcotic and amnesiac effect produced by administration of a combination of scopolamine and morphine during labor and delivery. In 1914–15 twilight sleep was a popular method of childbirth, and its use continued through most of the twentieth century until in recent years it was replaced by other drugs.

uterus

the hollow muscular organ that is the abode and place of nourishment of the embryo and fetus. In the unpregnant human, it is pear-shaped, approximately three inches in length. Its cavity opens into the vagina and is held in place by ligaments.

prolapsed uterus the falling down or sinking of the uterus, perhaps through the vaginal opening. In the nineteenth century, this condition was reported as a common postpartum problem.

gravid uterus the pregnant uterus.

subinvoluted uterus failure of the uterus to return to its normal size and condition following childbirth.

venesection

the opening of a vein for the purpose of letting blood. In obstetrics, bloodletting encouraged muscle relaxation and aided labor's progress. It was commonly used at the beginning of the nineteenth century.

version

turning the fetus within the uterus to facilitate vaginal delivery.

cephalic version turning the fetal head down into the maternal pelvis.

podalic version version in which the legs of the fetus are brought down into the maternal pelvis to be delivered first.

external version manipulation of the fetal body by force applied through the abdominal wall of the mother.

Index